Clinical Handbook
of Pediatric
Infectious Disease

INFECTIOUS DISEASE AND THERAPY

Series Editor

Burke A. Cunha

Winthrop-University Hospital
Mineola and
State University of New York School of Medicine
Stony Brook, New York

Clinical Handbook of Pediatric Infectious Disease

Third Edition

Russell W. Steele

Ochsner Children's Health Center
and
Tulane University School of Medicine
New Orleans, Louisiana, USA

CRC Press
Taylor & Francis Group
6000 Broken Sound Parkway NW, Suite 300
Boca Raton, FL 33487-2742

First issued in paperback 2019

ISBN-13: 978-1-4200-5150-6 (hbk)
ISBN-13: 978-0-367-38874-4 (pbk)

Library of Congress Cataloging-in-Publication Data

Steele, Russell W., 1942-
    Clinical handbook of pediatric infectious disease / Russell W. Steele. – 3rd ed.
        p. ; cm. – (Infectious disease and therapy ; v. 45)
    Rev. ed. of: The clinical handbook of pediatric infectious disease / edited by Russell W. Steele. 2nd ed. 2000.
    Includes bibliographical references and index.
    ISBN-13: 978-1-4200-5150-6 (hardcover : alk. paper)
    ISBN-10: 1-4200-5150-4 (hardcover : alk. paper) 1. Communicable diseases in children–Handbooks, manuals, etc. 2. Infection in children–Handbooks, manuals, etc. I. Clinical handbook of pediatric infectious disease. II. Title. III. Title: Pediatric infectious disease. IV. Series.
    [DNLM: 1. Communicable Diseases–Handbooks. 2. Child. 3. Infant. W1 IN406HMN v.45 2007 / WC 39 S814c 2007]
    RJ401.C545 2007
    618.92'9–dc22
                                                                  2007009439

Visit the Taylor & Francis Web site at
http://www.taylorandfrancis.com

and the CRC Press Web site at
http://www.crcpress.com

Preface

Physicians are expected to maintain, at their command, an extensive fund of knowledge. It is, of course, not realistic to commit all important information to memory or even to retain what will be considered essential aspects of diagnosis and treatment. We all, therefore, rely on reference sources for optimal patient care. Our personal libraries not only assure against omissions in medical management but also allow the most efficient method for keeping abreast of new developments in each subspecialty.

A major addition to the literature over the last ten years has been the publication of numerous guidelines for managing both the specific infections and clinical situations that predispose to infectious diseases. These guidelines have been written by experts under the direction of the American Academy of Pediatrics (*Red Book*®: *Report of the Committee on Infectious Diseases*), the Infectious Diseases Society of America, and the Centers for Disease Control and Prevention. A major change to the third edition of this handbook is inclusion of all current guidelines that pertain to the management of infectious diseases in children. These guidelines, based on evidence-based medicine, are not meant to define standards of care; rather, they offer a framework from which physicians can make final decisions.

In the care of pediatric patients, infectious diseases make up over half of all diagnostic considerations. For this reason, the pediatrician or primary care physician must particularly prepare him or herself with a basic understanding of infectious processes. In many cases, knowledge of the disease must be applied in the clinical setting with minimal delay. These situations may be best handled if the physician has at hand a reliable, concise manual that condenses essential information related to diagnosis and treatment, and that is the primary intent of this handbook. In most cases, it simply offers a rapid check of already planned management. In other cases, it may give guidance in an area less familiar to the clinician.

Most of the information in this book is presented in tabular or protocol form, which is essential for providing a quick reference in the broad area of pediatric infectious diseases. Where there is some difference of opinion, particularly for modalities of treatment, I have often elected to present just one approach. However, every effort has been made to use published guidelines and consensus recommendations.

Changes from the second edition, published in 2000, include not only updates on all infectious diseases but the addition of a number of published guidelines. All new antimicrobial agents approved since the last edition are included, and all new recommendations for therapies of choice have been updated.

Russell W. Steele

Contents

List of Tables

CHAPTER 12

CHAPTER 13

CHAPTER 14

1 | Congenital and Perinatal Infections

BACTERIAL INFECTIONS

Serious bacterial infections are more common in the neonatal period than at any other time in life, in large part a consequence of immature host-defense mechanisms. During the first 28 days of life, the incidence of sepsis is reported as high as 8 cases per 1000 live births with 20% to 25% of these having associated meningitis. With advances in neonatal intensive care and antibiotic therapy, mortality rate for such infections has been lowered to 5% from 10%.

Neonatal sepsis can be divided into early onset and late onset, each having distinct features. Late onset neonatal sepsis typically affects previously well infants who have been discharged from the hospital (Table 1).

Early clinical manifestations of neonatal sepsis are frequently non-specific and subtle, often showing overlap with noninfectious diseases. Perinatal factors can be helpful in identifying which infants are at greatest risk for infection. Prematurity markedly increases risk (Tables 2 and 3).

Clinical manifestations of neonatal sepsis are variable in their occurrence and involve many different organ systems (Table 4).

Laboratory studies can be helpful during initial clinical evaluation. Despite multiple attempts to develop more sensitive and specific rapid laboratory tests for infection, the WBC count and differential remain the most frequently used screening studies. Neutropenia, especially an absolute neutrophil count below $1800 \, \text{mm}^{-3}$, or an immature to total neutrophil ratio above 0.15 in the first 24 hours of life are suggestive of infection. Leukocytosis with WBC count above $25,000 \, \text{mm}^{-3}$ may also result from infection, but is more often associated with noninfectious causes. Other hematologic findings include thrombocytopenia, WBC vacuolization, and toxic granulations.

An elevation in the C-reactive protein has gained increasing clinical utilization as a predictor for infection. Rapid antigen tests, such as latex particle agglutination or countercurrent immunoelectrophoresis, can be helpful as supportive evidence for infection, but false positive results have limited their use.

Cultures of blood and cerebrospinal fluid should be obtained from all neonates with suspected sepsis, although clinical judgement must be used in determining the safety of lumbar puncture in infants at risk for respiratory compromise or preterm infants at risk for intraventricular hemorrhage. Blood cultures from two separate sites are recommended primarily to better interpret potential contamination in one of the cultures.

Tracheal aspirate cultures are useful when available in infants with respiratory symptoms, although endotracheal tube colonization is inevitable with prolonged intubation. Urine culture

TABLE 1   Common Features of Early Onset vs. Late Onset Neonatal Sepsis

Feature	Early onset	Late onset
Time	0–7 days	Beyond 7 days
Perinatal risk factors	++	+/−
Source of organism	Maternal genital tract	Environment, ?mother
Progress of infection	Fulminant	Insidious
Meningitis present	+	++
Fetal scalp electrodes	+	

++, prominent manifestation; +, occasionally seen; −, not a manifestation.

TABLE 2 Perinatal Risk Factors for Infection

Prematurity	Chorioamnionitis
Low birthweight	Maternal group B strep
Prolonged rupture of	colonization
membranes	Fetal distress
Maternal fever	Perinatal asphyxia
Maternal UTI	Male gender
Fetal scalp electrodes	Low socioeconomic
(Table 3)	status

TABLE 3 Infections Associated with Fetal Scalp Electrodes

Scalp abscesses
Mixed aerobes and anaerobes
E. coli
Mycoplasma hominis
Neisseria gonorrhoeae
Herpes simplex virus
Group B streptococcus

is of low yield in evaluation for early onset infection, but is very useful in late onset infection. Urine for culture should be obtained by suprapubic aspiration of the bladder when possible. Cultures of the gastric aspirate and skin may reflect the infant's bacterial colonization at birth, but do not always correlate with systemic infection. Chest X-ray is indicated in infants with respiratory distress as a screen for both pneumonia and noninfectious causes.

Normal values for cerebrospinal fluid in neonates differ from those in older infants. Cerebrospinal fluid WBC counts as high as $30\,\text{mm}^{-3}$, protein values as high as $170\,\text{mg/dL}$, and glucose values as low as $24\,\text{mg/dL}$ may be normal in the neonatal period.

Etiology

Early onset neonatal infections are typically transmitted vertically from the mother to the infant. Organisms can be acquired transplacentally, via infected amniotic fluid, or by direct contact in passage through the birth canal. Group B streptococci and *Escherichia coli* cause most infections, but a number of other organisms may be involved (Table 5).

Late onset infection typically involves group B streptococci, although gram-negative organisms and *Listeria* may also be involved.

Prevention of Group B Streptococcal Disease

Prior to the introduction of guidelines to prevent early onset group B streptococcal disease in neonates, this bacterium was the most common cause of neonatal sepsis with an attack rate of up to 4 per 1000 live births. The incidence was increased to 1 per 50 preterm infants weighing less than 2000 g. Serotype III is the predominant cause of early onset meningitis and most late onset infections in neonates and infants. While there is ongoing debate over the optimal method for prevention of early onset group B streptococcal disease, the American Academy of Pediatrics in conjunction with the American College of Obstetrics and Gynecology and others put forth a consensus statement on the use of intrapartum chemoprophylaxis in 1997 which was updated in 2006 (Table 6) (1).

TABLE 4 Clinical Manifestations of Sepsis

Temperature instability	Hypothermia, hyperthermia
Respiratory distress	Tachypnea, retractions, grunting, nasal flaring, apnea
Feeding disturbances	Poor suck, vomiting, gastric residuals, abdominal distention, diarrhea
CNS dysfunction	Lethargy, irritability, seizures
Cardiovascular	Tachycardia, bradycardia, cyanosis, pallor, hypotension
Hematologic	Bruising, petechiae, bleeding, jaundice

TABLE 5   Bacterial Etiology of Neonatal Infection

Organism	Percentage
Group B streptococci	35–40
Other gram-positive cocci	20–25
Staphylococcus sp.	
Enterococcus sp.	
Other streptococci	
Escherichia coli	20
Other gram-negative enterics	10–15
Klebsiella sp.	
Haemophilus sp.	
Pseudomonas sp.	
Listeria monocytogenes	1–2

TABLE 6   Two Prevention Strategies for Early Onset Group B Streptococcal Infection (1)

Screening method: maternal vaginal and rectal GBS cultures at 35–37 wks
Risk factors present. If yes to any, intrapartum penicillin:
Prior infant with GBS disease
GBS bacteriuria this pregnancy
Positive GBS screening culture (unless cesarean section done prior to labor and membrane rupture)
GBS screen results unavailable AND Maternal. If yes, intrapartum penicillin risk factors present:
Delivery <37 wks gestation
Temp >38°C
Membranes ruptured >18 hrs
GBS screen negative. No prophylaxis

Intravenous penicillin G (5 million units initially, then 2.5 million units every 4 hours) is the preferred method for intrapartum prophylaxis. Ampicillin or other broader spectrum drugs may be used based on additional maternal indications (urinary tract infection or chorioamnionitis). Intravenous clindamycin or erythromycin may be used for penicillin allergic mothers.

Management of the infant whose mother has received intrapartum prophylaxis for group B streptococcal infection should be individualized, but the algorithm in Table 6 of Chapter 2 has been suggested (Table 7).

Therapy of Neonatal Sepsis

Because of the high morbidity associated with delayed therapy for neonatal sepsis, empiric antibiotic therapy should be initiated for any neonate with suspected sepsis after appropriate cultures are obtained in a timely manner. Antibiotic administration should not be delayed due to difficulty or inability to obtain the appropriate specimens for culture. Because of the relatively low incidence of neonatal sepsis coupled with the uncertainties in making a definite diagnosis,

TABLE 7   Management of an Infant Born to a Mother Who Received Intrapartum Antimicrobial Prophylaxis (IAP)

Signs and symptoms of sepsis	Full diagnostic evaluation: CBC, differential, blood culture, consider chest X ray and lumbar puncture Empiric antibiotic therapy
Gestational age <35 wks or Duration of IAP antibiotics given to mother <4 hrs	Limited evaluation (CBC, differential, blood culture) Observe for 48 hrs; if sepsis suspected, full evaluation and therapy
2 or more doses of antibiotics given to mother	No evaluation, no therapy
<32 weeks gestation	Full diagnostic evaluation and therapy pending results of cultures

TABLE 8   Management of Suspected Neonatal Sepsis

Suspected sepsis based on clinical signs and perinatal risk factors	CBC, chest X-ray
	Blood and CSF cultures
	Tracheal and urine cultures (if appropriate)
	Empiric antibiotic therapy (see Chapter 20 for dosing)
Positive CSF cultures	Antibiotics for 21 days
Positive blood/urine cultures	Antibiotics for 10–14 days
Pneumonia	Antibiotics for 10–14 days
Negative cultures	
High suspicion remains	Antibiotics for 7–10 days
Low suspicion	Discontinue antibiotics at 48–72 hrs

a majority of infants who are treated for suspected sepsis will not have this condition. Empiric antibiotics are chosen to treat the most common pathologic organisms. Typical antibiotic choices are ampicillin to provide therapy against gram-positive organisms (group B streptococci, *Listeria*, and *Enterococcus*) coupled with an aminoglycoside (gentamicin most commonly) or a third generation cephalosporin (cefotaxime or ceftriaxone) to provide therapy against gram-negative organisms. Aminoglycoside concentrations must be monitored to prevent toxicity. Third generation cephalosporins have less toxicity, but present greater problems with alteration of normal flora and selection of resistant organisms. Ceftriaxone should be avoided in infants with significant hyperbilirubinemia as it may displace bilirubin from albumin binding sites (Table 8).

When culture and sensitivity results are available, antibiotic choices should be adjusted to provide more specific therapy.

In addition to antibiotic therapy, supportive care of the infected neonate is essential. Close attention to respiratory, cardiovascular, fluid and electrolyte, and hematologic support are essential to optimize outcome.

Adjunctive immunologic therapies continue to be investigated. WBC transfusions have been beneficial in some infants with severe neutropenia, but are often not readily accomplished. Therapy with granulocyte colony-stimulating factor (G-CSF, Filgrastim) in neonatal sepsis with associated neutropenia has resulted in increased neutrophil counts, but its effect on outcome requires further study. Similarly, the efficacy of intravenous immunoglobulin therapy to treat or prevent neonatal sepsis remains undetermined.

CONGENITAL INFECTIONS

Congenital infections with non-bacterial pathogens can result in significant morbidity and mortality. TORCH has been used as an acronym for what were once the more common pathogens involved in congenital infections—toxoplasma, rubella, cytomegalovirus (CMV), and herpes simplex virus (actually a perinatal infection). Changing incidence of the common pathogens involved in congenital infections, however, have made the TORCH acronym less useful. CMV is the most common agent involved in congenital infection, estimated to infect 1% to 2% of all newborns in the United States. Increased prevalence of sexually transmitted diseases such as syphilis and human immunodeficiency virus (HIV) has resulted in increasing numbers of newborns infected with these pathogens, while screening and immunization for rubella have all but eliminated this pathogen as a cause of congenital infection. Herpes only rarely manifests as a congenital infection with growth retardation and deep dermal scars, occurring almost always as a perinatally acquired infection.

Clinical manifestations of congenital infection are variable, but there is considerable overlap between different pathogens. As example the classical triad of jaundice, hepatosplenomegaly, and a petechial "blueberry muffin" rash (Fig. 1) is seen with many of the

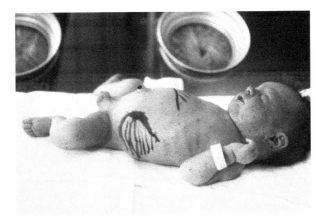

FIGURE 1 (*See color insert.*) The classical triad of jaundice, hepatosplenomegaly, and a petechial "blueberry muffin" rash is seen with congenital CMV, rubella, and toxoplasmosis.

TORCH agents. On the other hand, some characteristic features allow clinical differentiation of specific pathogens. Hydrocephalus with diffuse intracerebral calcifications is seen almost exclusively with toxoplasmosis (Fig. 2) and snuffles (Fig. 3) with congenital syphilis.

Clinical manifestations which should arouse suspicion for congenital infection include intrauterine growth retardation, microcephaly, hydrocephaly, hepatosplenomegaly, anemia, and thrombocytopenia. It should be noted, however, that most cases of intrauterine growth retardation and microcephaly are not caused by infection (Table 9).

When a congenital infection is suspected, appropriate laboratory studies should be performed. Because of the limited blood volume in a neonate, judicious use of the available laboratory studies is required. Prior to initiating such tests on the infant, a close review of available maternal history is essential (Table 10).

Toxoplasmosis

Congenital toxoplasmosis occurs in approximately 1 in 1000 deliveries in the United States as a result of transplacental acquisition of *Toxoplasma gondii* during maternal primary infection.

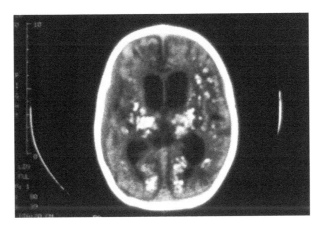

FIGURE 2 Hydrocephalus and diffuse calcifications, characteristic of congenital toxoplasmosis. With congenital cytomegalovirus, microcephaly and periventricular calcifications are more commonly seen.

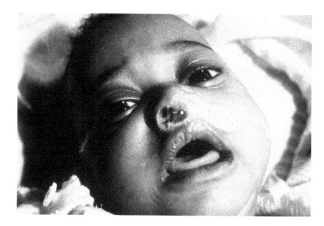

FIGURE 3 Thick nasal discharge termed snuffles is seen with congenital syphilis. This 2-mo-old infant also had frontal bossing, rhagades, and pneumonia on presentation.

Most infected infants are asymptomatic at birth, but may develop symptoms later in infancy. Chorioretinitis occurs in over 80% of infected infants. Other common clinical manifestations are listed in Table 8 of Chapter 2. Diagnosis can be confirmed by testing for Toxoplasma antigen and antibodies (Table 10); isolation of this protozoan is difficult.

Major sequelae of infection are neurologic problems including seizures, mental retardation, and deafness. Treatment of the infant may limit adverse sequelae (Table 11).

Hepatitis B Virus

Hepatitis B virus can be spread transplacentally, but the majority of affected infants are exposed at the time of birth. In the United States, almost 1% of pregnant women test positive for hepatitis B surface antigen (HBsAg). Hepatitis B infection in the neonate may result in acute hepatitis, but more worrisome is the very high likelihood of infected infants becoming chronic carriers with increased risks for cirrhosis and hepatocellular carcinoma.

Because of the high prevalence and chance for adverse outcome in infected neonates, universal screening of all pregnant women is recommended. All infants should receive the

TABLE 9   Clinical Manifestations of Congenital Infections

	CMV	Syphilis	Toxoplasmosis	Rubella
IUGR	++	+	+	++
Microcephaly	++	−	+	+
Hydrocephaly	+	+	++	+
Intracranial calcifications	++	−	++	−
Hepatosplenomegaly	++	++	++	++
Jaundice	++	++	++	+
Anemia	+	++	++	+
Thrombocytopenia	++	++	+	++
Petechiae/purpura	++	++	+	++
Cataracts	+	−	−	++
Chorioretinitis	+	+	++	+
Deafness	++	+	+	++
Cardiac defects	−	−	−	++
Bone lesions	−	+	−	++

++, prominent manifestation; +, occasionally seen; −, not a manifestation.

TABLE 10   Laboratory Evaluation of Suspected Congenital Infection

Initial general studies on neonate
CBC with differential, platelet count, liver function tests (bilirubin, GGT), urinalysis, serum creatinine, quantitative immunoglobulins, screening test for syphilis (VDRL, RPR, or ART); HIV-PCR if mother positive
Urine: CMV culture
CSF: cell count, protein, glucose, VDRL, Gram stain, bacterial, and viral cultures
Brain CT

Studies on mother
Blood: VDRL, HIV
Cervix: consider culture for herpes simplex and CMV

Additional studies when organism highly suspected
Toxoplasmosis
  Neonate's serum: Sabin-Feldman dye test (IgG), IgM ISAGA, IgA ELISA, IgE ISAGA/ELISA
  Neonate CSF: *T. gondii* IgG and IgM and quantitative IgG (to calculate antibody ratio)
  Maternal serum: same as neonate but substitute IgM ELISA for the IgM ISAGA; HS/AC (differential agglutination)
Syphilis
  Definitive tests: fluorescent treponemal antibody-absorption (FTA-ABS) or *T. pallidum* particle agglutination (TP-PA)
HIV
  Blood PCR-DNA or culture
Rubella
  Culture of placenta, pharynx, conjunctivae, urine, and CSF
  Cord serum rubella IgM
  Monitor rubella IgG for persistence
  CSF rubella IgM
CMV
  Culture of urine or saliva
  Blood PCR
  Serum CMV-IgM and serial IgG titers (low sensitivity and specificity)
  Biopsy and PCR or culture of involved organ (liver, lung)
Herpes simplex
  Cytologic exam of skin, eye or mouth vesicles (fluorescence or Tzanck smear)
  Culture of skin or mucosal lesions
  CSF: PCR
  Blood: PCR

hepatitis B vaccine and infants born to HBsAg positive mothers should also be passively immunized with hepatitis B immune globulin. After such passive and active immunization, breastfeeding for infants born to HBsAg positive mothers poses no additional risk for infection (Table 12).

TABLE 11   Treatment of Congenital Toxoplasmosis

Pyrimethamine: Loading dose 1 mg/kg q 12 hr × 4 followed by 1 mg/kg/day PO × 6 mo followed by 1 mg/kg 3 × weekly (M, W, F) × 6 mo plus
Sulfadiazine 100 mg/kg/day PO div. q 12 hr × 1 yr
Folinic acid (Leucovorin calcium) 10 mg three times weekly during and 1 wk after pyrimethamine therapy to prevent hematologic problems
Prednisone 1.0 mg/kg/day div q 24 hr during the inflammatory stages of this illness (CSF protein >1 g/dL, chorioretinitis)
No special isolation is required

TABLE 12   **Management of Hepatitis B in Neonates**

Hepatitis B vaccine to ALL infants at 0–2, 1–4, and 6–12 months
Hepatitis B immune globulin 0.5 mL IM and vaccine within 12 hrs of birth to
  infants born to HBsAg positive mothers and premature neonates <2000 g
  whose mother's HBsAg status is unknown

Hepatitis C Virus

Hepatitis C virus is transmitted in routes similar to hepatitis B virus. Seroprevalence of hepatitis C in pregnant women in the United States is 1% to 2%, with maternal–fetal transmission rates of 5%. Routine screening for hepatitis C in pregnancy is not recommended except for mothers with risk factors (blood transfusion, intravenous drug abuse, or other repeated exposure to percutaneous or mucosal blood). The risk of maternal–fetal transmission is increased for mothers with HIV infection.

Infants born to mothers with hepatitis C virus should be screened for infection at 18 months of age with an ELISA antibody assay. Those positive should have testing for active viral disease by obtaining a HCV RNA for antigen, liver enzymes to determine the extent of hepatic inflammation, and should be referred to a pediatric gastroenterologist. Transmission of hepatitis C by breastfeeding has not been documented.

Human Immunodeficiency Virus

Human immunodeficiency virus is the etiologic agent of acquired immunodeficiency syndrome and can be spread from an infected mother to her neonate. Transmission may occur by transplacental spread or by exposure to maternal blood and secretions at the time of delivery. While initial estimates were higher, it now appears that infection occurs in less than 25% of infants born to infected untreated mothers.

Transplacentally acquired antibody to HIV results in all infants born to seropositive mothers testing positive for HIV antibody at birth. Uninfected infants should be seronegative in follow-up testing by 15 months of age. More sensitive early diagnostic methods PCR, viral culture, and P24 antigen are currently recommended as methods for identifying infected infants (see Chapter 17).

Most infected newborns are normal at birth, with symptoms developing in the first year of life. The efficacy of pre- and postnatal antiviral therapy has now been well documented. Caesarian section delivery may result in an additive reduction to the risk of vertical transmission. Since HIV can be transmitted via breast milk, infants of infected mothers should be formula fed.

Syphilis

Congenital syphilis infections have had a resurgence in recent years due to the illicit drug epidemic. Transplacental passage of this spirochete may result in fetal wastage, non-immune hydrops, or postnatal manifestations such as snuffles, rash, hepatitis, and osteochondritis/periostitis. If untreated, late manifestations include neurosyphilis, deafness, and dental and bone abnormalities.

Infants may be infected with syphilis at birth and be asymptomatic, thus evaluation of maternal serology and therapy is essential to identify such infants and prevent subsequent complications. Serology may involve a non-treponemal test (e.g., VDRL, ART, and RPR) and a subsequent confirmatory treponemal test (e.g., TP-PA and FTA-ABS). Non-treponemal tests provide quantitative titers to correlate with disease activity; treponemal tests provide confirmation of positive non-treponemal results, but remain reactive for life despite adequate therapy (see Chapter 16) (Table 13).

Evaluation of infants at risk should include physical exam, non-treponemal screening assay, TP-PA or FTA-ABS, lumbar puncture, long-bone X-rays, and chest roentgenogram (see Chapter 15). Cerebrospinal fluid findings suggestive of neurosyphilis include leukocytosis, elevated protein, or positive VDRL (Table 14).

TABLE 13   Infants to be Evaluated for Congenital Syphilis

An infant should be evaluated for congenital syphilis IF
Infant symptomatic or with active disease as determined by radiographic
   studies
or
Mother has positive nontreponemal test confirmed by treponemal test
and
One or more of the following:
   Mother:
   Not treated
   Penicillin dose inadequate or unknown
   Treated with any antibiotic except penicillin
   Treated during the last month of pregnancy
   Less than 4-fold decrease in serologic screening assay following treatment

Treated infants and seropositive untreated infants of treated mothers should be followed closely with repeat non-treponemal serology at 3, 6, and 12 months of age for evidence of declining non-treponemal titers. Most infants who have been effectively treated will have negative non-treponemal serology by 6 months of age. If titers fail to decline, the infant should be re-evaluated and treated. Infants with abnormal CSF findings should have repeat CSF evaluations every 3 months until normal, with repeat treatment indicated for persistent evidence of neurosyphilis.

Varicella-Zoster Virus

Varicella-Zoster virus can result in congenital infection with variable expression depending on the timing of maternal infection. Maternal varicella infection in the first 20 weeks of pregnancy can infrequently result in fetal varicella syndrome manifested by growth retardation, cicatricial skin lesions, limb hypoplasia, and neurologic insults. Maternal chickenpox in the final 21 days of gestation can result in congenital chickenpox, with infants born to mothers with onset of rash from 5 days before to 2 days after delivery at highest risk for severe infection. Varicella-Zoster immune globulin (VZIG) 125 U IM should be given to these

TABLE 14   Treatment for Congenital Syphilis

Neonates with	
physical exam or X ray evidence of active disease, or	
abnormal CSF findings, or	
non-treponemal titers 4-fold or greater than mother's, or	
maternal treatment absent, unknown, undocumented, non-penicillin, or within 1 mo of delivery, or	
undocumented fall in maternal nontreponemal titers, or	
negative workup but uncertain follow-up after discharge	
Age <4 wks, normal CSF	Aqueous crystalline penicillin G 100–150,000 U/kg/day IV or IM div. b.i.d. (<7 days of age) or t.i.d. (>7 days) × 10 days
	or
	Procaine penicillin 50,000 U/kg/day IM div. qd × 10 days
Age <4 wks, abnormal CSF	Aqueous crystalline penicillin G 100,000–150,000 U/kg/day IV div. b.d. (<7 days) or t.i.d. (>7 days) × 10 days
Age >4 wks–yr normal CSF	Aqueous crystalline penicillin G 200,000 U/kg/day IV div. q.i.d. × 10 days
Age >4 wks–1 yr abnormal CSF	Aqueous crystalline penicillin G 200,000 U/kg/day IV div. q.i.d. × 10 days followed by benzathine penicillin G 50,000 *U*/kg IM weekly × 3
Age >1 yr normal CSF	Benzathine penicillin G 50,000 U/kg IM weekly × 3
Age >1 yr abnormal CSF	Aqueous crystalline penicillin G 200,000–300,000 U/kg/day IV or IM div. q.i.d. × 10 days followed by benzathine penicillin G 50,000 U/kg IM weekly × 3

high-risk infants. Infants born to mothers with chickenpox in the perinatal period should be isolated from susceptible infants until 21 days postnatally (28 days if VZIG given).

Infants who are exposed to chickenpox postnatally generally have a benign course, but preterm and other immunocompromised infants are at high risk for more severe infection (Table 15).

Rubella

Rubella virus, transplacentally acquired during the course of primary maternal infection, may result in growth retardation, heart defects, hepatosplenomegaly, thrombocytopenia, cataracts, and deafness. The incidence and severity of malformations increases with infection early in gestation. Diagnosis can be made by viral isolation or by testing for IgM to rubella. Treatment is supportive and infected infants require isolation because virus excretion may be prolonged.

Cytomegalovirus

Cytomegalovirus may be vertically transmitted to the fetus in primary or recurrent maternal infection. Approximately 10% of infected infants are symptomatic at birth with the classic manifestations; these infants have a mortality rate of 25% and almost all survivors have long-term morbidity. Of the 90% of infected infants who are asymptomatic at birth, up to 15% will develop significant late neurologic morbidity, sensorineural hearing loss being most common. Diagnosis is confirmed by urine culture for CMV.

Acquired CMV infection may be severe in premature and other immunocompromised infants. CMV is transmitted by blood products or by breast milk. Infected infants may develop pulmonary, hepatic, hematologic, and neurologic manifestations. Ganciclovir is active in vitro against CMV infection, but is only effective in preventing progressive hearing loss in neonates with congenital infection. Prevention is best accomplished by the use of CMV-negative or frozen deglycerolyzed blood for transfusion to infants at risk.

Herpes Simplex Virus

Herpes simplex virus (HSV) types 1 (15%) and 2 (85%) cause maternal herpes genitalis resulting in perinatally acquired neonatal infection. Neonatal disease may result from ascending infection prior to birth, acquisition from the birth canal during delivery, or postnatal acquisition from an infected caretaker. The incidence remains low at 0.2 to 0.5 cases per 1000 births. Infection is most likely with maternal primary HSV infection, but can also occur with recurrent infection. Most infected infants are born to mothers who are asymptomatic, but actively shedding virus from a genital infection at the time of delivery. Caesarian delivery should be performed within 4 hours of rupture of membranes for women with active lesions. Prenatal screening with serial cervical cultures for HSV to predict status at delivery is not effective and no longer recommended.

Infants at high risk for infection should be isolated initially until the results of viral cultures from the mother and infant are known. These infants should be closely observed in the hospital for evidence of infection with cultures obtained from the eyes, mouth, and any suspicious skin

TABLE 15   Management of Postnatal Varicella Exposure

VZIG 125 U IM should be given to these high-risk infants exposed postnatally to chickenpox
Infants born prior to 28 wks gestation or with birthweight less than 1000 gms
Preterm infants with negative maternal history of varicella
Immunocompromised infants
Isolation of exposed infants from other susceptible infants should be undertaken from 8–21 days postexposure (28 days if VZIG given)

lesions. Use of acyclovir during this observation period should be individualized. Infants at lower risk for infection should also be isolated while hospitalized and caretakers should be educated about the early signs of infection.

Neonatal herpes infection presents in the first 42 days of life as a rapidly evolving disease with clinical symptoms similar to those of bacterial sepsis. Disease may subsequently be categorized into one of three classifications: localized infection of the skin, eyes, or mouth (S.E.M.); central nervous system infection with or without skin, eye, or mouth involvement; and disseminated infection. Mortality is highest for infants with disseminated infection, while morbidity is high for infants with disseminated or central nervous system infection.

Diagnosis can be confirmed by culture of the virus from skin vesicles, mucosal lesions, blood, or CSF and with PCR identification of HSV antigen in CSF or blood. Cytologic exam with fluorescent or Tzanck smears of lesion scrapings may be helpful in early diagnosis. Early therapy with acyclovir 60 mg/kg/day IV div TID for 14 days for S.E.M. disease or 21 days for disseminated and CNS infection has resulted in improved outcome.

Most experts recommend starting acyclovir in neonates and infants younger than 42 days with CSF findings suggestive of aseptic meningitis or pneumonia unresponsive to broad spectrum antimicrobial therapy.

COMMON FOCAL INFECTIONS

Conjunctivitis

Conjunctivitis in the newborn is common, with chemical irritation from prophylactic silver nitrate the most common cause. Chemical conjunctivitis occurs in the first 48 hours of life and is self-limited. Conjunctivitis beginning after 48 hours of life is usually of infectious origin and of greater clinical significance. Gram stain and appropriate cultures are required to identify the pathogen involved (Table 16).

Omphalitis

Omphalitis is characterized by purulent discharge from the umbilical stump with erythema and induration of the periumbilical area. Etiologic bacteria include *Staphylococcus aureus*, group A and B streptococci, diphtheroids, and gram-negative enteric bacilli. Complications include sepsis, umbilical arteritis or phlebitis, peritonitis, and necrotizing fasciitis. Recommended initial therapy is intravenous methicillin plus an aminoglycoside or third generation cephalosporin.

Scalp Abscess

Fetal monitoring with internal scalp electrodes may result in a break in skin continuity with subsequent abscess formation. Treatment consists of local antiseptic care, incision, and

TABLE 16   Common Neonatal Eye Infections

Infecting organism	Age of onset	Clinical features	Therapy
Staphylococcus aureus	2–5 days	Unilateral crusted purulent discharge	Topical sulfacetamide, neomycin erythromycin, or tetracycline
Neisseria gonorrhoeae	3 days–3 wks	Bilateral hyperemia and chemosis, copious thick white discharge	Ceftriaxone IV or IM, 50 mg/kg (max. 125 mg) as a single dose; Saline irrigation; Contact isolation
Chlamydia trachomatis	2–20 wks	Unilateral or bilateral mild conjunctivitis, copious purulent discharge	Oral erythromycin 50 mg/kg/day div. q.i.d. × 14 days

drainage. Culture and sensitivity of the abscess drainage should be performed. If there is evidence of extension or systemic illness, intravenous vancomycin plus an aminoglycoside or third generation cephalosporin should be administered. Consideration should be given for scalp electrode site infection with herpes simplex virus or *Neisseria gonorrhoeae* when the mother is infected with these organisms.

HEALTH CARE–ASSOCIATED INFECTIONS

Health care–associated (formerly called "nosocomial") infection in the newborn is defined as an infection that was neither present nor incubating at birth, generally occurring after 48 hours of life. The incidence of such infections in normal newborn nurseries is around 1% while in neonatal intensive care units the incidence may be as high as 20%, especially in very low birthweight infants. Factors that contribute to higher rates of health care-associated infection include immature host-defense mechanisms, prolonged hospitalization, invasive supportive measures, and crowding.

Organisms responsible for these infections in the NICU include coagulase-negative staphylococci, *Staphylococcus aureus*, gram-negative enteric bacilli, and *Candida* species. Health care–associated infection should be considered in any hospitalized infant who exhibits unexplained clinical deterioration. As with early onset neonatal disease, clinical manifestations of infections are frequently subtle and non-specific.

Empiric antibiotic therapy for these suspected infections should be based on the pathogens most prevalent in that nursery and the hospital organism susceptibility profile. Vancomycin in combination with a third generation cephalosporin offers broad-spectrum coverage of the most frequent pathogens. Empiric therapy should be changed to more specific therapy when culture and sensitivity results are available. Antifungal therapy is usually not begun empirically, but this choice should be individualized.

Health care–associated viral infections are also of clinical significance. Respiratory syncytial virus (RSV) infections are associated with high morbidity and mortality in preterm infants and infants with underlying cardiorespiratory disease. Spread is by direct contact and droplet contamination. Hospital outbreaks are common during community epidemics which may occur from late fall to early spring. Therapy with ribavirin may be beneficial for high-risk infants. Infected infants should be isolated. Passive immunization with palivizumab, a monoclonal antibody product against RSV, reduces the frequency and severity of infection in high-risk groups such as infants with severe prematurity and those with bronchopulmonary dysplasia.

The incidence of health care–associated infections can be reduced with close attention to infection control measures and special emphasis on strict handwashing practices.

Coagulase-Negative Staphylococci

Coagulase-negative staphylococci, typically *Staphylococcus epidermidis*, have become the most common cause of health care–associated bacterial infection in the NICU. These organisms are present on skin and mucosal surfaces and are especially prone to cause infection in infants with foreign bodies in place such as umbilical catheters, central venous lines, and shunts. *Staphylococcus epidermidis* produces a slime layer on the foreign body that serves to isolate the bacteria from both host defenses and antibiotics. While some strains may be susceptible to penicillinase-resistant penicillins such as naphcillin or oxacillin, most infections require treatment with vancomycin. Rifampin or gentamicin may offer synergy with vancomycin. Serious infections often require the removal of the colonized foreign body.

CANDIDA SPECIES

Candida species, typically *Candida albicans*, are a ubiquitous group of fungal organisms that colonize the skin and mucous membranes. In the absence of competing, bacterial flora as may occur with broad-spectrum antibiotic use or in immunocompromised patients, infections with *Candida* may occur. Superficial infections such as thrush or diaper dermatitis may be treated with oral or topical nystatin preparations.

Candida invasive disease is a more serious infection that is more difficult to diagnose and treat. Infants with such invasive infections may present with features similar to bacterial sepsis. Diagnosis requires isolation of *Candida* from a normally sterile body site, such as the blood, CSF or tissue. Urine culture positive for *Candida* may represent contamination, depending on the method by which the specimen was obtained. Ophthalmologic exam to assess for *Candida* endophthalmitis may be useful initially and is recommended for anyone with candidemia 3 months after treatment is completed.

For infection in otherwise stable neonates, fluconazole is the preferred antifungal therapy because of its low toxicity and excellent activity against the predominant species. Amphotericin B is the agent of choice for *Candida* invasive disease, although its toxicities have resulted in an ongoing search for alternative therapies. Many clinicians use combination amphotericin B plus fluconazole initially, discontinuing the amphotericin B when neonates are improved. Flucytosine may be synergistic with amphotericin B for very severe infections but rarely can sick neonates tolerate P.O. medications. Liposomal forms of amphotericin B should be used in patients with impaired renal function. The duration of therapy can be individualized, but more severe infections in high-risk newborns generally require treatment for 4 to 6 weeks.

Intravenous or indwelling catheters should always be removed once vascular catheter-associated candidemia is documented.

With less severe infections associated with an indwelling catheter, prompt therapy and catheter removal may allow for shorter courses of therapy.

Judicious use of antibiotics and indwelling catheters are important in the prevention of health care–associated infections with both coagulase-negative *Staphylococci* and *Candida* species.

2 | Infectious Disease Emergencies with Multiorgan Involvement

INTRODUCTION

Some infectious disease presentations must be diagnosed and treated rapidly to prevent mortality and optimize the opportunity to reduce morbidity. These are true emergencies and fortunately only a few such entities are commonly encountered in pediatric patients. Sepsis, pneumonia with respiratory failure, diarrhea with severe dehydration, and meningitis are the most common. In the majority of cases, culture specimens should be obtained before treatment is begun. Most generally involve multiple organs/systems. Such infections in infants and children associated with a high mortality are included in this chapter. In most cases, therapy is instituted before a diagnosis can be confirmed.

In some instances, only supportive therapy is available, either because antimicrobial treatment has not been developed (enteroviral encephalitis and myocarditis) the clinical progression is the consequence of a post-infectious process (chickenpox encephalitis, Guillain-Barré syndrome) or because eradication of the invading pathogen is unnecessary, e.g., infant botulism.

Most infectious disease emergencies should be managed in a well-equipped intensive care unit, at least during the acute phase of illness. Progression of disease may require advanced life-support including endotracheal intubation or other specialized support procedures. For this reason, transport to tertiary care centers should be considered if local facilities do not have intensive care capabilities.

BACTEREMIA

Occult Bacteremia

Spontaneous or occult bacteremia now occurs in only one of 200 children who present with acute high fever [temperature of 102.2°F (39°C) or higher], no apparent focus of infection, and a WBC count of >15,000 mm^{-3}. Pneumococcus is still the most common cause and *H. influenzae* type b has virtually disappeared following the routine administration of *H. flu vaccine* (Table 1).

TABLE 1 Etiology of Bacteremia in Otherwise Normal Febrile Infants and Children

Organism	% of total
Pneumococcus	90–95
Salmonella	5
Group A streptococcus	1
Meningococcus	1
Group B streptococcus	1
Staphylococcus aureus	<1
Gram (−) coliforms	<1

TABLE 2   Treatment of Patients with a Positive Blood Culture and No Focus of Infection

Streptococcus pneumoniae
  If the patient is febrile and/or has a toxic appearance:
    Hospitalize
    Repeat blood cultures
    Perform lumbar puncture
    Administer IV antibiotics
  If the patient is afebrile and asymptomatic:
    Repeat blood cultures
    Begin PO antibiotics if not given initially
    Continue observation at home and follow-up if indicated
    May continue oral antibiotics if parenteral or PO antibiotics were begun at the initial visit

Salmonella
  Intravenous antibiotics until afebrile
  PO antibiotics to complete 14 days

Neisseria meningitidis
  If patient is either febrile or afebrile:
    Hospitalize
    Repeat blood cultures
    Perform lumbar puncture
    Administer IV antibiotics

TABLE 3   Etiology of Bacteremia Associated with Intravascular Catheters

Staphylococcus epidermidis	85%
Staphylococcus aureus	7%
Candida albicans	3%
Enterococcus spp.	2%
Others	3%
Escherichia coli	
Klebsiella spp.	
Pseudomonas aeruginosa	
Viridans streptococci	
Other gram-negative bacilli	

When there is no evidence of toxicity, occult bacteremia is a benign, self-limited event in >90% of cases. Because of the extremely low yield and because two-thirds of all recovered organisms are contaminants, blood cultures are no longer warranted in children aged 3 to 36 months who have no obvious source of infection. Empiric antibiotics for febrile children is not appropriate. However, if a child remains febrile or worsens clinically, further diagnostic evaluation and treatment with antimicrobial agents pending results of cultures may be considered.

Management of the child with a positive blood culture for an organism which is likely a true pathogen depends partly on the infective organism (Table 2). Pneumococcal bacteremia exhibits spontaneous resolution in over 94% of cases and an infrequent rate of subsequent focal infection such as otitis media or pneumonia; therefore, for patients who are afebrile and clinically stable following the initial exam, most experts recommend a follow-up visit, repeat blood cultures, and PO antibiotics. Because meningococcal bacteremia is much more likely to progress to severe infection, particularly meningitis, a more aggressive approach is necessary.

Intravascular Catheter-Related Bacteremia

Intravascular line infections are increasingly seen because the use of such devices for critical care patients as well as patients with chronic diseases is presently so routine. Likely organisms are listed in Table 3. Guidelines for the management of central venous line infections (1), published by the Infectious Diseases Society of America, the Society of Critical Care Medicine, and the Society for Healthcare Epidemiology of America are summarized in Figures 1 and 2. Antibiotics for specific pathogens are listed in Chapter 20.

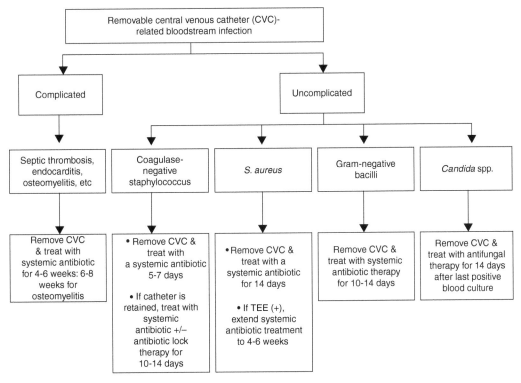

CVC = central venous catheter
TEE = transesophageal echocardiogram

FIGURE 1 Management of patients with nontunneled central venous catheter (CVC)—related bacteremia.

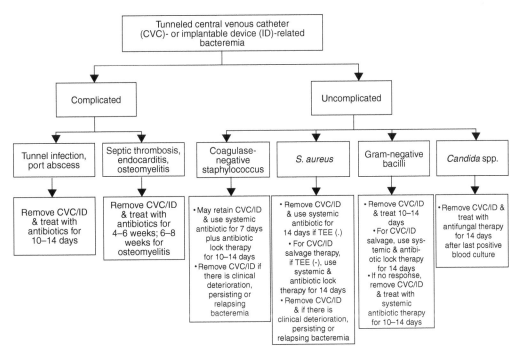

FIGURE 2 Management of patients with a tunneled central venous catheter (CVC)—or a surgically implanted device (ID)—related bacteremia.

TABLE 4   Clinical Diagnosis of Infant Botulism

Early symptoms	Later clinical findings
Constipation	Floppiness
Generalized	Drooping eyelids
hypotonia	Respiratory distress
Poor feeding	Absent deep tendon reflexes
Weak cry	Dilated reactive pupils
Muscle weakness	Poor suck
	Decreased to absent gag
	reflex
	Ptosis

TABLE 5   Laboratory Diagnosis of Infant Botulism

Toxin in stools is diagnostic
Stool culture for *Clostridium botuilinum*
Electromyography with repetitive stimulation
Lumbar puncture to exclude other diagnoses

BOTULISM

Botulism is caused by ingestion of the organism, *Clostridium botulinum*, or its performed neurotoxin. There are three forms of disease: food-borne, wound, and infant botulism. The only form commonly seen in pediatrics is infant botulism. Disease in infants is caused by the release of toxin from organisms that have gained entry to the gastrointestinal tract.

Onset of illness is usually 8 to 11 weeks of age with a reported range of 1 week to 10 months. Constipation and poor feeding are the first indications of disease with more suggestive neurologic signs beginning a few days later (Table 4). Diagnosis is best confirmed by identification of botulinus toxin in the stool (Table 5). Culture of the stool for *C. botulinum* should also be attempted but, because the organism is ubiquitous, it is not unusual to find it as normal flora in an infant's intestinal tract. Botulinus toxin has rarely been observed in the serum of infantile cases although the presence of toxin is fairly consistent in cases of food poisoning and wound botulism.

The differential diagnosis is rather limited (Table 6). Lumbar puncture should be performed to rule out other infectious etiologies. A negative response to edrophonium (Tensilon) (1 mg IV or 2 mg IM) and electromyographic studies will differentiate myasthenia gravis.

Treatment for botulism is primarily supportive but studies have demonstrated benefit of human derived antitoxin (Table 7). Aminoglycosides should be avoided because these agents can potentiate the neuromuscular blockade resulting in respiratory arrest and sudden death.

Specific pre-disposing factors to infant botulism remain speculative. A practical approach to prevention, however, might best focus on methods of reducing exposure to spores (Table 8), which infants might ingest.

CARDIAC INFECTIONS

Infections of the heart in children generally present as life-threatening disease requiring management by a pediatric cardiologist.

TABLE 6   Differential Diagnosis of Infant Botulism

Sepsis
Guillain-Barré syndrome
Myasthenia gravis
Aseptic meningitis
Polio
Diphtheria
Tick paralysis

TABLE 7   Treatment of Infant Botulism

Antitoxin for types A and B—human derived (BIGIV)
Supportive care
  Monitor cardiac and respiratory function
  Endotracheal intubation and assisted ventilation
    nutrition
Avoid aminoglycosides

TABLE 8 Prevention of Infant Botulism

Infants under 1 year of age
    Wash objects placed to infants' mouths (pacifiers, toys, etc.)
    Wash or peel skin of fruits and vegetables
    Avoid honey

Endocarditis

Endocarditis is the consequence of bacteremia in children with congenital anatomic cardiac abnormalities and occasionally in patients, most commonly neonates, with indwelling venous catheters. Infection is characteristically subacute in its onset and presentation (Table 9).

Criteria for diagnosis have been established at Duke University Medical Center based on blood culture, echocardiogram, and clinical findings (Table 10) (2). These criteria were modified and published as guidelines (Table 11) by the Committee on Rheumatic Fever, Endocarditis, and Kawasaki Disease, Council on Cardiovascular Disease in the Young, and the Councils on Clinical Cardiology, Stroke, and Cardiovascular Surgery and Anesthesia, American Heart Association; endorsed by the Infectious Disease Society of America (3).

TABLE 9 Pediatric Endocarditis: Clinical and Laboratory Findings

Bacterial etiology
    Streptococcus viridans
    Staphylococcus aureus
    Enterococcus
    Streptococcus bovis
    Staphylococcus epidermidis (neonates)
Other etiology
    Acute rheumatic fever (ARF)
    Systemic lupus erythematosus (SLE)
    Libman-Sacks syndrome
Clinical findings
    Underlying congenital or valvular heart defect (neonate-associated central hyperalimentation lines)
    Presents slowly over weeks/months with fever, malaise, fatigue (occasionally acute with febrile illness, toxicity, congestive heart failure)
    Associated findings of ARF or SLE
    Examination may reveal prominent murmur (may have new murmur, usually valve insufficiency, findings of congestive heart failure)
    Embolic findings include petechiae, Roth spots, Osler nodes, splinter hemorrhages, Janeway lesions, embolic pneumonias, splenomegaly
    Chest X-ray may show enlarged heart or embolic pneumonias
    ECG findings are non-specific (ARF may have increased PR interval)
    Echocardiography shows vegetations on valves or chambers
Laboratory findings
    Bacterial endocarditis-positive blood culture
    Anemia
    Elevated white blood cell count
    Left shift
    Elevated sedimentation rate (may be lowered with CHF)
    Increased acute-phase reactants
    Hematuria
    ARF-Jones criteria
    Elevated acute phase reactants, white blood cell count, sedimentation rate
    ASO or streptozyme confirmation of streptococcal infection

TABLE 10   Infective Endocarditis—Duke Criteria (2)

Major criteria
  Blood cultures positive for typical pathogens: Viridans streptococci, *Staphylococcus aureus,* enterococci, *Streptococcus bovis*
    2 cultures 12 hrs apart
    3 of 3 positive
    Majority of >3 cultures positive
  Echocardiogram positive
Minor criteria
  Predisposing heart lesions or intravenous drug use
  Fever
  Vascular lesions: major arterial emboli, septic pulmonary infarcts, mycotic aneurysm, intracranial hemorrhage, conjunctival hemorrhages, and Janeway's lesions
  Immunologic phenomena: glomerulonephritis, Osler's nodes, Roth's spots, and rheumatoid factor
  Microbiological evidence: positive blood culture but does not meet a major criterion as noted above or serological evidence of active infection with organism consistent with endocarditis

Treatment of endocarditis is summarized in Table 12 (viridans streptococci and *Streptococcus bovis*), Table 13 (*Staphylococcus aureus*), Table 14 (*Enterococcus*), and Table 15 (culture negative and *Bartonella henselae*). General care during and after completion of antimicrobial therapy for endocarditis is summarized in Table 16.

Myocarditis and Pericarditis

Myocarditis is more likely to have a viral etiology (Table 17), whereas endocarditis and pericarditis are more commonly caused by bacterial agents (Table 18). Intravenous immunoglobulin (IVIG) is recommended for the treatment of myocarditis and pericardial drainage for pericarditis. Broad spectrum antimicrobial therapy is appropriate for all patients with these life threatening cardiac infections pending results of cultures and other diagnostic evaluation.

DIPHTHERIA

Diphtheria, an acute illness caused by the organism *Corynebacterium diphtheriae,* is relatively rare in the United States, but is still occasionally seen among the non-immunized population. The incubation period for diphtheria is 1 to 6 days and may present in a number of clinical

TABLE 11   Definition of Endocarditis: Modified Duke Criteria

Definite infective endocarditis
  Pathological criteria
    Microorganisms demonstrated by culture or histological examination of a vegetation, a vegetation that has embolized, or an intracardiac abscess specimen; or
    Pathological lesions; vegetation or intracardiac abscess confirmed by histological examination showing active endocarditis
  Clinical criteria (Table 9)
    2 major criteria, or
    1 major criterion and 3 minor criteria, or
    5 minor criteria
  Possible endocarditis
    1 major criterion and 1 minor criterion, or
    3 minor criteria
  Rejected firm alternative diagnosis explaining evidence of endocarditis; or resolution of suspected endocarditis with antibiotic therapy for <4 days; or no pathological evidence of endocarditis at surgery or autopsy, with antibiotic therapy for <4 days; or does not meet criteria for possible endocarditis

TABLE 12 Therapy of Endocarditis Caused by Viridans Group Streptococci and *Streptococcus bovis*

Regimen	Dosage and route	Duration (wks)	Comments
Native valve			
Highly penicillin-susceptible (MIC-minimum inhibitory concentration <0.12 μg/mL)			
Aqueous crystalline penicillin G sodium	200,000 U/kg per 24 hrs IV in 4–6 equally divided doses;	4	
or			
Ceftriaxone sodium	Ceftriaxone 100 mg/kg per 24 hrs IV/IM in 1 dose	4	
Aqueous crystalline penicillin G sodium	Either continuously or in 6 equally divided doses	2	Two-week regimen not intended for patients with known cardiac or extracardiac abscess or for those with creatinine clearance of <20 mL/min, impaired 8th cranial nerve function, or *Abiotrophia, Granulicatella*, or *Gemella* spp. infection; gentamicin dosage should be adjusted to achieve peak serum concentration of 3–4 μg/mL and trough serum concentration of <1 μg/mL when 3 divided doses are used; nomogram used for single daily dosing
or			
Ceftriaxone sodium		2	
plus			
Gentamicin sulfate	3 mg/kg per 24 hrs IV/IM in 1 dose or 3 equally divided doses	2	
Vancomycin hydrochloride	40 mg/kg per 24 hrs IV in 2–3 equally divided doses not to exceed 2 g per 24 hrs unless concentrations in serum are inappropriately low	4	Vancomycin therapy recommended only for patients unable to tolerate penicillin or ceftriaxone; vancomycin dosage should be adjusted to obtain peak (1 hour after infusion completed) serum concentration of 30–45 μg/mL and a trough concentration range of 10–15 μg/mL
Relatively resistant to penicillin (MIC >0.12 μg/mL but <0.5 μg/mL)			
Aqueous crystalline penicillin G sodium	Penicillin 300,000 U/24 hrs IV in 4–6 equally divided doses	4	Patients with endocarditis caused by penicillin-resistant (MIC >0.5 μg/mL) strains should be treated with regimen recommended for enterococcal endocarditis (see Table 14)
or			
Ceftriaxone sodium	100 mg/kg per 24 hrs IV/IM in 1 dose;	4	
plus			
Gentamicin sulfate	3 mg/kg per 24 hrs IV/IM in 1 dose or 3 equally divided doses	2	

(Continued)

TABLE 12   Therapy of Endocarditis Caused by Viridans Group Streptococci and *Streptococcus bovis* (*Continued*)

Regimen	Dosage and route	Duration (wks)	Comments
Vancomycin hydrochloride	40 mg/kg 24 hrs in 2 or 3 equally divided doses not to exceed 2 g/24 hrs, unless serum concentrations are inappropriately low	4	Vancomycin therapy recommended only for patients unable to tolerate penicillin or ceftriaxone therapy
Prosthetic valves or other prosthetic material			
Penicillin-susceptible strain (minimum inhibitory concentration ≤0.12 μg/mL)			
Aqueous crystalline penicillin G sodium	300,000 U/kg per 24 hrs IV in 4–6 equally divided doses	6	Penicillin or ceftriaxone together with gentamicin has not demonstrated superior cure rates compared with monotherapy with penicillin or ceftriaxone for patients with highly susceptible strain; gentamicin therapy should not be administered to patients with creatinine clearance of <30 mL/min
or Ceftriaxone with or without	100 mg/kg IV/IM once daily	6	
Gentamicin sulfate	3 mg/kg per 24 hrs IV/IM, in 1 dose or 3 equally divided doses	2	
Vancomycin hydrochloride	40 mg/kg per 24 hrs IV or in 2 or 3 equally divided doses	6	Vancomycin therapy recommended only for patients unable to tolerate penicillin or ceftriaxone
Penicillin relatively or fully resistant strain (minimum inhibitory concentration >0.12 μg/mL)			
Aqueous crystalline penicillin sodium	300,000 U/kg per 24 hrs IV in 4–6 equally divided doses	6	
or Ceftriaxone plus	100 mg/kg IV/IM once daily	6	
Gentamicin sulfate	3 mg/kg per 24 hrs IV/IM, in 1 dose or 3 equally divided doses	6	
Vancomycin hydrochloride	40 mg/kg per 24 hrs IV or in 2 or 3 equally divided doses	6	Vancomycin therapy is recommended only for patients unable to tolerate penicillin or ceftriaxone

forms. These various presentations indicate that numerous etiologies must be considered in the differential diagnosis.

Diagnosis is confirmed by culture of material from beneath the pharyngeal membrane. Treatment, however, must be instituted as early as possible, usually based on clinical suspicion rather than culture results. The treatment prescribed varies with severity of disease as well as duration of symptoms prior to starting treatment (Table 19). Prognosis depends on the patient's age, the location and extent of the diphtheritic membrane, and the promptness with which antitoxin is given.

Consideration must also be given to other persons exposed to the index case; treatment varies with the immune status of these individuals (Table 20).

(*Text continues on page 26*)

TABLE 13   Therapy for Endocarditis Caused by *Staphylococcus aureus*

Regimen	Dosage and route	Duration	Comments
In the absence of prosthetic materials			
Oxacillin-susceptible strains			
Nafcillin or oxacillin	200 mg/kg per 24 h IV in 4–6 equally divided doses;	6 wk	For complicated right-sided IE and for left-sided IE; for uncomplicated right-sided IE, 2 wk (see text)
with			
Optional addition of gentamicin sulfate	3 mg/kg per 24 h IV/IM in 3 equally divided doses	3–5 d	Clinical benefit of aminoglycosides has not been established
For penicillin-allergic (nonanaphylactoid type) patients:			Consider skin testing for oxacillin-susceptible staphylococci and questionable history of immediate-type hypersensitivity to penicillin
Cefazolin	6 g/24 h IV in 3 equally divided doses	6 wk	Cephalosporins should be avoided in patients with anaphylactoid-type hypersensitivity to β-lactams; vancomycin should be used in these cases
with			
Optional addition of gentamicin sulfate	3 mg/kg per 24 h IV/IM in 2 or 3 equally divided doses *Pediatric dose*: cefazolin 100 mg/kg per 24 h IV in 3 equally divided doses; gentamicin 3 mg/kg per 24 h IV/IM in 3 equally divided doses	3–5 d	Clinical benefit of aminoglycosides has not been established
Oxacillin-resistant strains			
Vancomycin	30 mg/kg per 24 h IV in 2 equally divided doses	6 wk	Adjust vancomycin dosage to achieve 1-h serum concentration of 30–45 µg/mL and trough concentration of 10–15 µg/mL (see text for vancomycin alternatives)
	Pediatric dose: 40 mg/kg per 24 h IV in 2 or 3 equally divided doses		
Prosthetic valve			
Oxacillin-susceptible strains			
Nafcillin or oxacillin	200 mg/kg per 24 h IV in 4–6 equally divided doses;	≥6	Penicillin G 24 million U/24 h IV in 4 to 6 equally divided doses may be used in place of nafcillin or oxacillin if strain is penicillin susceptible (minimum inhibitory concentration ≤0.1 µg/mL) and does not produce β-lactamase; vancomycin should be used in patients with immediate-type hypersensitivity reactions to β-lactam antibiotics; cefazolin may be substituted for nafcillin or oxacillin in patients with non-immediate-type hypersensitivity reactions to penicillins

(Continued)

TABLE 13 Therapy for Endocarditis Caused by *Staphylococcus aureus* (*Continued*)

Regimen	Dosage and route	Duration	Comments
plus Rifampin	20 mg/kg per 24 h IV/PO in 3 equally divided doses;	≥6	
plus Gentamicin	3 mg/kg per 24 h IV/IM in 3 equally divided doses		
Oxacillin-resistant strains Vancomycin	40 mg/kg per 24 h IV in 2 or 3 equally divided doses;	≥6	Adjust vancomycin to achieve 1-h serum concentration of 30–45 μg/ mL and trough concentration of 10–15 μg/mL (see text for gentamicin alternatives)
plus Rifampin	20 mg/kg per 24 h IV/PO in 3 equally divided doses (up to adult dose);	≥6	
plus Gentamicin	3 mg/kg per 24 h IV or IM in 3 equally divided doses	2	

TABLE 14 Therapy for Native Valve or Prosthetic Valve *Enterococcal* Endocarditis

Regimen	Dosage and route	Duration (wks)	Comments
Caused by strains susceptible to penicillin, gentamicin, and vanconmycin			
Ampicillin sodium	300 mg/kg per 24 hr IV in 4–6 equally divided doses;	4–6	Native valve: 4-wk therapy recommended for patients with symptoms of illness ≤3 mo; 6-wk therapy recommended for patients with symptoms >3 mo
or Aqueous crystalline penicillin G sodium	Penicillin 300,000 U/kg per 24 hr IV in 4–6 equally divided doses	4–6	Prosthetic valve or other prosthetic cardiac material: minimum of 6 wk of therapy recommended
plus Gentamicin sulfate	3 mg/kg per 24 hr IV/IM in 3 equally divided doses	4–6	
Vancomycin hydrochloride	40 mg/kg per 24 hr IV in 2 or 3 equally divided doses	6	Vancomycin therapy recommended only for patients unable to tolerate penicillin or ampicillin
plus Gentamicin sulfate	3 mg/kg per 24 hr IV/IM in 3 equally divided doses	6	6 wk of vancomycin therapy recommended because of decreased activity against enterococci

(Continued)

TABLE 14 Therapy for Native Valve or Prosthetic Valve *Enterococcal* Endocarditis (*Continued*)

Regimen	Dosage and route	Duration (wks)	Comments
Caused by strains susceptible to penicillin, streptomycin, and vancomycin and resistant to gentamicin			
Ampicillin sodium	300 mg/kg per 24 hrs IV in 4–6 equally divided doses;	4–6	Native valve: 4-wk therapy recommended for patients with symptoms of illness <3 mo; 6-wk therapy recommended for patients with symptoms >3 mo
or Aqueous crystalline penicillin G sodium	penicillin 300,000 U/kg per 24 hrs IV in 4–6 equally divided doses;	4–6	
plus Streptomycin sulfate	streptomycin 20–30 mg/ kg per 24 hrs IV/IM in 2 equally divided doses	4–6	Prosthetic valve or other prosthetic cardiac material: minimum of 6 wk of therapy recommended
Vancomycin hydrochloride	40 mg/kg per 24 hrs IV in 2 or 3 equally divided doses	6	Vancomycin therapy recommended only for patients unable to tolerate penicillin or ampicillin
plus Streptomycin sulfate	20–30 mg/kg per 24 hrs IV/IM in 2 equally divided doses	6	
Caused by strains resistent to pencillin and susceptible to aminoglycoside and vancomycin			
β-Lactamase–producing strain			
Ampicillin-sulbactam	300 mg/kg per 24 hrs IV in 4 equally divided doses	6	Unlikely that the strain will be susceptible to gentamicin; if strain is gentamicin resistant, then >6 wk of ampicillin-sulbactam therapy will be needed
plus Gentamicin sulfate	3 mg/kg per 24 hrs IV/IM in 3 equally divided doses	6	
Vancomycin hydrochloride	40 mg/kg per 24 hrs in 2 or 3 equally divided doses;	6	Vancomycin therapy recommended only for patients unable to tolerate ampicillin-sulbactam
plus Gentamicin sulfate	3 mg/kg per 24 hrs IV/IM in 3 equally divided doses gentamicin 3 mg/kg per 24 hrs IV/IM in 3 equally divided doses	6	
Intrinsic penicillin resistance			
Vancomycin hydrochloride	40 mg/kg per 24 hrs IV in 2 or 3 equally divided doses	6	Consultation with a specialist in infectious diseases recommended
plus Gentamicin sulfate	3 mg/kg per 24 hrs IV/IM in 3 equally divided doses	6	

(*Continued*)

TABLE 14 Therapy for Native Valve or Prosthetic Valve *Enterococcal* Endocarditis (*Continued*)

Regimen	Dosage and route	Duration (wks)	Comments
Caused by strains resistant to penicillin, aminoglycoside, and vancomycin			
E faecium			
Linezolid	Linezolid 30 mg/kg per 24 hrs IV/PO in 3 equally divided doses;	≥8	Patients with endocarditis caused by these strains should be treated in consultation with an infectious diseases specialist; cardiac valve replacement may be necessary for bacteriologic cure; cure with antimicrobial therapy alone may be <50%; severe, usually reversible thrombocytopenia may occur with use of linezolid, especially after 2 wk of therapy; quinupristin-dalfopristin only effective against *E faecium* and can cause severe myalgias, which may require discontinuation of therapy; only small no. of patients have reportedly been treated with imipenem/cilastatin-ampicillin or ceftriaxone + ampicillin
or			
Quinupristin-dalfopristin	22.5 mg/kg per 24 hrs IV in 3 equally divided doses;	≥8	
E faecalis			
Imipenem/cilastatin	60–100 mg/kg per 24 hrs IV in 4 equally divided doses;	≥8	
plus			
Ampicillin sodium	300 mg/kg per 24 hrs IV in 4–6 equally divided doses;	≥8	
or			
Ceftriaxone sodium	100 mg/kg per 24 hrs IV/IM once daily	≥8	
plus			
Ampicillin sodium		≥8	

GUILLAIN-BARRÉ SYNDROME

Guillain-Barré syndrome (GBS), or acute idiopathic polyneuritis, is one of the most serious pediatric neurologic disorders. Although the majority of cases of GBS are mild and self-limited, at times the disorder may progress to complete respiratory paralysis and severe autonomic dysfunction. The overall incidence is 1 or 2 cases per 100,000 population. Although GBS generally peaks during the winter and spring, it may occur at any time of year. Factors, associated with onset of disease are listed in Table 21.

The underlying pathology is a nearly symmetrical, segmental demyelination of the peripheral nervous system distal to the ventral and dorsal root ganglia. Lymphocytic and macrophagic infiltration is characteristic, but the inflammatory mechanism resulting in infiltration has not been determined.

The clinical presentation of GBS is notoriously variable and diagnosis complex (Table 22). The classic case includes an ascending paralysis with sensory symptoms such as muscle cramps but few sensory signs. However, GBS may present atypically with a

TABLE 15 Therapy for Culture-Negative Endocarditis Including *Bartonella* Endocarditis

Regimen	Dosage and route	Duration, wk	Comments
Native valve			
Ampicillin-sulbactam	300 mg/kg per 24 h IV in 4–6 equally divided doses;	4–6	Patients with culture-negative endocarditis should be treated with consultation with an infectious diseases specialist
plus			
Gentamicin sulfate	3 mg/kg per 24 h IV/IM in 3 equally divided doses;	4–6	
Vancomycin	40 mg/kg per 24 h in 2 or 3 equally divided doses	4–6	Vancomycin recommended only for patients unable to tolerate penicillins
plus			
Gentamicin sulfate	3 mg/kg per 24 h IV/IM in 3 equally divided doses;	4–6	
plus			
Ciprofloxacin	20–30 mg/kg per 24 h IV/PO in 2 equally divided doses;	4–6	
Prosthetic valve (early, ≤1 y)			
Vancomycin	40 mg/kg per 24 h IV in 2 or 3 equally divided doses;	6	
plus			
Gentamicin sulfate	3 mg/kg per 24 h IV/IM in 3 equally divided doses	2	
plus			
Cefepime	150 mg/kg per 24 h IV in 3 equally divided doses;	6	
plus			
Rifampin	20 mg/kg per 24 h PO/IV in 3 equally divided doses	6	
Prosthetic valve (late, >1 y)		6	Same regimens as listed above for native valve endocarditis
Suspected Bartonella, culture negative			
Ceftriaxone sodium	100 mg/kg per 24 h IV/IM once daily;	6	Patients with *Bartonella* endocarditis should be treated in consultation with an infectious diseases specialist
plus			
Gentamicin sulfate	3 mg/kg per 24 h IV/IM in 3 equally divided doses	2	
with/without			
Doxycycline	2–4 mg/kg per 24 h IV/PO in 2 equally divided doses;	6	
Documented Bartonella, culture positive			
Doxycycline	2–4 mg/kg per 24 h IV/PO in 2 equally divided doses	6	
plus			
Gentamicin sulfate or Rifampin	3 mg/kg per 24 h IV/IM in 3 equally divided doses rifampin 20 mg/kg per 24 hr PO/IV in 2 equally divided doses	2	If gentamicin cannot be given, then replace with rifampin, 600 mg/24 h PO/IV in 2 equally divided doses

TABLE 16   Care During and After Completion of Antimicrobial Treatment

Initiate before or at completion of therapy
  Obtain transthoracic echocardiogram to establish new baseline
  Drug rehabilitation referral for patients who use illicit injection drugs
  Educate regarding signs of endocarditis, need for antibiotic prophylaxis for certain dental/surgical/invasive
      procedures
  Thorough dental evaluation and treatment if not performed earlier in evaluation
  Prompt removal of IV catheter at completion of antimicrobial therapy
Short-term follow-up
  Obtain at least 3 sets of blood cultures from separate sites for any febrile illness and before initiation of
      antibiotic therapy
  Physical examination for evidence of congestive heart failure
  Evaluate for toxicity resulting from current/previous antimicrobial therapy
Long-term follow-up
  Obtain at least 3 sets of blood cultures from separate sites for any febrile illness and before initiation of
      antibiotic therapy
  Evaluation of valvular and ventricular function (echocardiography)
  Scrupulous oral hygiene and frequent dental professional office visits

TABLE 17   Pediatric Myocarditis

Viral etiology
  Coxsackie
  ECHO
  Polio
  Influenza
  Adenovirus
  Mumps
  Rubella
Bacterial etiology
  Staphylococcus aureus
  Neisseria meningitidis
  Corynebacterium diphtheriae (toxin)
  Rickettsia rickettsii (Rocky Mountain–spotted fever)
Other etiology
  Acute rheumatic fever (pancarditis)
  Kawasaki disease
  Toxemia
  Chagas disease
Clinical findings
  Febrile illness with chest pain followed by shortness of breath, malaise, fatigue over several weeks to months,
      may present as an arrhythmia or with a sudden fulminating course (especially in young infants) or with
      sudden collapse (sudden death), often associated with pericarditis (myopericarditis)
  Bacterial and rickettsial etiologies develop fulminant illness with sepsis, shock, and congestive heart failure
  Acute rheumatic fever-associated findings (Jones criteria) valvulitis (pancarditis)
  Kawasaki disease etiology during the acute phase manifesting diffuse myocarditis and small vessel arteritis
  Clinical examination gives findings of congestive heart failure
Laboratory findings
  Chest X-ray shows enlarged heart (left atrium and ventricle) and pulmonary edema
  ECG shows diffuse ST-T changes, low voltage, arrhythmias, left ventricular hypertrophy with strain pattern (late)
  Acute-phase reactants helpful only early in illness
  Laboratory studies for rheumatic or Kawasaki disease helpful but nonspecific
  Viral cultures usually negative; acute and convalescent viral titers (>4-fold increase)
  Echocardiography shows enlarged left atrium and left ventricular poor contractility
  Multi-gated acquisition scan shows increased uptake by the heart
  Endomyocardial biopsy is diagnostic

(Continued)

TABLE 17   Pediatric Myocarditis (*Continued*)

Course of disease
Variable course: may show spontaneous improvement with time or progress to chronic cardiomyopathy
Bacterial and rickettsial etiologies have a severe course with high mortality despite early diagnosis and
appropriate antibiotic coverage
Treatment
IVIG, 2 g/kg over 24 hr
Supportive therapy
Inotropes and diuretics
Afterload-reducing agents
Extracorporeal support (ECMO, LVAD)
Failure to respond or deterioration, may consider steroids and/or immunosuppressive agents

descending paralysis, ophthalmoplegia, or a "locked-in" state with complete motor paralysis in which the patient appears comatose.

The course of severe GBS may be influenced by early recognition and the availability of intensive care, in particular ventilatory support (Table 23). With such support, all children with GBS should survive with a favorable outcome. The most common pediatric complications of GBS are respiratory arrest, aspiration pneumonia, autonomic dysfunction, and iatrogenic complications of prolonged ventilation. Intravenous immunoglobulin has been shown to prevent progression of more severe disease and decrease the development of late-stage GBS.

Management of children with GBS (Table 24) requires physicians, nurses, respiratory therapists, and physical and occupational therapists who are acquainted with the course and evolution of the disorder. In general, any patient with suspected GBS should be admitted to a pediatric intensive care unit or ward in which meticulous observation and neurologic re-examination is possible. Guillain-Barré syndrome may evolve acutely from minimal motor weakness to complete respiratory paralysis in some cases. Pulmonary function testing should be included for the evaluation of prognosis and to identify candidates for intravenous immunoglobulin therapy.

HANTAVIRUS PULMONARY SYNDROME

Hantavirus pulmonary syndrome (HPS) defines an acute respiratory illness caused by Sin Nombre, a hantavirus endemic in the Southwestern United States. Disease is characterized by a short prodrome of fever and myalgia followed by interstitial pneumonia with massive pulmonary capillary leak, non-cardiogenic pulmonary edema, cardiovascular collapse, and death in almost 50% of infected individuals. Additional clinical characteristics are summarized in Table 25.

First recognized in the spring of 1993 during a cluster outbreak in New Mexico, an additional 200 cases were reported over the next 4 years predominantly in southwestern and southeastern states. Etiologic confirmation can now be achieved with a number of highly specific serologic assays for hantavirus serum antibody or antigen identification in respiratory secretions and tissue (Table 26), available through diagnostic services at CDC.

Treatment of HPS is largely supportive with careful attention to fluid balance and cardiopulmonary support (Table 27). Assisted ventilation is usually required. Inhaled nitric oxide has been shown to provide significant benefit to patients with a persistent oxygenation index above 20 and evidence of pulmonary hypertension. Extracorporeal membrane oxygenation has also been used successfully in patients believed to have a 100% mortality risk.

MENINGOCOCCEMIA

The organism *Neisseria meningitidis* causes illness in humans with a variety of clinical presentations, ranging from benign upper respiratory infection to acute endotoxemia and vasculitis. Chronic disease has also been described. The common signs and symptoms of acute

TABLE 18 Pediatric Pericarditis

Viral etiology
   Coxsackie
   ECHO
   Adenovirus
   Influenza
   Mumps
   Cytomegalovirus
   Epstein-Barr virus
Bacterial etiology
   Staphylococcus aureus
   Streptococcus pneumoniae
   Neisseria meningitidis
Other etiologies
   Uremia
   Postpericardiotomy
   Collagen vascular disease
   Systemic lupus erythematosus, acute rheumatic fever
   Mycoplasma
   Tuberculosis
   Parasitic disease
Clinical findings
   Chest pain (precordial) referred to back and shoulder, relieved by sitting
     upright
   Dyspnea
   Fever, malaise (bacterial etiology with increased toxicity)
   Presents as sepsis associated with meningitis and septic arthritis (young
     infant)
   Examination reveals tachycardia, decreased heart sounds, rub, Kussmaul's
     sign (distension of neck veins with inspiration), paradoxical pulse
     >10 mmHg early tamponade)
   Associated illnesses include renal failure, previous heart surgery, systemic
     lupus erythematosus, juvenile rheumatoid arthritis, acute rheumatic
     fever, meningitis, pneumonia
Laboratory findings
   Chest X-ray shows enlarged, water bottle-shaped heart (initially may show
     just a straightened left-heart border)
   ECG shows diffuse ST-T changes, low voltage
   Elevated white blood cell count
   Left shift
   Elevated sedimentation rate
   Abnormal renal and collagen vascular studies if autoimmune etiology
   Positive blood cultures with bacterial etiology
   Echocardiography is diagnostic
   Pericardial fluid exudate has protein >3 g/100 mL, inflammatory cells
     (bacterial), polymorphonuclear leukocytes, low glucose, specific gravity
     >1.015
   Pericardial fluid transudate has protein <2 g/100 mL, few cells (mesothelial),
     normal glucose, specific gravity <1.015
Course and treatment
   Bacterial etiology: requires adequate drainage (repeated pericardiocentesis,
     tube drainage, or pericardial windows)-most patients have organisms
     recovered via blood or pericardial fluid—appropriate antibiotics
     (14–21 days)
   Viral etiology: 2–6 wk course, pain usually controlled with aspirin or non-
     steroidal; viral cultures usually negative, can progress occasionally to
     constriction; tamponade requires pericardiocentesis
   Other etiologies: usually follows course of other illness unless tamponade
     occurs

TABLE 19   Treatment of Diphtheria

Drug/support	Dosage/duration
Antitoxin	Dilute 1:20 in isotonic sodium chloride and infuse IV not exceeding 1 mL/min
Pharyngeal and laryngeal disease symptom duration <48 hr	20,000–40 000 U antitoxin
Nasopharyngeal	40,000–60,000 U
Extensive disease of symptom Duration >3 days or diffuse swelling of the neck	80,000–120,000 U
Diphtheria toxoid	First dose at end of 1st week of illness Second dose 1 mo later Third dose 1 mo after second dose
Antibiotics Penicillin or	100,000 U/kg/ day IV div. q 6 hr for 10 days
Erythromycin	20–50 mg/kg/day for IV div. q 6 hr for 10 days
Supportive intensive	Airway protection with endotracheal intubation as needed to assure patent airway and prevent aspiration Mechanical ventilation for respiratory failure associated with paralysis of muscles of respiration Support for failing circulation Bedrest (minimum 2–3 wk) until risk of myocarditis passes Prednisone 1–1.5 mg/kg/day for 2 wk for myocarditis Provision for nutrition and hydration (enteral or parenteral) Isolation after completion of antibiotic therapy until three cultures of nose and throat (taken 24 hr apart) are negative for toxigenic diphtheria bacilli

and chronic meningococcemia may initially be subtle, but fever accompanied by a petechial rash should always suggest meningococcal infection.

Diagnosis of meningococcemia is made by a characteristic clinical presentation (Fig. 3) and is usually confirmed by culture (Table 28). Care must be taken to differentiate meningococcemia from other febrile illnesses with rashes. These include septicemia and disseminated intravascular coagulation (DIC) due to other bacteria, endocarditis, Rocky Mountain–spotted fever, and enteroviral infections.

TABLE 20   Management of Contacts of Index Cases

Contact	Management
Household contacts	Surveillance for 7 days Culture for *C. diphtheriae* follow-up cultures in positives after completing therapy PO erythromycin 40–50 mg/kg/ days × 10 days or benzathine penicillin 1.2 × 10⁶ U.IM
Immunized household contacts	Booster dose of diphtheria toxoid vaccine

TABLE 21   Factors Associated with Onset of Guillain-Barré Syndrome

Infectious agents or postinfectious factors (60%)
  Viral
    Non-specific upper respiratory or gastrointestinal infections
    Epstein-Barr virus
    Cytomegalovirus
  Rickettsia
  Mycoplasma
  Bacterial
Noninfectious factors (10%)
  Vaccinations
  Immune disorders
  Endocrine disturbances
  Pregnancy
  Neoplasms
  Toxic exposures
  Surgery

TABLE 22   Diagnostic Criteria for Guillain-Barré Syndrome

Criteria required for diagnosis
  Progressive motor weakness of more than one limb and/or truncal or bulbar
    weakness
  Areflexia
Criteria strongly suggestive of diagnosis
  Minimal sensory findings
  Relative symmetry of weakness
  Progressive motor involvement (2–4 wk) followed by a plateau and gradual
    complete recovery
  Cranial nerve involvement, especially bifacial paralysis
  Autoimmune system involvement
  Absence of fever at onset
  Elevated cerebrospinal fluid protein at some point of illness
Factors inconsistent with diagnosis
  Marked asymmetry of weakness
  Persistent bladder dysfunction
  Sudden onset of bowel or bladder dysfunction
  Over 50 mononuclear cells/mm^3 cerebrospinal fluid (or presence of any
    polymophonuclear leukocytes)
  Sharp sensory level
Factors that exclude diagnosis
  History of toxic hydrocarbon or lead exposure, acute intermittent porphyria,
    diphtheria, botulism, poliomyelitis, or other well-recognized causes of
    neuropathy
  Purely sensory symptoms
  Electromyographic findings

Treatment of meningococcemia includes antibiotics and intensive supportive care when shock is present (Table 29). In addition, prophylactic treatment of family members and other close contacts of the index case is indicated (Tables 30 and 31).

ORBITAL CELLULITIS

Orbital subperiosteal abscesses with resulting eyelid and periorbital skin cellulitis in children, inclusively termed orbital (or postseptal) cellulitis, have previously been considered acute surgical emergencies by pediatricians (Fig. 4). More recently, a conservative medical approach for most orbital infections is appropriate, including those associated with subperiosteal abscesses secondary to sinusitis. Management of orbital infections is based primarily on clinical staging of infection as summarized in Table 32.

PERITONITIS

Acute bacterial peritonitis occurs in two distinct forms as determined by the source of infection (Table 33 and 34). Peritonitis should be suspected from the clinical presentation (Table 35) and confirmed by laboratory evaluation (Table 36).

(Text continues on page 36)

TABLE 23   The Course of Guillain-Barré Syndrome

Development	Incidence (%)
Requirement of ventilatory support	20
Relapse	5–10
Complete recovery	50
Residual neurologic or orthopedic sequelae	10
Fatal pulmonary or cardiac (adults) complications	5

TABLE 24 Management of Guillain-Barré Syndrome

Chronic care
  Prevention of urinary tract infection
  Prevention of decubiti
  Prevention of immobilization hypercalcemia and renal/bladder calculi
  Prevention of contractures
  Recognition and treatment (in some cases) of autonomic dysfunction
Respiratory care
  Admission of intensive care unit setting
  Recognition of deteriorating respiratory ability through clinical observation, pulmonary function tests, and
    arterial blood gas analysis
  Endotracheal intubation and mechanical ventilation should be considered:
    Forced vital capacity <15–20 mL/kg
    Maximum negative inspiratory pressure <20–30 cm H_2O p_aCO_2 >50 Torr
    Weakness of protective reflexes (cough and gag)
  Pharmacologic management
    Severe disease: Intravenous immunoglobulin (IVIG) 400 mg/kg per day for 5 days or until improvement is
      significant; no proven efficacy for mild disease, i.e., those with no or little respiratory involvement
    Corticosteroids have no proven efficacy in acute cases
    Treatment of autonomic dysfunction (rarely indicated)
      Antihypertensives (diuretic agents)
      Fludrocortisone (Florinef) for marked orthostatic hypotension
      Plasmapheresis (controlled studies underway) appropriate for severe cases not responding to IVIG

TABLE 25 Common Clinical Characteristics of Hantavirus

Rodent exposure; appropriate geographic regions
Fever >38.3°C
Interstitial pneumonia
Rapidly progressive respiratory failure
Intubation 1–14 days (median 4 days) after onset of
  symptoms
Hemoconcentration (elevated Hgb, Hct)
Thrombocytopenia

TABLE 26 Diagnosis of Hantavirus

Compatible clinical course
Hantavirus-specific serology
  IgG, IgM
Lower respiratory tissue or secretions
  PCR for hantavirus RNA
  Immunohistochemical identification of
    hantavirus antigen

TABLE 27 Management of Hantavirus-Related Acute Respiratory Distress Syndrome (ARDS)

Symptoms
  Rapid onset ARDS
  Neurologic disturbance
  Hemoconcentration (elevated hemoglobin)
  Coagulopathy including disseminated intravascular coagulation
  Renal failure
  Hepatic failure
Definition of ARDS
  Antecedent event (e.g., infection with hantavirus)
  Hypoxemia (p_aO_2/FIO$_2$ < 200)
  Exclusion of left heart failure
  Bilateral diffuse infilitrates
  Non-cardiogenic pulmonary edema
Treatment of ARDS
  Intravenous ribavirin may be of benefit if given early
  Supportive treatment
  Extracorporeal life support

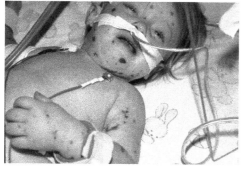

FIGURE 3 (*See color insert.*) The rash of meningococcemia is usually a combination of petechiae, ecchymoses, and purpura as seen in this 13-mo-old. Larger purpura have a straked appearance as contrasted with the purpura with Henoch-Schonleion disease which are round. Severe infection with disseminated intravascular coagulation caused by many other bacterial pathogens may look identical to meningococcemia.

TABLE 28   Laboratory Diagnosis for Meningococcemia

Complete blood count characteristically shows leukocytosis and
  thrombocytopenia
Cultures (blood, cerebrospinal fluid, skin lesion, nasopharynx)
Cerebrospinal fluid analysis for evidence of meningitis
Latex agglutination of blood, CSF and urine
Clotting studies for evidence of DIC: low-prothrombin time, fibrinogen, and
  fibrin split products with disseminated intravascular coagulation

TABLE 29   Treatment of Meningococcemia

Ceftriaxone 80 mg/kg per day IV div. qd for 5 days
Aggressive fluid resuscitation for patient in shock to
  replete intravascular volume (see Table 57) for
  supportive care
Platelet or clotting factor replacement therapy for
  patient with disseminated intravascular
  coagulation and hemorrhage
Activated protein C (Xigris) for severe sepsis—
  24 mcg/kg/hr infusion × 96 hrs
Steroids not shown to improve survival
Burn-type wound care for skin sloughs in areas of
  thrombosis
Hyperbaric oxygen may be useful in wound
  management

TABLE 30   High-Risk Contacts of Meningococcal Disease

All household contacts
Nursery or day care center contacts
Hospital personnel and individual who had intimate
  exposure to oral secretions from the index case

TABLE 31   Antibiotics for Meningococcal Prophylaxis

Antibiotic prophylaxis	Dosage	Comments
Rifampin	<1 mo: 5 mg/kg twice daily PO for 2 days	Contraindicated for pregnant women
	>1 mo: 10 mg/kg twice daily PO for 2 days (max, 600 mg/dose)	Orange-red urine Stains contact lenses
Ceftriaxone	<12 yr: 125 mg IM as single dose	Safe for pregnant women
	>12 yr: 250 mg IM as a single dose	Better compliance
Ciprofloxacin	Single adult PO dose 500 mg	Contraindicated for pregnant women and children younger than 18 yrs

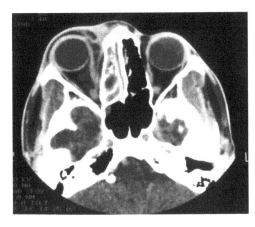

FIGURE 4 CT of the orbit in a child with orbital cellulitis who presented with proptosis, chemosis, and limitation of extraocular movement. There is opacification of the right retro-bulbar space, displacing the eye and orbit contents forward to account for the proptosis.

TABLE 32   Staging and Management of Orbital Cellulitis

Stage I	More likely preseptal (periorbital). Eyelid swelling with sinusitis. Occasionally febrile. CT scan normal except for periorbital swelling. Management: Outpatient antibiotics (IM followed by PO)
Stage II	Edema of orbital lining, chemosis, proptosis, limitation of extraocular movement, fever. CT scan: no subperiosteal abscess. Might see mucosal edema or swelling. Management: Inpatient IV antibiotics
Stage III	Occasional visual loss. Progression of changes seen in Stage II. CT scan: subperiosteal abscess; globe displacement; intraconal involvement of extraocular muscles. Management: Inpatient IV antibiotics. Surgical drainage if not clinically improving after 24 hr
Stage IV	Ophthalmoplegia with visual loss. CT scan: proptosis; abscess formation involving the extraocular muscles and orbital fat. Periosteal rupture. Management: IV antibiotics and surgical drainage.

TABLE 33   Characteristic Forms of Peritonitis

Primary form
    Focus of infection outside of abdominal cavity
    Infection is blood- or lymph-borne
    Commonly seen in children with ascites secondary to nephrosis or cirrhosis
Secondary form
    Infection disseminated by extension from or rupture of an intra-abdominal
        viscus or abscess of an intra-abdominal organ

TABLE 34   Bacteriology of Peritonitis

Primary peritonitis
  Streptococcus pneumoniae
  Streptococci
  Gram-negative rods
  Mycobacterium tuberculosis
  Haemophilus influenzae
Secondary peritonitis
  Aerobic bacteria
    Escherichia coli
    Streptococci
    Enterococci
    Staphylococcus aureus
	Enterobacteriaceae
	    Klebsiella
	    Proteus
	    Pseudomonas
	    Candida
	  Anaerobic bacteria
	    Bacteroides fragilis
	    Eubacteria
	    Clostridia
	    Peptostreptococci
	    Peptococci
	    Propionibacteria
	    Fusobacteria

TABLE 35   Signs and Symptoms of Generalized Peritonitis

Abdominal pain and tenderness
Edema
Ascites
Fever
Anorexia, vomiting, constipation, or diarrhea
Ileus
Lethargic, toxic-appearing child
Abdominal wall cellulites

TABLE 36   Laboratory Diagnosis of Peritonitis

Leukocytosis
Ultrasonographic examination of abdomen
Radiographic examination of abdomen
Dilation of large and small intestines
Edema of small intestinal wall
Peritoneal fluid
Obliteration of psoas shadow
Free air within peritoneal cavity (secondary peritonitis)
Paracentesis (see Chapter 7)
Elevated protein concentration
Pleocytosis (>800 leukocytes/mm^3, more than 25% of which are polymorphonuclear leukocytes)
Positive Gram smear and culture of fluid

Note: The treatment for bacterial peritonitis is nonoperative for primary peritonitis and operative for secondary peritonitis (Table 37). Common postoperative complications include formation of adhesions with subsequent intestinal obstruction and intra-abdominal abscess formation.

TABLE 37   Treatment of Peritonitis

Primary peritonitis	
Systemic antibiotics	Ceftriaxone
	Cefotaxime
Secondary peritonitis	
Preoperative disturbances	Correct hypovolemia and stabilize electrolytes to re-establish adequate urine output
	Correct hypoxemia with supplemental oxygen and mechanical ventilation if necessary
	Decompress gastrointestinal tract using nasogastric suction or long intestinal tube
Antibiotic therapy	Ampicillin
	plus
	Clindamycin
	plus
	Meropenem, ceftriaxone, cefotaxime or gentamicin (dosing increments vary for neonates)
Operative therapy	Close, exclude, or resect perforated viscus, followed by either
	Complete exposure of peritoneal cavity with radical debridement of peritoneum, followed by massive irrigation with or without antibiotics
	or
	Placement of drains after repair of perforation without further exploration or irrigation
Postoperative management	Continued administration of systemic antibiotics
	Intraperitoneal lavage with antibiotic solution
	Attention to repletion of intravascular fluid volume
	Observation for autonomic hyperreflexia when draining peritoneum
	Nutritional support to meet high metabolic demands
	Close observation for intraabdominal abdominal abscess formation

RABIES

Rabies is an acute encephalitis caused by a rhabdovirus. Transmitted via secretions, urine or saliva following the bite of an infected animal, the virus passes along peripheral nerves to the central nervous system where neuronal necrosis occurs, principally in the brainstem and medulla. Incubation varies from 10 days to as long as 2 years, with mean onset being within 2 months of the bite (Table 38). In the United States, most human rabies cases are transmitted by bats as determined by viral strain analysis. There is rarely a known history of exposure to infected animals.

There are two basic presentations of rabies in humans, classic and paralytic. The classic symptom of hydrophobia (Table 39) is caused by inspiratory muscle spasms, a consequence of

TABLE 38   Factors Affecting Time-to-Onset of Symptoms in Rabies

Distance of site of initial inoculum from central nervous system
Amount of inoculum
Virulence of virus
Resistance of host

destruction of brainstem neurons inhibitory to neurons of the nucleus ambiguous, which control inspiration.

Diagnosis may be confirmed by demonstration of the antigen, antibody, or viral complexes (Table 40). The differential diagnosis of rabies includes other causes of encephalitis and ascending neuritis.

Prevention of rabies includes measures to control the virus reservoir in the animal population as well as vaccination of domestic animals (95% effective). Postexposure treatment of humans also includes human rabies immunoglobulin and human diploid cell vaccine (Table 25). The only true protection, however, is immunity acquired pre-exposure.

Once a victim is clinically symptomatic, the prognosis is grim; there have only been four reported survivors. Treatment centers around intensive supportive care so should be provided in facilities able to provide optional intervention to control the airway and assure ventilation in the patient with hydrophobia or obtundation, as well as circulatory system support. Antiviral therapy was also used in one 15-year-old girl who survived (Table 41).

RHEUMATIC FEVER

This nonsuppurative sequela of group A beta-hemolytic streptococcal infections (GABHS) can be prevented by treatment of the antecedent strep throat or other GABHS disease (see Chapter 8) even if given as late as 9 days after the onset of symptoms. Once a diagnosis of

TABLE 39   Symptoms of the Classic Form of Rabies

Prodrome (2 days to 2 wks)	Malaise, anorexia, headache, fever, irritability, pain, numbness or tingling at site of bite spreading upward. Later symptoms; jerky movements, pupillary dilatation, increased tearing and salivation
Acute neurologic phase (2–7 days)	Dysphagia, hydrophobia, mania (alternating with lethargy), increased salivation, abnormal biting and chewing, excitement, fear, apathy, terror, convulsive movements, choking, distended bladder, constipation, penile pain
Final phase (7–10 days)	Coma, dysrhythmias, hypotension, heart block, bradycardia, respiratory muscle spasm, hypoventiliation, disturbance in fluid balance metabolic upsets, cardiorespiratory arrest

TABLE 40   Diagnosis of Rabies

Identification of antigen on cell culture
Electron microscopy
Immunofluorescent rabies–antibody staining
Antibody titers
Diagnostic in non-vaccinated persons
Cerebrospinal fluid titers to diagnose post-vaccination encephalomyelitis
Viral complexes
Corneal touch preparations
Fluorescent antibody staining of parafollicular neurons of neck skin biopsy

TABLE 41   Treatment of Rabies

Induction of coma
Ketamine
Midazolam
Antiviral therapy
Ribavirin
Amantadine

rheumatic fever is made, children should be placed on antibiotic prophylaxis to prevent recurrences as outlined in Table 42.

RICKETTSIAL INFECTIONS

Rocky Mountain Spotted Fever

Rocky Mountain spotted fever is a disease caused by inoculation with *Rickettsia rickettsii*, transmitted via the bite of a tick. The organisms replicate within the endothelial lining and smooth muscle cells of blood vessels, causing generalized vasculitis. Vasculitic changes of various organ systems account for the observed clinical findings (Table 43).

The incubation period in children is 1 to 8 days. When early nonspecific symptoms appear in a child with a history of a tick bite, xRocky Mountain spotted fever should be seriously considered and early treatment instituted. Most laboratory findings in Rocky Mountain spotted fever are nonspecific until positive convalescent titers appear (Table 44). The exception to this is the appearance of the organism on skin lesion stains or by use of immunofluorescent biopsy of skin for early specific diagnosis.

It is difficult to differentiate Rocky Mountain spotted fever from the myriad other causes of febrile exanthemas. Its diagnosis is also frequently overlooked in patients who do not present with the typical rash (Fig. 5) or in whom a history of tick bite cannot be elicited (Table 45).

Treatment of Rocky Mountain spotted fever should be instituted as soon as the diagnosis is suspected clinically (Table 46). In addition to antibiotic therapy, careful supportive intensive care is needed with aggressive intervention necessary to stabilize the most severely ill patients.

TABLE 42 Prophylaxis for Rheumatic Fever

Antibiotic
  Benzathine penicillin G: 1.2 million U q 4 wk IM
  or
  Penicillin V: 250 mg b.i.d. PO
  or
  Sulfadiazine or sulfisoxazole: <27 kg 500 mg qd PO
                             >27 kg 1 g qd PO
  Allergic to penicillin and sulfonamides: erythromycin 250 mg b.i.d. PO

TABLE 43 Clinical Findings in Rocky Mountain Spotted Fever

History of tick bite (70–80% of cases)
Fever
Headache
Anorexia
Chills
Sore throat
Nausea and vomiting
Abdominal pain
Mild diarrhea
Arthralgias and myalgias
Rash
  Petechial but may begin as macular or maculopapular rash, blanching lesions, affects extremities first, spreads
    centripetally, occasionally appears later (or not at all)
Noncardiogenic pulmonary edema
Occasionally manifestations
  Edema (periorbital early, generalized later), splenomegaly in one-third of cases, hepatomegaly, pneumonitis,
    mycocardial involvement, conjunctivitis, photophobia, papilledema, transient deafness, meningismus,
    delirium, seizures, coma

TABLE 44   Laboratory Studies in Rocky Mountain Spotted Fever

Type of study	Result
White blood cell count	Normal or slightly decreased with left shift in 1st week; leukocytosis in 2nd week
Platelet count	Depressed
Fibrogen	Depressed with disseminated intravascular coagulation
Electrolytes	Hyponatremia and hypochloremia
Liver function tests	Elevated AST (asparate aminotransferase), ALT (alanine aminostransferase), and bilirubin; depressed total protein and albumin
Creatinine	Increased
Lactate dehydrogenase	Increased
Urinalysis	Hematuria
Cerebrospinal fluid	White blood cell count <300 mm^{-3}, predominantly lymphocytes in most cases; normal glucose; mildly elevated protein
Well-Felix reaction	Proteus OX-19 and OX-2 single titer >1:160 or 4-fold rise in titer diagnostic
Rocky Mountain spotted fever complement fixation titers	Convalescent titers may increase after 14 days of illness
Giemsa stain of skin lesion	May demonstrate organism
Immunofluorescent biopsy of skin	Possible to make diagnosis using this technique

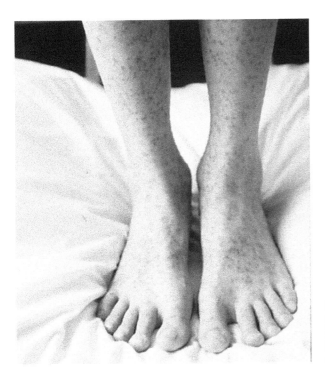

FIGURE 5   A centrifugal, petechial rash with fever is characteristic of Rocky Mountain spotted fever but is also seen with enteroviral infections and with human monocytotrophic ehrlichiosis.

Ehrlichiosis

In the United States, there are 3 forms of human ehrlichiosis: monocytotrophic caused by *Ehrlichia chaffeensis*, granulocytotrophic anaplasmosis caused by *Anaplasma phagocytophilum*, and *E. ewingii* ehrlichiosis caused by *Ehrlichia ewingii*. Most common is the monocytotrophic form. All present clinically as acute, systemic, febrile illnesses very similar to Rocky Mountain spotted fever, but are less likely to have a rash. A striking laboratory

TABLE 45   Differential Diagnosis of Rocky Mountain Spotted Fever

Ehrlichiosis
Meningococcemia
Measles
Enteroviral infections
Typhoid fever
Endemic murine typhus
Rickettsialpox
Colorado tick fever
Tularemia
Immune-complex vasculitis
Collagen vascular diseases
Thrombotic thrombocytopenic purpura
Idiopathic thrombocytopenic purpura

TABLE 46   Treatment of Rocky Mountain Spotted Fever

Doxycycline 4 mg/kg/day div. q 12 hr for 7–10 days; must be afebrile at least 3 days prior to stopping antibiotics
Fluid management with replacement (as needed) of intravascular volume, lost to 3rd spacing, in order to restore circulation
Mechanical ventilation and positive end expiratory pressure may be needed to correct hypoxemia from noncardiogenic pulmonary edema
Replacement of platelets and clotting factors in cases with disseminated intravascular coagulation and associated hemorrhage
Present and future understanding of the role of nitric oxide and endothelial defects caused by Rocky Mountain spotted fever may lead to new treatment regimens

TABLE 47   Diagnosis and Treatment of Human Ehrlichiosis

Diagnosis: Isolation of organisms from blood or CSF
    Antibody titer by indirect immunofluorescence assay (IFA) 4-fold or greater increase in antibody titer
    PCR-DNA
    Intraleukocytoplasmic microcolonies on peripheral smear along with an IFA titer = or >64
Treatment: Doxycycline 4 mg/kg/day div. b.i.d. until afebrile × 3 days, but a minimum of 10 days

TABLE 48   Clinical Findings in Presumed Septicemia

Fever and chills (or hypothermia)
Toxic appearance
Poor peripheral perfusion (cold extremities)
Shock
Disseminated intravascular coagulation
Multiorgan failure
Documented source of infection
Host predisposition

feature is profound leukopenia, particularly neutropenia. As with Rocky Mountain spotted fever, thrombocytopenia and hyponatremia are common.

SEPTIC SHOCK

No other problem is encountered as commonly in pediatric intensive care as sepsis. The diagnosis of sepsis in the child, particularly without an obvious source of infection, requires a high degree of suspicion (Table 48 and 49).

Progressing sepsis usually results in multiple organ system involvement and subsequent system failure (Table 50). Septic shock is encountered in a number of severe cases of sepsis,

TABLE 49   Clinical Syndromes Commonly Associated with Sepsis in Children

Primary bacteremia	
Newborns	
Compromised host	Malignancy, immunodeficiency syndrome, immunosuppressive drug therapy
Normal children	Meningococcemia, pneumococcemia, *Staphylococcus aureus* or β-hemolytic streptococcal septicemia
Secondary bacteremia	
Secondary to remote infection	Meningitis, osteomyelitis, septic arthritis, pneumonia, orbital cellulitis, wound infection, intestinal obstruction, pyelonephritis, burns, diarrhea
Secondary to operation or instrumentation	

TABLE 50   Effects of Sepsis on Organ Systems

Organ/system	Effect of sepsis
Hematologic	Granulocytosis, thrombocytopenia, disseminated intravascular coagulation
Pulmonary	Acute respiratory distress syndrome
Renal	Oliguria, acute renal insufficiency
Cardiac	Hypotension, myocardial depression (late)
Hepatic	Elevation of serum glutamic oxalo-acetic transaminase, glutamic pyruvic transaminate and bilirubin
Brain	Altered level of consciousness or confusion (especially with hypotension)

TABLE 51   Incidence of Shock with Bacteremia

Organism causing bacteremia	Percentage with shock (1%)
Gram-negative bacilli	40–45
Staphylococcus aureus	25–35
Streptococcus pneumoniae	10–15

TABLE 52   Progression of Septic Shock

Early symptoms
  Fever
  Increased VO_2[a]
  Increased cardiac output
  Normal A VdO_2[b]
Followed by
  "Warm" shock
  Vasodiliation
  Decreased systemic vascular resistance
  Redistribution of blood volume
  Decreased ventricular preload
  Increased cardiac output
  Hypotension
  Wide pulse pressure
  Oliguria
  Hypoxemia
Progressing to
  Generalized capillary leak
  Further decreased ventricular preload
	Hypotension
	Edema
	Acute respiratory distress syndrome
	Multiple organ system dysfunction
	Late symptoms
	  Oxygen extraction failure
	  Decreased VO_2[a] and A VdO_2[b]
	  Increased cardiac output
	Progressing to
	  "Cold" shock
	  Vasoconstriction
	  Increased systemic vascular resistance
	  Release of myocardial depressant factor
	  Poor coronary perfusion
	  Decreased cardiac output
	  Increased A VdO_2
	  Lactic acidosis
	  Progressing to death

[a]VO_2, oxygen consumption.
[b]A VdO_2, arteriovenous dissolved oxygen.

TABLE 53   Management of Septicemia in Children

Attempt to identify source of infection
  Careful physical examination, cultures, and radiographs as needed
Antibiotics
Surgical exploration and/or drainage if indicated
Monitoring for development of multiple organ system failure
  Arterial blood pressure monitoring
  Accurate recording of fluid balance (hourly)
  Neurological checks to assess level of consciousness (hourly)
  Frequent arterial blood gas determination and observation for signs of respiratory distress
  Determination of white blood cell and platelet count, hematocrit, and liver and renal function tests may be desirable daily during acute phase of illness

TABLE 54   Initial Antibiotic Therapy for Presumed Septicemia of Unknown Source

Patient	Therapy
Neonatal	Ampicillin
	plus
	cefotaxime, ceftriaxone, or gentamicin
Pediatric	Ceftriaxone or cefotaxime
	plus vancomycin plus
	Clindamycin[a] (when group A strep suspected)
Immunocompromised host	Ticarillin
	plus
	Tobramycin
	plus
	Vancomycin

[a] See Tables 10 and 11 of Chapter 20 for antibiotic dosages.

most commonly with gram-negative infections (Table 51). The cause and progression of unchecked septic shock are outlined in Table 52.

Management of septicemia in children and empiric antibiotic therapy for presumed septicemia of unknown etiology are summarized in Table 53 and 54. A general outline for treatment for septic shock should follow the familiar ABCs of cardiopulmonary resuscitation (Table 55).

TABLE 55   Treatment of Septic Shock

Airway oxygenation
   Endotracheal intubation
   Mechanical ventiliation with supplemental oxygen
   Positive end expiratory pressure as needed to correct hypoxemia if adult respiratory distress syndrome is
     present
   Goal is maintenance of over 95% arterial oxyhemoglobin saturation
Cardiac output
   Transfusion of packed red blood cells as needed to assure optimal red cell mass for adequate tissue oxygen
     delivery
   Optimize ventricular preload using fluid resuscitation with isotonic crystalloid solution or colloid (20 mL/kg over
     20 min) repeated as needed until circulation has stabilized or CVPz[a] >10 mmHg or PCWP[b] >12 mmHg
   Correct acidosis with bicarbonate if pH <7.2 [0.3 × base deficit × weight (kg)]
   Correct hypocalcemia if present
   Inotropic support indicated if ventricular preload has already been optimized and cardiac output is still
     insufficient to meet tissue oxygen demands
   Vasoactive agents as needed to maintain normal systemic vascular resistance
Steroids
   Efficacy in septic shock still not established in children
Activated protein C (Xigris) 24 mcg/kg/hr infusion × 96 hr
Access and monitoring lines
   Intravenous line
   Intra-arterial line
   CVP or PCWP lines
   Urinary catheter
   Nasogastric tube (to buffer gastric pH)
Developing treatments
   Antitumor necrosis antibody
   Nitric oxide scavengers/nitric oxidase inhibitors
   Pentoxyphyline
   Naloxone and other opiate antagonist

Abbreviations: CVP, central venous pressure; PCWP, pulmonary capillary wedge pressure.

TABLE 56   Clinical Manifestations of Tetanus

Localized tetanus
   Pain, continuous rigidity and spasm of muscles in proximity to site of injury
Generalized tetanus
   Trismus
   Dysphagia
   Restlessness
   Irritability
   Headache
   Risus sardonicus
   Tonic contractions of somatic musculature
   Opisthotonus
   Tetanic seizures
   Spasm of laryngeal and respiratory muscles with airway obstruction
   Urinary retention
   Fever
   Hyperhydrosis
   Tachycardia
   Hypertension
   Cardiac arrhythmias
Cephalic tetanus
   Dysfunction of cranial nerves III, IV, VII, IX, X, and XI
Tetanus neonatorum
   Difficulty in sucking
   Excessive crying
   Dysphagia
   Opisthotonus
   Spasms

TETANUS

Tetanus is caused by inoculation with the organism *Clostridium tetani*, which exists in both vegetative and sporulated forms. Spores introduced into a wound may convert into the vegetative form that produce a potent exotoxin, tetanospasmin, which affects the nervous system in several ways.

TABLE 57   Treatment of Tetanus

Antitoxin
   Tetanus immunoglobulin (500 U IM); infiltrate part around the wound
Antibiotics
   IV or PO metronidazole, 30 mg/kg day ÷ q.i.d. × 10–14 days
   Alternative: parenteral penicillin G, 100,000 U/kg/day ÷ q.i.d. × 10–14 days
      to eliminate vegetative forms of *Clostridium tetani*
Surgical wound care
Supportive measures
   Decrease external stimuli (noise, light)
   Endotracheal intubation or tracheostomy as needed to protect against
      laryngospasm and aspiration
   Sedation
   Barbiturates, muscle relaxants, or non-polarizing neuromuscular blocking
      agents to decrease severity of muscle spasms
   Assure adequate ventilation, using mechanical ventilator if needed
   Treatment of sympathetic nervous system over-activity (extreme
      hypertension and tachycardia) with cautious use of β- and/or
      α-adrenergic blockers
   Nutritional support

TABLE 58   Incubation Period for Staphylococcal Toxic Shock Syndrome

Clinical setting	Onset of symptoms
Menstruation	1–11 days after vaginal bleeding begins
Surgical wounds	2 days after surgery
Skin, subcutaneous soft tissue, wound, or osseous infection	1 day to 8 wks after inoculation
Postpartum and post-abortion	1 day to 8 wks after delivery/abortion

TABLE 59   Clinical Manifestations of Toxic Shock Syndrome

Signs	Symptoms
Rash	Myalgia
Desquamation	Vomiting
Fever	Dizziness
Hypotension	Sore throat
Pharyngitis	Headache
Strawberry tongue	Diarrhea
Conjunctivitis	Arthralgia
Vaginitis	Cough
Edema	
Confusion	
Agitation	
Somnolence	
Polyarthritis	

TABLE 60   Criteria for Diagnosis of Toxic Shock Syndrome

Body temperature ≥38.9°C
Diffuse macular erythroderma or polymorphic maculopapular rash
Desquamation of palms or soles 1–2 wks after onset of illness
Hypotension: systolic BP ≤90 mmHg (adults) or <5th percentile by age
   (children under 16 years), or orthostatic dizziness or syncope
Involvement of three or more of the following organ systems:
   Gastrointestinal
      Vomiting or diarrhea at onset of illness
   Hepatic
      Total bilirubin, SGOT, or SGPT over twice upper normal value
   Hematologic
      Platelet count ≤100,000 mm^{-3}
   Mucous membrane
      Conjunctival, pharyngeal, or vaginal hyperemia
   Muscular
      Severe myalgia or creatine phosphokinase over twice upper normal value
   Renal
      ≥5 White blood cells per high power field, or blood urea nitrogen or
      creatinine over twice upper normal value
   Neurologic
      Disorientation or altered level of consciousness without focal neurologic
      signs when fever and hypotension absent
   Metabolic
      Decreased total serum protein, albumin, calcium, and/or phosphorus
Reasonable evidence for absence of other bacterial, viral, or rickettsial
   infections, drug reactions, or autoimmune disorders.

Abbreviations: SGOT, serum glutamic oxalo-acetic transaminase; SGPT, serum glutamic pyruvic transaminase.

The incubation period for the development of tetanus varies from 3 days to 3 weeks. There are four forms of the disease with distinct presentations (Table 56). Generalized tetanus is the most common. Cephalic tetanus is unusual and is seen following otitis media or injuries to the head and face. Neonatal tetanus usually presents in the first week of life in neonates born to unimmunized mothers after a contaminated delivery.

The diagnosis of tetanus is essentially a clinical diagnosis with a history of injury, followed by development of the symptoms described in Table 56. Laboratory findings are nonspecific in most cases of tetanus.

TABLE 61   Laboratory Abnormalities in Toxic Shock Syndrome

High serum creatinine
Elevated serum creatine phosphokinase
Low serum calcium
Low serum phosphorus
Low total serum protein
Hypoalbuminemia
Leukocytosis with left shift
Anemia
Thrombocytopenia
Elevation of liver function results [bilirubin, AST
   (aspartate aminotransferase), ALT (alanine
   aminotransferase), prothrombin time]
Pyuria

TABLE 62   Factors Associated with Increased Risk for Toxic Shock Syndrome

Staphylococcal
   Previous history of vaginal infection
   Similar illness during a previous menstrual period
   Use of tampons, particularly highly absorbent
      brands
Streptococcal
   Fasciitis
   Chickenpox
   Pharyngitis
   Pelvic infection

TABLE 63   Treatment for Toxic Shock Syndrome

Supportive intensive care—see septic shock (Table 55)
Antibiotics (clindamycin plus penicillin or cephalosporin for *Streptococcus*;
   vancomycin or linezolid for *Staphylococcus*)
Discontinue tampon use
IVIG 2 g/kg as single infusion

Treatment of tetanus focuses on removal of the source of toxin, neutralization of toxin, and supportive case until the toxin (which is fixed to neural tissue) is metabolized (Table 57). The average mortality of tetanus is 50% with even greater morality for neonates. Recovery from tetanus does not confer immunity and prevention is best accomplished by active immunization.

TOXIC SHOCK SYNDROME

Group A, β-hemolytic streptococci and *Staphylococcus aureus*, including methicillin-resistant *S. aureus* are causative agents of this syndrome. Toxic shock syndrome is an illness seen in all age groups, though it is more commonly found in the clinical settings of antecedent fasciitis (GABHS), chickenpox (GABHS) or in young menstruating women (*S. aureus*). Shock is the result of exotoxins produced by GABHS and enterotoxins prodused by *S. aureus*.

TUBERCULOSIS

Most children are diagnosed because they have a positive tuberculosis skin test and are in high risk groups for disease or have an illness compatible with tuberculosis, usually pneumonia. Early morning gastric aspirates may recover *Mycobacterium tuberculosis* for diagnosis and sensitivity testing, but organisms recovered from adult contacts are more commonly used to guide therapy.

Short-course chemotherapy has now been shown to be equal to previous regimens of one year or longer (Table 64) (4).

Screening for Tuberculosis in Infants and Children

Routine skin testing for tuberculosis in children with no risk factors residing in low-prevalence communities is not indicated. In such settings, skin reactions are most likely to be falsely positive.

TABLE 64   Recommended Treatment Regimens for Tuberculosis in Infants, Children, and Adolescents

Tuberculous infection/ disease	Regimens	Remarks
Asymptomatic infection (positive skin test, no disease)		If daily therapy is not possible, twice a week may be substituted. HIV-infected children should be treated for 12 mos
Isoniazid-susceptible	6–9 mos of I daily	
Isoniazid-resistant	6–9 mos of R daily	
Isoniazid- Rifampin-resistant	Consult a TB specialist	
Pulmonary	6 mos (standard) 2 mos of I, R, and Z daily, followed by 4 mos of I and R daily	If drug resistance is possible, another drug (ethambutol or streptomycin) is added to the initial therapy until drug susceptibility is determined
	or	
	2 mos of I, R, and Z daily, followed by 4 mos of I and R twice a week	Drugs can be given 2 or 3 times per week under direct observation in the initial phase if nonadherence is likely
	9-mos alternative regimens (for hilar adenopathy only); 9 mos of I and R once a day	Regimens consisting of 6 mos of I and R once a day, and 1 mo of I and R once a day, and 1 mo of I and R daily, followed by 5 mos of I and R twice a week, have been successful in areas where drug resistance is rare
	or	
	1 mo of I and R daily, followed by 8 mos of I and R twice a week	
Extrapulmonary meningitis, disseminated (miliary), bone/joint disease	2 mos of I, R, and Z and S once a day, followed by 10 mos of I and R once a day (12 mos total)	S is given with initial therapy until drug susceptibility is known
	or	
	2 mos of I, R, Z, and S daily, followed by 10 mo of I and R twice a week (12 mos total)	For patients who may have acquired tuberculosis in geographic locales where resistance to S is common, capreomycin (15–30 mg/kg/day) or kanamycin (15–30 mg/kg/day) may be used instead of S
Other (e.g., cervical lymphadenopathy)	Same as pulmonary	See pulmonary

Abbreviations: I, isoniazid; R, rifampin; S, streptomycin; Z, pyrazinamide.

Children at high risk (Table 65) should be tested annually using Mantoux tuberculin tests. All results (positive or negative) should be routinely read by qualified medical personnel (Table 66). Children with no risk factors but residing in high-prevalence regions and children whose risk factor history is incomplete or unreliable may be screened periodically such as at 1, 5, and 15 years of age. Such a decision should be made at the local level.

Tuberculosis—Scrofula

Tuberculosis of lymph nodes and overlying skin is called scrofula. Cervical lymph nodes are most frequently involved. *Mycobacterium tuberculosis* or atypical mycobacteria (*M. kansasii* or *M. marinum*) are all causative agents.

Scrofula may resolve spontaneously without therapy. The treatment of choice for persistent nodes is excisional biopsy. Specific chemotherapy depends upon the sensitivity of isolated agents. Often these microorganisms are resistant to standard antituberculous therapy. Clarithromycin, rifampin, and ethambutol have been used with some success.

TABLE 65   Infants, Children, and Adolescents at High Risk for Tuberculosis Infection: Immediate and Annual Skin Testing Recommended

Contact with adults with infectious tuberculosis
Those from, or whose parents have emigrated from, high-prevalence regions of the world
Abnormalities on chest radiograph
Clinical evidence of tuberculosis
HIV seropositive
Immunosuppressed
Other medical risk factors: Hodgkin's disease, lymphoma, diabetes mellitus, chronic renal failure, malnutrition
Children frequently exposed to the following adults:
  HIV infected
  Homeless persons
  Users of intravenous and other street drugs
  Poor and medically indigent city dwellers
  Residents of nursing homes
  Migrant farm workers
Incarcerated adolescents

TABLE 66   Definition of a Positive Mamtoux Skin Test (5TU-PPD) in Children

Reaction size of ≥5 mm
  Children in close contact with known or suspected infectious cases of tuberculosis:
    Households with active cases
    Households with previously active cases if:
      treatment cannot be verified as adequate prior to the exposure
      treatment was initiated after period of child's contact
      reactivation is suspected
  Children suspected to have tuberculous disease:
    Chest roentgenogram consistent with active or previously active tuberculosis
    Clinical evidence of tuberculosis
  Children with underlying conditions which put them at high risk of acquiring severe tuberculosis:
    Immunocompromised conditions
    HIV infection
Reaction size of ≥10 mm
  Children at increased risk of dissemination:
    Young age: <4 years of age
    Other medical risk factors: Hodgkin's diseases, lymphoma, diabetes mellitus, chronic renal failure, malnutrition
  Increased environmental exposure:
    Those from or whose parent have emigrated from high-prevalence regions of the world
    Children frequently exposed to the following adults:
      HIV infected
      Homeless persons
      Users of intravenous and other street drugs
      Poor and medically indigent city dwellers
      Residents of nursing homes
      Migrant farm workers
Reaction size of ≥15 mm
  Children 4 years of age without any risk factors

TULAREMIA

Infection with *Franciscella tularensis* presents as one of 6 different primary manifestations (Table 67) but all cases usually begin with the abrupt onset of high fever, chills, headache, cough, generalized myalgia, and vomiting. Disease is most prevalent in the mid southern states: Arkansas, Missouri, Tennessee, and Oklahoma. Organisms are transmitted through tick bites or exposure to infected animals/carcasses, particularly skinning rabbits.

TABLE 67 Clinical Syndromes of Tularemia

Ulceroglandular	65%
Glandular	25%
Oculoglandular	<5%
Typhoidal	<5%
Pneumonic	<5%
Oropharyngeal	<1%

Diagnosis is made by serologic testing with a serum titer of = or >1:128 by microagglutination or = or >1:160 by tube agglutination being confirmatory. However, positive titers may not be seen until 3 to 4 weeks into the illness.

Treatment is a 7 to 10 course of an aminoglycoside: streptomycin b.i.d., gentamicin t.i.d, or amikacin t.i.d. There is more experience with streptomycin and the b.i.d. dosing is more convenient for outpatient therapy.

REFERENCES

1. Mermel LA, Farr BM, Sherertz RJ, et al. Guidelines for the management of intravascular catheter-related infections. Clin Infect Dis 2001; 32:1249–72.
2. Durack DT, Lukes AS, Bright DK. New criteria for diagnosis of infective endocarditis: Utilization of specific echocardiographic findings. Duke Endocarditis Service. Am J Med 1994; 96:200–9.
3. Baddour LM, Wilson WR, Bayer AS, et al. AHA scientific statement: Infective endocarditis, diagnosis, antimicrobial therapy, and management of complications: Endorsed by the Infectious Diseases Society of America. Circulation 2005; 111:e394–e434.
4. American Thoracic Society, CDC, and Infectious Diseases Society of America. Treatment of tuberulosis. Am J Resp Crit Care Med 2003; 167:603–62.

3 | Common Outpatient Infections

INTRODUCTION

Most infections can be managed on an outpatient basis and these comprise, by most estimates, 50 to 60% of unscheduled pediatric office or emergency room visits. Approximately 90% of febrile episodes in children are caused by viruses rather than bacteria and are usually accompanied by upper respiratory signs and symptoms. Reassurance and medication for fever or congestion are the only interventions warranted. Distinguishing more severe infectious processes remains the most important aspect of outpatient evaluation.

ABSCESSES (CUTANEOUS)

Organisms most frequently recovered from skin and soft tissue abscesses are *Staphylococcus aureus*, particularly methicillin-resistant *S. aureus* (MRSA), and group A β-hemolytic streptococci. Among these infections, cutaneous abscesses should be distinguished from impetigo, cellulitis, and wound infections where treatment is somewhat different. All fluctuant abscesses should be incised and drained. When there is a question as to whether a lesion is fluctuant, anesthetic cream, e.g., EMLA®, can be applied to the skin and an 18-G needle and syringe used to aspirate material or probe the abscess. An incision can then be made and a wick placed to assure continued drainage. This is all that is necessary for *S. aureus* and most other organisms. Group A streptococci require penicillin or an appropriate alternative oral antibiotic to penetrate the larger areas of cellulitis. Bacteremia from cutaneous abscesses is extremely rare but should be considered with extensive involvement, high fever, or in the immunocompromised host (Table 1).

Methicillin-Resistant *S. aureus*

Empiric antibiotic therapy is selected to cover *S. aureus* and group A strep and cephalosporins or semi-synthetic penicillins were previously the drugs of choice. However, the recent increase in strains of *S. aureus* resistant to methicillin (MRSA) causing infections has greatly modified choices of initial therapy for skin and skin structure abscesses, since penicillins and cephalosporins are ineffective against MRSA. More than 90% of MRSA are susceptible to

TABLE 1   Organisms Recovered from Cutaneous Abscesses in Children

Aerobes (65%)
Staphylococcus aureus (40%)
Group A β-hemolytic streptococci (20%)
Enterobacteriaceae
Escherichia coli
Anaerobes (10%)
Bacteroides melaninogenicus
Bacteroides fragilis
Fusobacterium
Mixed aerobes and anaerobes (15%)
No organism (10%)

TABLE 2   Management of Recurrent Subcutaneous Abscesses

For infected patients
   Incise and drain all abscesses
   P.O. clindamycin or TMP/SMX × 10 days
   "Swimming pool" baths twice weekly (2 tsps. clorox/gallon of water in bath)
Patients and their families
   Nasal mupuricin (Bactroban) b.i.d. × 5 days for patient and all family
     members

clindamycin and most to trimethoprim/sulfamethoxazole now making these antibiotics preferred choices. Almost all strains are susceptible to intravenous vancomycin and to linezolid which has an oral formulation.

Recurrent Skin Infections

Recurrent subcutaneous abscesses in all age groups are an increasingly common problem, primarily attributable to the emergence of MRSA. Often a member of the family has eczema. Table 2 offers suggestions for managing individuals and families with recurrent skin infections.

Abscesses in the perirectal region are almost always associated with anaerobic bacteria. As with other cutaneous abscesses, incision with drainage is the most important aspect of therapy. In contrast to infection in other anatomic areas, simple drainage may be inadequate. Fistulae must be identified, opened, and excised. Perirectal abscesses therefore require surgical consultation (Tables 3 and 4).

ADENITIS

Adenitis should be distinguished from adenopathy (see Chapter 12) although considerable clinical overlap exists. Adenitis is usually painful, hot, and occurs more frequently (75%) in the 1- to 4-year-old age group. Untreated, these nodes will suppurate and occasionally progress to cellulitis and bacteremia. When there is no primary focus such as pharyngitis or tonsillitis, fever, and other systemic symptoms imply such progression. Pitting edema strongly suggests the presence of a suppurative node that requires drainage. Ultrasonography is a useful tool in determining the consistency of the node and in helping identify localized exudate. This test should be most strongly considered for the child who is toxic or has significant pain since he is more likely to benefit from early drainage. Cervical adenitis with minimal tenderness or persistence following 10 days of antimicrobial therapy increases the likelihood of atypical mycobacterial and *Mycobacterium tuberculosis* infection. This should be evaluated by intradermal testing with intermediate PPD (5 tuberculin units). Adenitis in all locations is caused most commonly by either *S. aureus* or group A streptococci and therapy is directed against these two pathogens.

TABLE 3   Organisms Recovered from Perirectal Abscesses in Children

Anaerobes (85%) *Staphylococcus aureus* (35%) *Escherichia coli* (20%) Streptococci (10%) Other aerobes (10%)

TABLE 4   Treatment of Perirectal Abscesses

Incision and drainage	
Antibiotics	Clindamycin and a third generation cephalosporin (or as directed by Gram stain and culture); only for extensive involvement, systemic symptoms, compromised host

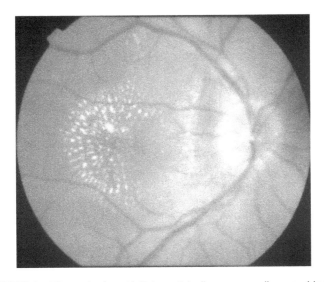

FIGURE 1 (*See color insert.*) Cat scratch disease was diagnosed in this adolescent male with a large, tender, axillary node and flu-like illness of three weeks duration. Ophthalmologic examination when he experienced decreased vision in his right eye revealed papilledema and white spots in the macula in a unique configuration, giving this finding the name "macular star."

The most common cause of chronic (>3 weeks) adenitis or adenopathy is cat-scratch disease. Other manifestations of this infection include prolonged fever, Parinaud's oculoglandular syndrome (conjunctivitis and preauricular adenitis), hepatic and splenic peliosis (granulomas), erythema nodosum, and retinitis, i.e., papilledema with a macular star (Fig. 1, Tables 5 and 6).

ANIMAL AND HUMAN BITES

Animal bites account for 1% of emergency room visits with 80% to 90% caused by dogs, 10% by cats, and 1% by rodents (rabbits, squirrels, hamsters, and gerbils). Approximately 90% are pets owned by the family or neighbors which suggests that better education of children (and parents) might reduce these all too common injuries. Human bites require similar management and are therefore included in this discussion.

A major focus of treatment concerns prevention of wound infection. Human bites most commonly become infected (greater than 50%), followed by cat (30%), whereas dog and rodent bites are associated with a 5% incidence of cellulitis or abscess formation. Such infection is usually clinically apparent within 24 hours after the injury. Upper extremity injuries become infected more commonly than those to the face, scalp, or lower extremities. This is because debridement and irrigation of the compartments of the hand are more difficult. In contrast to animal attacks, human inflicted bites are commonly associated with infection caused by *Eikenella corrodens* (Table 7).

Gram stains or cultures immediately following the injury are not predictive of organisms subsequently associated with infection. Therefore, these laboratory studies should only be obtained once cellulitis or abscess formation occurs.

Every effort should be made primarily to close lacerations, both for cosmetic reasons and to reduce local bacterial colonization. Large wounds, those associated with extensive tissue destruction, or ones requiring optimal cosmetic repair may best be managed under general anesthesia in the operating room (Table 8).

TABLE 5   Bacterial Etiology of Adenitis

All locations	*Staphylococcus aureus* 40–50%
	Group A streptococci 30–40%
Other organisms by location	
Cervical	Atypical mycobacteria
	Mycobacterium tuberculosis
	Gram-negative enterics
	H. influenzae
	Anaerobes
	Actinomyces israelii
	Tularemia
Preauricular	Tularemia
Occipital	Tinea capitis
Axillary	*Bartonella henselae* (cat scratch disease)
	Sporotrichosis
Inguinal	Anaerobes
	Gram-negative enterics
	Tularemia
Generalized	Infectious mononucleosis
	Toxoplasmosis
	CMV
	Other viruses
	Kawasaki disease
	Syphilis
	Hepatitis
	Brucellosis
	Sarcoidosis
Chronic (>3 wks)	*Bartonella henselae* (cat scratch disease)
	Atypical mycobacteria
	M. tuberculosis

BACTEREMIA

Bacteremia occurs in fewer than 1% of febrile infants who do not appear toxic and have received *Hib* and conjugate pneumococcal vaccines. The most common predisposing infections are otitis media, pneumonia, and *Salmonella* gastroenteritis. The majority of patients, however, have no obvious focus. Unique are children with sickle cell disease who exhibit a high incidence of pneumococcal bacteremia. These children, when febrile, require close observation (Table 9).

Febrile neonates less than 28 days of age should be hospitalized and evaluated for sepsis. This includes two blood cultures, lumbar puncture, and urine for culture obtained by catheterization or bladder tap. Older infants are managed on an individual basis with decision for hospitalization based on physical assessment rather than any laboratory parameters. The decision to obtain a blood culture should usually be accompanied by one for observation in the hospital setting.

TABLE 6   Treatment of Adenitis

Needle drainage when fluctuant
Prescribe any of the following:
Cephalexin
Cloxacillin or dicloxacillin
Erythromycin
Cephradine, cefadroxil, or cefuroxime axetil
Amoxicillin/clavulanate

TABLE 7   Organisms Recovered from Infected Animal Bites

Pasteurella multocida
Staphylococcus intermedius
Streptococcus sp.
Anaerobic bacteria

TABLE 8   Treatment of Animal and Human Bites

Cleansing and debridement
Extensive wound irrigation
Suturing for closure of face and other cosmetically
  sensitive areas
Antibiotics: amoxicillin/clavulanate
Tetanus prophylaxis when indicated
Rabies prophylaxis when indicated
Reexamine in 24 hr

TABLE 9   Bacteremia in Infants

S. pneumoniae (92%)
Salmonella sp. (6%)
N. meningitidis (1%)
Group A streptococci (1%)
S. aureus (<1%)

If pneumococcal bacteremia is documented from an outpatient culture, the patient must be reexamined. If improved but showing no focus of infection, penicillin or an alternative antibiotic for penicillin-resistant strains should be given for 10 days. Specific infections seen on follow-up such as otitis media or pneumonia are managed in the usual fashion.

Salmonella bacteremia is usually associated with gastroenteritis. Although there is no direct evidence that bacteremic cases should be managed differently from those with simple intestinal infection most experts recommend antimicrobial therapy, either parenteral or oral, depending on the severity of illness.

CELLULITIS

Infection of the skin and subcutaneous tissue is most commonly the result of local trauma or the extension of an underlying abscess. Periorbital cellulitis more likely follows conjunctival colonization with pneumococcus or other potential pathogens, whereas orbital cellulitis is a consequence of ethmoid sinusitis with penetration into the retrobulbar space. Buccal cellulitis is frequently associated with ipsilateral otitis media.

There are some features that help differentiate more likely etiologic agents and these should be used as guides to therapy. A painful cellulitis with well-demarcated raised borders on the face is characteristic of erysipelas caused by group A β-hemolytic streptococci (Fig. 2, Table 10).

Selection of antibiotics is guided by an understanding of pathogens most likely to cause cellulitis. Any abscess should first be incised and drained. In most cases, a penicillinase-resistant cephalosporins or penicillin is used to cover staphylococci and group A streptococci. When S. pneumoniae is a likely agent, such as with facial cellulitis, a third generation cephalosporin is most appropriate. Blood and when practical, an aspirate of the advancing margin of the cellulitis, should be cultured (Table 11).

CONJUNCTIVITIS

Causes of conjunctivitis are largely age dependent and include sensitivity to environmental agents (allergic conjunctivitis) as well as viral and bacterial pathogens. Microscopic examination of exudate with Gram stain (N. gonorrhoeae) and Giemsa stain (Chlamydia trachomatis) when appropriate will help differentiate the varied etiologies. Cultures should be obtained prior to treatment (Table 12).

DERMATOPHYTOSES AND CANDIDIASIS

Dermatophytes have the unique ability to colonize skin, hair, and nails, but almost never invade deeper tissues. Diagnosis is made clinically by noting characteristic patterns such as a ring with central clearing or kerion formation. Occasionally, a geographic tongue will have the appearance of thrush (Fig. 3). If there is a question in diagnosis, confirmation is best achieved with a KOH preparation of a tongue scraping.

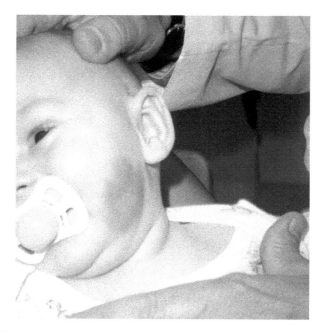

FIGURE 2 (*See color insert.*) This 5-month-old had a temperature of 104.5°F and a hot, painful area of cellulitis on the cheek with well-demarcated borders characteristic of erysipelas. A blood culture grew group A β-hemolytic streptococcus.

Wood light examination of skin lesions of tinea corporis will occasionally demonstrate the characteristic apple green fluorescence of *Microsporum* and some other organisms. Currently, 37 species of dermatophytes have been identified. It is more practical to approach diagnosis and selection of antifungal agents according to clinical presentation. Cultures are most useful for infections that do not respond to initial therapy (Table 13).

FEVER AND OCCULT BACTEREMIA

Neonates, 0 to 28 days of age, with fever should be hospitalized and undergo a full sepsis workup, which includes cultures of blood (2), CSF, and urine (collected by bladder catheterization or suprapubic aspiration). Infants 28 to 60 days may be followed on an outpatient basis if they are non-toxic and fulfill laboratory criteria for being at low risk for having severe bacterial infection as defined in Table 14.

TABLE 10   Cellulitis: Clinical Features Associated with Specific Bacteria

Clinical feature	Organism
Neonatal cellulitis	
Facial	Group B streptococci
Funicitis (periumbilical)	Group A streptococci
Predisposing trauma	*S. aureus*, group A streptococci
Foot (puncture wound)	*Pseudomonas* sp.
Burn	Group A streptococci
Chickenpox	Group A streptococci, *S. aureus*
Infant cellulitis	
Facial, periorbital	*S. pneumoniae*
Ascending lymphangitis	Group A streptococci
Erysipelas (distinct borders)	Group A streptococci

TABLE 11 Treatment of Cellulitis

Neonate	Ceftriaxone or cefotaxime + clindamycin
1 mo–5 yrs	Ceftriaxone or cefotaxime
Predisposing trauma	Clindamycin
Ascending lymphangitis	Penicillin

Although children 3 to 36 months of age with fever $\geq$39.0°C, WBC >15,000 mm^{-3} and no focus of infection are at increased risk for having pneumococcal occult bacteremia, antimicrobial treatment is only warranted for those who appear toxic. The preferred antibiotic for outpatient treatment is ceftriaxone 50 to 75 mg/kg (max. 1 g) as a single dose.

The vast majority resolve their fever without subsequent focal or systemic infection. If the child's condition worsens, he/she should be admitted to the hospital for a sepsis work-up and begun on parenteral antibiotics (Table 15).

Much more important than fever per se is its underlying cause. Once this has been determined, antipyretics may be used for the child's comfort and to help prevent febrile convulsions in the susceptible age group. Newer pharmacokinetic data offer better guidelines for administration of acetaminophen or aspirin (Table 16).

FEVER OF UNKNOWN ORIGIN

Fever of unknown origin (FUO) is a convenient term used to classify patients who warrant a particular systematic approach to diagnostic evaluation and management. Criteria first proposed for adult patients by Petersdorf and Beeson in 1961 have been used for over three decades for all ages, but may not be applicable today. In contrast to adults, prognosis for children who fulfill criteria for FUO is much better since they are less likely to have malignancies or autoimmune processes as the cause of prolonged fever.

Definition is generally the following: An immunologically normal host with oral or rectal temperature $\geq$38.0°C (100.4°F) at least twice a week for more than 3 weeks, a non-contributory history and physical examination, and one week of outpatient investigation. Early diagnostic studies would normally include a complete blood cell count, lactic dehydrogenase (LDH), uric acid, urinalysis and culture, chest roentgenogram, tuberculin skin test, erythrocyte sedimentation rate (ESR) and, in the older child, an antinuclear antibody titer.

Certain medical circumstances would greatly influence both diagnostic and management approaches. These include patients with acquired or congenital immunodeficiency, neutropenic patients, and those whose fevers have occurred during prolonged hospital stays.

TABLE 12 Etiology and Treatment of Conjunctivitis

Age	Etiology	Treatment
<3 days	Chemical (silver nitrate)	None
3 days–3 wks	*N. gonorrhoeae*	Ceftriaxone IV/IM 25–50 mg/kg, max. 125 mg × 1 dose
2–20 wks	*C. trachomatis*	Erythromycin PO × 14 days or Sulfonamide eye drops
>12 wks	*H. influenzae*/("pink eye")	Polymyxin/trimethoprim opth soln or Polymyxin/bacitracin/ neospoin opth oint. × 7 days
	Pneumococcus	
	S. aureus	Topical bacitracin
	S. pneumoniae	Sulfonamide eye drops
	Moraxella lacunata	Sulfonamide eye drops
	Streptococci	Sulfonamide eye drops
	Adenoviruses	Cold soaks
	Enterovirus 70	Cold soaks
	Herpes simplex	Trifluridine eye drops or idoxuridine opth soln, adenine arabinoside ointment for 1 wk after healing
	P. aeruginosa	Ticarcillin or Ceftazidime and Tobramycin IM or IV for 7 days

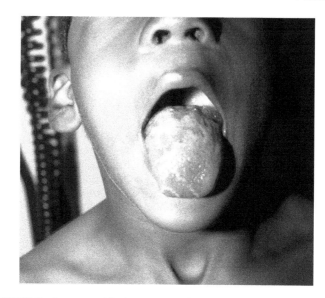

FIGURE 3 A geographic tongue may be confused with thrush if the history does not clearly indicate its chronic persistence with waxing and waning appearance. It is found in 1% to 2% of the population, with a predisposition in atopic individuals. In this young boy, a scraping was negative for the pseudo-branching hyphae of *Candida*.

The greatest clinical concern in evaluating FUO is identifying patients whose fever has a serious or life-threatening etiology for whom a delay in diagnosis could jeopardize successful intervention. Cancer and severe bacterial infections are the causes most frequently discussed and likely to influence diagnostic and management approaches. However, it should be emphasized that a vast majority of children with prolonged FUO resolve their illnesses without a diagnosis and do not exhibit long-lasting effects. Therefore, it appears appropriate for most children to delay extensive diagnostic evaluation until the child has remained febrile for at least 6 weeks.

TABLE 13   Treatment of Dermatophytoses

Clinical disease	Therapy
Tinea capitis	Griseofulvin microsized 20–25 mg/kg/day once daily PO for 1 mo or longer or Griseofulvin ultramicrosized 10 mg/kg/day or Itraconazole 5 mg/kg/day PO qd or
Kerion	As above plus prednisone 1–2 mg/kg/day for 1 wk or Selenium shampoo 2 times weekly
Black-dot ringworm Gray-patch ringworm	Griseofulvin 20–25 mg/kg/day PO div. q 24 hr × 4–8 wk
Tinea corporis	Topical butenafine, ciclopirox, clotrimazole, econazole, haloprogin, ketoconazole, miconazole, naftifine, oxiconazole, sulconazole, terbinafine or tolnaftate bid × 4 wk
Tinea cruris	Topical (as above) × 4–6 wk
Tinea pedis	Topical (as above) × 6–12 wk; oral griseofulvin for *Trichophyton rubrum*
Onychomycosis Candidiasis	Oral griseofulvin × 3–4 mo
Thrush	Nystatin PO 200,000 U q.i.d. × 10–14 days or fluconazole 6 mg/kg on the first day followed by 3 mg/kg daily × 6 days
Diaper rash	Nystatin cream q.i.d.

TABLE 14   Laboratory Criteria for Infants 28–60 Days of Age for Being at Low Risk for Severe Bacterial Infection

Blood: WBC <20,000 mm^{-3}; immature/mature PMNs
   <0.2
CSF: WBC <8 mm^{-3}
Urine: UA WBC <10 mm^{-3}, few or no bacteria
X ray: Normal chest plain film

TABLE 15   Laboratory Studies for Children Two Months to Three Years of Age with Fever and No Apparent Source

Urinalysis—all children
Urine culture—uncircumcized males; females <2 yrs
Optional
   Complete blood count
   Chest roentgenogram (with respiratory symptoms)
   Stool culture (with GI symptoms)

Diagnostic evaluation should begin with basic studies done during outpatient observation as summarized in Table 17.

The initial outpatient evaluation generally requires 1 week to complete laboratory testing and to obtain final results. After this time the physician must decide whether simple continued observation or progressive laboratory investigation is more appropriate. Decisions are based primarily on the clinical status of the child and results of initial evaluation. For most patients, observation is most prudent since the majority will become afebrile by 6 weeks. A practical approach to continued evaluation once this appears necessary is summarized in Table 18.

OROPHARYNGEAL INFECTION

Almost all "upper respiratory infections" are caused by viral agents and require only symptomatic therapy. Pharyngitis or tonsillitis without nasal involvement is more commonly associated with group A streptococci and a throat culture or test for streptococcal antigen is essential for determining this bacterial etiology. Epstein-Barr virus infectious mononucleosis is a common cause in older children. Often, documentation of an outbreak of oropharyngeal infection caused by a particular viral pathogen offers guidance to management of subsequent cases. Rare but important bacterial pathogens causing pharyngitis are *Arcanobacterium hemolyticum*, *Neisseria gonorrhoeae*, *Corynebacterium diphtheriae*, and *Francisella tularensis* with other groups of streptococci, particularly C and G, accounting for isolated outbreaks of disease (Table 19).

OTITIS EXTERNA (SWIMMER'S EAR)

Otitis externa is caused by retention of water in the external canal with resulting bacterial replication and inflammation. Recovered bacterial pathogens are those which commonly colonize skin and thrive in moist environments (Table 20).

TABLE 16   Antipyretic Therapy

Acetaminophen	Loading dose: 22 mg/kg
	Maintenance: 13 mg/kg q6 hr
Aspirin	Loading dose: 18 mg/kg
	Maintenance: 8.5 mg/kg q 6 hr

TABLE 17   Initial Evaluation of Children with FUO and Rationale for Screen

History and physical (all causes)
Complete blood cell count (leukemia and infections)
Lactic dehydrogenase (LDH), uric acid (leukemia and lymphomas)
Urinalysis and culture (infection)
Chest roentgenogram (infections and malignancies)
Tuberculin skin test (tubercuosis)
Antinuclear antibody titer—older child (autoimmune)
ESR or CRP (all causes)

TABLE 18   Protocol for Continued Evaluation of Children with FUO

```
Phase 1. Outpatient (after 3–6 wks of fever)
   Complete blood cell count (repeat)
   Erythrocyte sedimentation rate
   Urinalysis and culture (repeat)
   Epstein-Barr Virus serology
   Chest roentgenogram (review if already obtained)
   Blood culture
   Anti-streptolysin O
   Human immunodeficiency virus antibody (if there are risk factors)
   Twice daily temperature recordings (by parents at home)
Phase 2. Inpatient (after 6 wks of fever)
   Hospitalize for observation
   Lumbar puncture (partial treatment or any toxicity in a young infant)
   Repeat blood cultures
   Sinus radiographs
   Ophthalmologic examination for iridocyclitis
   Liver enzymes
   Serologic tests
      Cytomegalovirus
      Toxoplasmosis
      Hepatitis A, B, and C
      Tularemia (in endemic regions)
      Brucellosis (with risk factors)
      Leptospirosis
      Salmonellosis
Phase 3. Inpatient (after 6 wks of fever if condition worsens)
   Abdominal ultrasonography
   Abdominal CT scanning
   Gallium or indium scanning
   Upper gastrointestinal tract X-ray series with follow-through (older child
      with any abdominal symptoms)
   Bone marrow (if any abnormalities in complete blood cell count)
   Technetium bone scanning
```

Therapy is directed at eradication of probable organisms with broad spectrum topical antibiotics which can be accomplished with a brief 10-day course. Children who swim frequently or have had repeated bouts of otitis externa should instill an acidified alcohol solution into the external canals after swimming or showering (Table 21).

OTITIS MEDIA

It has been estimated that pediatricians spend as much as 30% of their time in the management of otitis media, second only to well child care in clinical responsibilities. Early and aggressive intervention is essential for the child's comfort as well as prevention of severe suppurative complications such as mastoiditis and meningitis. As important is prevention of the persistent conductive hearing loss which has been shown to delay speech development and cognitive function.

Definitions

A diagnosis of acute otitis media (AOM) requires the presence of middle ear effusion along with the rapid onset of clinical signs and symptoms, specifically fever, pain, irritability, anorexia, or vomiting. This definition separates AOM from otitis media with effusion (OME) which is not associated with symptoms, and from chronic suppurative otitis media which is a persistent inflammatory process with a perforated tympanic membrane and draining exudate for longer than 6 weeks.

TABLE 19   Upper Respiratory Infections—Common Etiologic Agents and Treatment

Classification	Etiology	Treatment
Common cold	Rhinovirus Parainfluenza RSV	Symptomatic

Nasopharyngitis	Adenovirus
	  Enteroviruses (e.g.,
	    herpangina)
	  Rhinoviruses
	Parainfluenza
	Influenza
	RSV
		Symptomatic

Pharyngitis-tonsillitis	Viruses (as with
	  nasopharyngitis)
	Bacteria
	  Group A streptococci
	Streptococci C and G
	*Arcanobacterium
	  hemolyticum*
	N. gonorrhoeae
	F. tularensis
		
		Penicillin
		Penicillin
		Erythromycin
		
		Ceftriaxone
		Streptomycin or
		  gentamicin

Peritonsillar abscesses	Group A streptococci *S. aureus*	Penicillin Clindamycin Incision and drainage

Identification of AOM is made by direct visualization of the tympanic membrane, using a pneumatic otoscope so that movement of the membrane can be fully evaluated. With AOM, the eardrum may be bulging or retracted, landmarks are distorted and most importantly, movement is markedly decreased. In difficult to diagnosis cases, particularly in children with scarred tympanic membranes from previous infection, tympanometry and acoustic reflectometry offer simple and accurate means of confirming the presence of fluid. One of these devices should be available to every primary care physician who manages children with otitis media, not only as an aid in the diagnosis of AOM but also to follow children with persistent effusion.

Microbiology

The organisms causing AOM have changed considerably during the last 5 years following the routine administration of conjugate pneumococcal vaccine; non-typeable *Haemophilus influenzae* is now the most common pathogen with the vaccine strains of pneumococcus reduced by 60% in immunized children (Table 22).

TABLE 20   Organisms Causing Otitis Externa

S. aureus
Pseudomonas aeruginosa
Proteus vulgaris
Streptococcus pyogenes
Enterobacteriaceae
Aspergillus

TABLE 21   Treatment of Otitis Externa

Acute treatment: otic drops
  Floxacin or ofloxacin 5 drops b.i.d. × 10 days
  Cortisporin (polymyxin B, neomycin, and
    hydrocortisone) or
  Otobiotic (polymyxin B and hydrocortisone) q.i.d.
    × 10 days
Prophylaxis: (swimmer's ear drops) after swimming
  or showering

TABLE 22   Etiology of Otitis Media in Infants and Children

Pathogen	Mean (%)	Range (%)
H. influenzae (non-typeable)	39	27–52
S. pneumoniae	27	16–52
M. catarrhalis	10	2–27
S. pyogenes	3	0–11
None or non-pathogens	30	12–45

The aspect of these pathogenic bacteria which has changed dramatically is their susceptibility to previously recommended antimicrobial therapy, particularly increasing resistance to amoxicillin. Beginning a decade ago clinicians were warned that the prevalence of β-lactamase production by nontypeable *H. influenzae* and *M. catarrhalis* was increasing and presently 60% and 95–100% of these organisms respectively are not susceptible to penicillin by this mechanism. More importantly, *S. pneumoniae* has now developed amoxicillin resistance via an alteration in penicillin-binding proteins, which also renders these organisms non-susceptible to penicillin/β-lactamase inhibitor combinations such as amoxicillin-clavulanate and ticarcillin-clavulanate.

Selection of first-line therapy for otitis media must be made by the individual physician based on regional susceptibility data of bacterial pathogens and more importantly, treatment failure rates of previous regimens. Regional differences for these variables make it difficult to offer recommendations that are appropriate for all locations. If a decision is made to change from amoxicillin as first-line therapy, there are many options (Fig. 4). Other considerations for selection might include cost and compliance issues. Compliance is enhanced for antibiotics that are better tasting, given once or twice rather than 3 or 4 times a day, and those given for briefer durations.

A change to other classes of antibiotics for most outpatient infections also offers the theoretic advantage of reversing the trend to penicillin resistance among these organisms by eliminating the pressure for mutation which always occurs with excessive use of a single agent.

Acute Otitis Media

Spontaneous resolution of signs and symptoms after 48 hours of treatment for AOM in approximately 50% of cases is somewhat organism dependent, lowest for pneumococcus (10% to 20%), highest for Moraxella (70%) and intermediate for *H. influenzae* (50%). Because there is no way of predicting which children do not require antibiotics, they should be offered to all cases. Withholding therapy for more than 48 hours, an option to management used by some physicians has been associated with an increase in the incidence of mastoiditis.

Antimicrobial therapy alleviates symptoms within 48 hours in more than 90% of children. Persistence of symptoms at this timepoint is an indication for empiric change to another class of antibiotics. In young children the effusion persists for 1 month in 40% of patients, 2 months in 20% and 3 months in 10%. Therefore, additional management is not indicated until after 12 months of follow-up for those with persistent effusion at which time tympanometry should be obtained. Children with a tympanogram showing a C2, C3, or B pattern should undergo audiometry. If this testing demonstrates a 20 dB loss or greater, tympanostomy tubes should be considered. This may be necessary in as many as 2% of all AOM cases, representing 10% of all children less than 3 years of age.

Otitis Media with Effusion

A clinical practice guideline for OME was published jointly by the pediatric, family physician, and otolaryngology academies with the review and approval of the Agency for Health Care Policy and Research of the U.S. Department of Health and Human Services. The algorithm in Figure 5 is adapted from this document with some modifications.

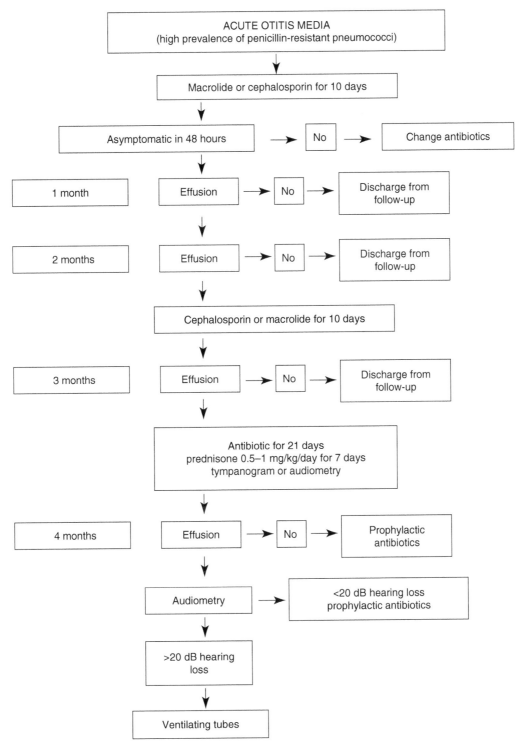

FIGURE 4 Algorithm for management of acute otitis media (AOM) including follow-up of persistent middle ear effusion.

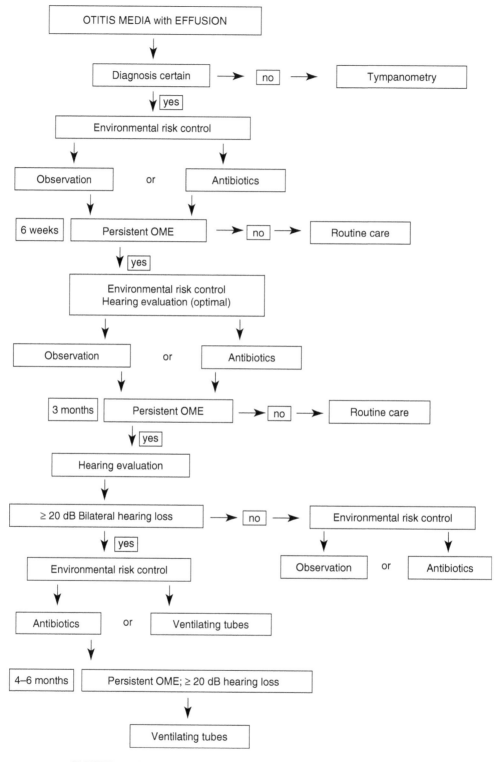

FIGURE 5 Algorithm for managing otitis media with effusion in an otherwise healthy child aged one through three years.

The option for using antibiotics both initially and after 2 months of persistent effusion was chosen and the addition of steroids at 2 months is included although the practice guideline does not support their use. In the latter decision, although clinical trials have been inconclusive, current practice and the absence of adverse consequences support this modification. The use of antihistamines or decongestants is not recommended at any stage of management because clinical trials have never demonstrated efficacy. Likewise, the association between allergy and OME is not clear from available evidence and therefore no recommendation can be made relevant to allergy testing or treatment. The most problematic intervention step pertains to the indications and timing of tympanostomy tube placement. Decisions are guided by the likelihood of persistent effusions resulting in delayed speech and reduction in cognitive development. Age and duration of effusion are both important variables in this assessment. With all data considered, it appears prudent to recommend ventilating tubes in children with effusion of greater than 4 to 6 months duration who have a hearing loss of ≥ 20 dB and for children less than 3 years of age with effusion >3 months who have recurrent infection while on prophylactic antibiotics.

Chronic Suppurative Otitis Media (CSOM)

Chronic suppurative infection is a sequelae of poorly responsive recurrent AOM, particularly when a perforation has occurred. As the perforation heals, squamous epithelium may grow into the organizing abscess material producing a sac-like structure called a cholesteatoma. This frequently disrupts the ossicular chain resulting in a severe conductive hearing loss. It is essential, therefore, to differentiate CSOM without cholesteatoma which requires aggressive medical management from CSOM with cholesteatoma which is a surgical disease. Otomicroscopic evaluation by an otolaryngologist of all patients with a perforated drum and otorrhea for more than 6 weeks, particularly with ear pain and hearing loss, is warranted to identify the presence or absence of a cholesteatoma. Risk factors for CSOM, in addition to recurrent AOM are family history of chronic ear disease, crowded family living conditions, and large group day care. The incidence has been estimated at one case per 2500 children 0 to 15 years of age.

An algorithm for the management of CSOM is presented in Figure 6.

The goal of treatment is a dry ear and healing tympanic membrane. Parenteral therapy may be required in more difficult patients who have failed oral or topical ear drop therapy, selected primarily to eradicate *Pseudomonas aeruginosa*, almost always the causative pathogen, and to a lesser extent to treat *Staphylococcus aureus*. Cultures of exudate will help establish appropriate antimicrobial therapy. Patients require frequent suctioning and debridement of the external auditory canal, usually provided by an ENT consultant.

Parenteral antibiotic therapy in an outpatient setting is preferred, both for cost and convenience and the option of once daily gentamicin at a dose of 5 to 7 mg/kg is suggested. With normal renal function, monitoring serum antibiotic concentrations is not necessary. There are no adequate oral agents for CSOM alternatives, but topical quinolones (floxacin and ofloxacin), which represent the only class of antibiotics with adequate anti-pseudomonal activity, are available for use in children. Many oral antibiotics are available to treat *S. aureus* and most other potential pathogens. Treatment failures following these outpatient options may require combination parenteral antibiotics in an in-patient setting. Tympanomastoid surgery is recommended for the 25% of patients who do not respond to medical management and for any patient who develops a cholesteatoma.

Prevention

Risk factors for recurrent otitis media include many which cannot be controlled, namely male sex, selected racial groups (American Indians, Alaskan and Canadian Eskimos, and Africans), winter season, crowded households and age less than 6 months for the first episode of AOM. Other epidemiologic factors however, can be adjusted for the infant who is felt to be otitis

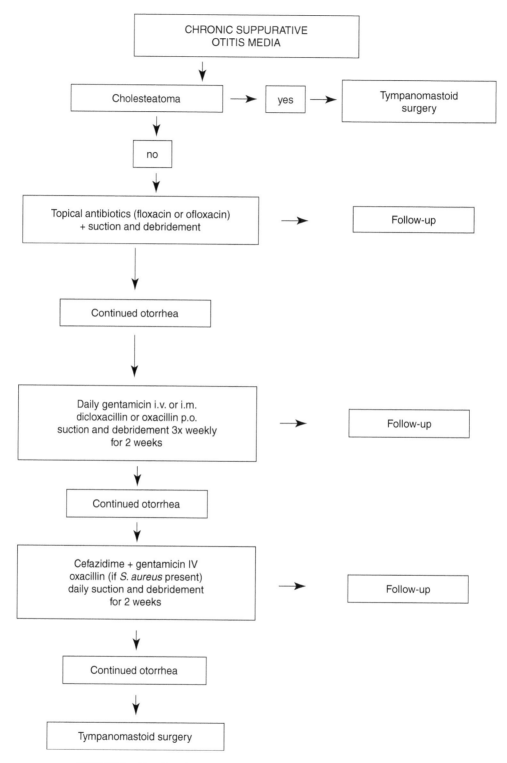

FIGURE 6   Algorithm for management of chronic suppurative otitis media (CSOM), including option of once-daily gentamicin outpatient therapy and indications for tympanomastoid surgery.

media prone and might be considered for the routine care of any child. Large group day care attendance for more than 20 hours per week is perhaps the greatest risk factor for frequent infection. Although this cannot be circumvented for many children, alternatives such as care by family members and small group care options could be pursued. Breast feeding is protective and is particularly recommended for the child whose sibling was otitis media prone. The easiest factor to control is exposure to tobacco smoke, which not only increases the incidence of AOM but is also associated with other respiratory infections in children.

Prior to the introduction of conjugate pneumococcal vaccine, *Streptococcus pneumoniae* was the leading pathogen for AOM. Today, in immunized children, AOM caused by vaccine strains of pneumococcus is reduced by 60% and the overall incidence of AOM is 6% to 7% lower than in unimmunized children. Protection from severe pneumococcal disease in infants is even greater.

Chemoprophylaxis has been shown to reduce the incidence of AOM in children who are otitis media prone. The accepted criteria for this intervention is 3 episodes of acute disease within 6 months or 4 in 12 months. Sulfisoxazole may be administered at one-half the usual therapeutic dose, 50 to 75 mg/kg/day, divided once or twice a day. The recommendation for chemoprophylaxis is included in the algorithm for AOM. Studies have suggested benefit with 3 different strategies: (1) chemoprophylaxis during the winter months, (2) for 90 days after the third episode of AOM within 6 months, or (3) antibiotics during the course of each new viral respiratory infection.

Otitis Media in Neonates

Bacteria causing otitis media in the first 6 weeks of life include Gram-negative coliforms, which are frequently resistant to amoxicillin. A diagnostic tympanocentesis is therefore required to guide therapy. In addition, these patients should be carefully evaluated for evidence of systemic disease including meningitis (Table 23).

PARASITIC INFECTIONS

Most parasitic diseases have virtually disappeared in developed countries as a result of concentrated efforts to improve sanitary conditions. Only pinworm (enterobiasis) and giardiasis are seen with any frequency in pediatric practice with occasional cases of ascariasis, amebiasis, strongyloidiasis, toxocariasis, hookworm, and whipworm (trichuriasis) requiring management. Presenting manifestations are summarized in Table 24. This section includes only these more common parasites. Giardiasis and amebiasis are discussed in Chapter 9 because they present with predominantly gastrointestinal symptoms (Table 24).

The most common parasitic disease, pinworm, should be treated if itching or discomfort interfere with sleep and other activities (Table 25). Reinfection is very common but the

TABLE 23   Etiology of Otitis Media in Neonates

Gram-negative enterics (*E. coli, Klebsiella, Pseudomonas, Proteus*)	60%
H. influenzae	15%
S. pneumoniae	15%
S. aureus	15%
Others	10%

TABLE 24   Presenting Manifestations of Common Parasitic Infections

Pinworm	Perianal pruritis
Ascariasis	Passage of adult worms
Strongyloidiasis	Marked eosinophilia
	Immunosuppression
	Diarrhea
Toxocariasis	Marked eosinophilia
	Visceral larval migrans
Hookworm	Usually asymptomatic
	anemia
Whipworm (trichuriasis)	Chronic diarrhea

TABLE 25   Treatment of More Common Parasitic Infections

Ascariasis	Albendazole 400 mg × 1 dose
	Mebendazole 100 mg b.i.d. × 3 days or 500 mg × 1 dose
	Ivermectin 150–200 mcg/kg × 1 dose
Hookworm (*Ancylostoma duodenale* and *Necator americanus*)	Albendazole 10 mg/kg (max. 400 mg) × 1 dose
	Mebendazole 100 mg b.i.d. × 3 days or 500 mg × 1 dose
	Pyrantel pamoate 11 mg/kg (max. 1 g/day) qd × 3 days
Pinworm	Pyrantel pamoate 11 mg/kg × 1 dose (max. 1 g); repeat in 2 wks
	Mebendazole 100 mg × 1 dose; repeat in 2 wks (treat all household members)
	Albendazole 400 mg × 1 dose; repeat in 2 wks
Note: Treat all household members	
Strongyloidiasis	Invermectin 200 mcg/kg qd × 2 days
	Albendazole 400 mg b.i.d. × 7 days
	Thiabendazole 50 mg/kg/24 hrs div. q 12 hrs × 2 days; max. 3 g/day
Toxocariasis	Albendazole 400 mg b.i.d. × 5 days
	Mebendazole 100–200 mg b.i.d. × 5 days
Whipworm (trichuriasis)	Mebendazole 100 mg b.i..d. × 3 days or 500 mg × 1
	Albendazole 400 mg × 3 days
	Ivermectin 200 mcg/kg qd × 3 days

presence of *Enterobius* is usually of minor clinical consequence. Most important is reassurance of the family that these nematodes are not the result of poor hygiene.

Strongyloides infection in the immunocompromised patient is associated with a high degree of parasitemia, dissemination, and significant mortality even with early administration of thiabendazole (Table 25).

Unusual parasitic infections are more likely to be seen in immigrants and individuals who have traveled to endemic areas. Presenting symptoms are commonly diarrhea, weight loss, rash, eosinophilia, skin ulcers, or fever. Treatment programs for unusual parasitic infections are summarized in Chapter 20, Table 20.

TABLE 26   Postexposure Rabies Management

Routine treatment of animal bites (see Table 8)
Rabies management
Healthy domestic animal: observe animal for 10 days
Wild rodent (mouse, rat, rabbit, squirrel, etc.): rabies prophylaxis is not indicated
Wild animal (skunk, raccoon, bat, fox, etc.) or escaped domestic animals (dog or cat): HRIG 20 IU/kg total dose
All infiltrated around wound if possible
HDC vaccine
1 mL IM on day 0, 3, 7, 14, and 28
Follow-up rabies antibody titer on day 42 only for patients who are immunocompromised

TABLE 27 Emergency Treatment of Snakebites

Apply tourniquet loosely, proximal to edema
Splint
Transport to medical facility
For large snakes where transport will take >1 hr
  Clean the bite
  Make 5 mm incision over fang marks
  Apply suction, DO NOT
    Use tight tourniquet
    Pack on ice

TABLE 28 In-Hospital Treatment of Snakebites

Admit for observation
Laboratory studies
  CBC, U/A, electrolytes
  Blood type and crossmatch
  Clotting studies monitored frequently
Antivenin IV for significant envenomation
  Begin within 2 hr of bite
  Skin test for hypersensitivity
  Dose is individualized
    Moderate cases—3 to 5 vials
    Severe cases—10 to 20 vials
  Children—relatively higher doses
    Monitor for allergic reactions
    Serum sickness common at 4–7 days
Fasciotomy if neuromuscular function compromised
Tetanus prophylaxis
Severe cases
  Volume expanders, respiratory support, dialysis

RABIES PROPHYLAXIS

Postexposure rabies management has become much easier now that immunotherapeutic agents of extremely low toxicity have become available (Table 26). Rabies immune globulin is prepared from the plasma of human volunteers hyperimmunized with rabies vaccine thereby eliminating serum sickness episodes so common with animal rabies serum, and human diploid cell vaccine is not associated with the encephalitic reactions so characteristic of duck embryo vaccine. The only drawback to this present treatment is the high cost.

SNAKEBITES

Most snakebites are inflicted by nonpoisonous species or result in minimal envenomation where pit vipers (rattlesnakes, water moccasins, and copperheads) are involved. Simple observation for progression of local or systemic symptoms during a 4-hour period following the bite is the only therapy usually required. Emergency procedures are given in Table 27. Coral snake bites should always be considered potentially fatal. Large rattlesnakes and water moccasins account for the largest number of serious or fatal bites. The greatest number of poisonous bites, however, are inflected by copperheads, which are small and whose bites almost never result in fatal consequences. A conservative approach is therefore indicated when this species is identified.

Initial assessment of the patient is directed at determining the amount of envenomation and time lapse between the bite and institution of definitive therapy. Antivenin therapy (Table 28) should be started within 2 hours of the bite to assure maximum benefit. Guidelines for amount of antivenin are detailed in the package insert. Surgical consultation should be obtained if the bite is on a distal extremity because a fasciotomy may become necessary to preserve neurovascular function.

4 | Immunizations

ACTIVE IMMUNIZATION

Routine Vaccination

The ultimate goal in medicine is not treatment but prevention of disease and vaccine administration represents the most efficacious and cost effective measure for accomplishing this goal. Success is best supported by the worldwide eradication of smallpox, elimination of polio in the western hemisphere and control of previously common severe infections such as measles (Fig. 1), diphtheria, tetanus (Fig. 2), and pertussis (Fig. 3). Fourteen diseases can be prevented with vaccines that should be routinely administered to all children prior to beginning school. The diseases include hepatitis B, *H. influenzae*, pneumococcus, diphtheria, tetanus toxoid, pertussis, trivalent polio, rotavirus, influenza, hepatitis A, measles, mumps, rubella and Varicella-Zoster. In addition, 3 immunizations are recommended for administration in preadolescents, aged 11 to 12 years. They are the conjugate meningococcal (Menactra©), booster pertussis—TdaP (Adacel© or Boostrix©), and for girls, human papilloma virus (Gardasil©) vaccines. The current recommendations from the Committee on Infectious Diseases, American

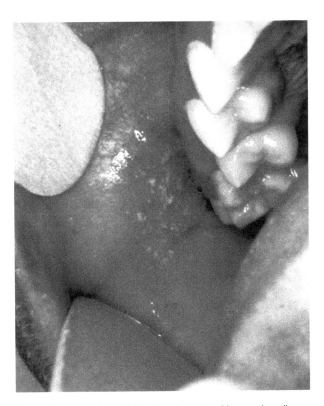

FIGURE 1 (*See color insert.*) The Koplik spots with measles allow an early definitive diagnosis. They appear on the buccal mucosa opposite the upper and lower premolar teeth 24 to 48 hours before onset of the rash and may persist for 48 to 72 hours after the rash begins. If the spots are not present 24 hours before and after onset of the rash, the diagnosis of measles is unlikely.

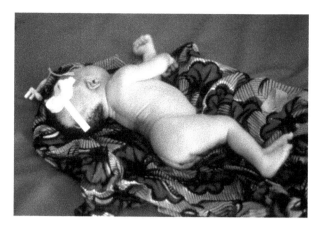

FIGURE 2 This neonate developed opisthotonus on the fourth day of life following an unsterile delivery. The greatest factor accounting for this case of neonatal tetanus is failure of the mother to receive tetanus immunization.

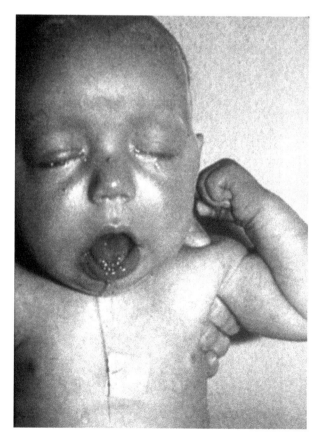

FIGURE 3 This 3-month-old infant with culture proven pertussis was cyanotic during this episode of a severe coughing paroxysm. Mortality is 1% to 2% in neonates and infants one to three months of age.

Academy of Pediatrics (Report of the Committee on Infectious Diseases, 27th ed., 2006) for immunization in children are outlined in Table 1. Additional vaccines and vaccine combinations available in the United States are itemized in Table 2.

TABLE 1 Routine Immunization Schedule

Vaccine	Age for administration
Hepatitis B	0–2 mos, 1–4 mos, 6–18 mos
H. influenzae	2 mos, 4 mos, (6 mos), 12–15 mos
Pneumococcus (PCV)	2, 4, 6, 12–18 mos
DTaP	2 mos, 4 mos, 6 mos, 15–18 mos
Polio (IPV)	2 mos, 4 mos, 6–18 mos, 4–6 yrs
Rotavirus	6 wks–2 mos, 10–16 wks, 14–32 wks
Influenza	6 mos and yearly thereafter
Hepatitis A	12–23 mos, 18–41 mos
MMR	12–15 mos, 4–6 yrs
Varicella	12–18 mos, 4–6 yrs
Meningococcus (MCV4)	11–12 yrs
TdaP	11–12 yrs
Human papilloma virus	11–12 yrs (girls)

Recommended immunizations by age	
Age	**Vaccine**
Birth	Hepatitis B (based on risk)
2 mos	Hepatitis B
	DTaP
	H. influenzae type b
	Polio (IPV)
	Pneumococcus (PCV)
	Rotavirus
4 mos	Hepatitis B
	DTaP
	H. influenzae type b
	Polio (IPV)
	Pneumococcus (PCV)
	Rotavirus
6 mos	Hepatitis B
	DTaP
	H. influenzae type b (if needed)[a]
	Polio (IPV)
	Pneumococcus (PCV)
	Rotavirus
	Influenza (and yearly)
12 mos	*H. influenzae* type b
	MMR-VZ
	Pneumococcus (PCV)
	Hepatitis A
18 mos	DTaP
	Hepatitis A
5 yrs	DTaP
	MMR-VZ
	Polio (IPV)
11–12 yrs	TdaP
	Meningococcus (MCV4)
	HPV (girls)

[a] PedVax hib requires just 2 primary doses.
Abbreviations: DTaP, diptheria, tetanus and pertussis; HPV, human papillomavirus; IVP, inactivated polio vaccine; MCV4, meningoccal conjugated vaccine; PCV, pneumococcus conjugated vaccine.

TABLE 2 Vaccines Available in the United States

Vaccine	Type	Route
BCG (Bacillus of Calmette and Guérin)	Live bacteria	Intradermal or subcutaneous
Diphtheria-tetanus (DT, Td)	Toxoids	Intramuscular
Diphtheria–tetanus–acellular pertussis DTaP	Toxoids and inactivated bacterial components	Intramuscular
Diphtheria–tetanus–acellular pertussis—booster TdaP	Toxoids and inactivated bacterial components	
Hepatitis A	Inactivated viral antigen	Intramuscular
Hepatitis B	Recombinant viral antigen	Intramuscular
Hib conjugates	Polysaccharide-protein conjugate	Intramuscular
Hib conjugate-DTaP (PRP-T reconstituted with DTaP)	Polysaccharide–protein conjugate with toxoids and inactivated bacterial components	Intramuscular
Hib conjugate (PRP-OMP) hepatitis B	Polysaccharide-protein conjugate with inactivated virus	Intramuscular
Human papilloma virus (HPV)	Recombinant (viral-like particle)	Intramuscular
Influenza	Inactivated virus (whole-virus), viral components	Intramuscular
Influenza	Live-attenuated virus	Intranasal
Japanese encephalitis	Inactivated virus	Subcutaneous
Measles	Live virus	Subcutaneous
Meningococcal	Polysaccharide	Subcutaneous
Meningococcal	Polysaccharide-protein conjugate	Intramuscular
MMR and MMRV	Live viruses	Subcutaneous
Mumps	Live virus	Subcutaneous
Pneumococcal	Polysaccharide	Intramuscular or subcutaneous
Pneumococcal conjugate	Polysaccharide-protein conjugate	Intramuscular
Poliovirus (IPV)	Inactivated virus	Subcutaneous or intramuscular
Rabies	Inactivated virus	Intramuscular
Rotavirus	Live reassortment viruses	Oral
Rubella	Live virus	Subcutaneous
TdaP	Toxoids and inactivated bacterial components	Intramuscular
Tetanus	Inactivated toxin (toxoid)	Intramuscular
Tetanus-diphtheria (Td, DT)	Inactivated toxins	Intramuscular
Typhoid		
Parenteral	Capsular polysaccharide	Intramuscular
Oral	Live-attenuated bacteria	Oral
Varicella-zoster	Live-attenuated virus	Subcutaneous
Yellow fever	Live virus	Subcutaneous
Zoster (shingles)	Live-attenuated virus	Subcutaneous

Methods for providing these vaccines are certainly simple, essentially requiring only a concerned attitude on the part of parents and physicians. It is, therefore, unfortunate that many children in the United States are inadequately immunized against these infectious agents. Recent surveys of private pediatric practices have indicated that, even under optimal circumstances, 30% to 40% of preschool children were not appropriately vaccinated.

Other Recommendations for Vaccine Use. If the immunization program for a young child is begun but not completed, the physician can simply continue where the program was interrupted. Original doses do not have to be repeated. There are, however, a few alterations. Rotavirus vaccine is not recommended if immunization cannot be completed prior to 32 weeks of age. If the child is past the 7th birthday, pertussis vaccine should be eliminated and the adult form of diphtheria vaccine (Td) should be substituted. Td vaccine contains approximately 15% of material included in childhood diphtheria. Otherwise, diphtheria–tetanus–acellular pertussis (DTaP) or adult tetanus diphtheria (Td) are given at 2-month intervals with measles–mumps–rubella (MMR) administered as soon as is practical.

Tetanus prophylaxis in wound management is simple if patients have received their primary immunization doses. Under these circumstances, tetanus toxoid, usually along with diphtheria, is given for a tetanus prone wound if the patient has not received tetanus toxoid within 5 years of the accident. If the individual has received three doses of tetanus toxoid during his or her lifetime, this is considered adequate and tetanus immune globulin need not be given. Fewer than three doses of tetanus toxoid is considered inadequate for protection and, under these circumstances for a tetanus prone wound, 250 U of tetanus immunoglobulin should be given along with tetanus toxoid, and the immunization procedure should be completed during long-term management with the next dose of DTaP or Td given 4 weeks later.

The simultaneous administration of vaccines, particularly when "catching-up" on immunization programs, is a common practice. A great deal of clinical data now support the efficacy of vaccines administered on the same day if circumstances make this the only practical approach. The one drawback is that simultaneously administered vaccines are more likely to cause local or systemic side effects and, if any reaction is severe, the clinician would not know which agent was responsible.

Additional vaccines are generally administered only to individuals traveling to foreign countries where other infectious agents are endemic. This is discussed in Chapter 5. Additional information for these travelers is available in the periodic publication of a supplement to *Morbidity and Mortality Weekly Report* entitled "Health Information for International Travel," which can be obtained from the Superintendent of Documents, U.S. Government Printing Office, Washington, D.C. 20402, U.S.A. or from state health departments.

Local side effects, such as erythema and induration with tenderness, are common after the administration of all vaccines, but particularly with tetanus. This represents an Arthus reaction in individuals with pre-existing high levels of tetanus antibody. Reactions are self-limited and do not require specific therapy, although most physicians routinely administer acetaminophen prior to offering immunizations. A nodule may appear at the injection site and persist for several weeks but this should not be considered a significant reaction. Rarely, systemic reactions occur and these necessitate the alteration of immunization programs (Table 3).

If reactions occur with DTaP injections, the physician can usually assume that the pertussis antigen is the causative agent and immunizations should then be completed with TD or Td. The only contraindication to tetanus and diphtheria toxoids is the history of a neurologic or a severe hypersensitivity reaction following a previous dose when pertussis had been excluded. When the causative agent cannot be determined, skin testing (prick and intradermal) may be useful with tetanus and diphtheria toxoids to document immediate hypersensitivity. Tetanus toxoid should not be routinely given more frequently than every 10 years since with more frequent injections a percentage of recipients will develop major local reactions (Arthus reactions).

Other contraindications to pertussis vaccine. Hypersensitivity to vaccine components, presence of an evolving neurologic disorder, or a history of a severe reaction (usually within

TABLE 3 Contraindications to Immunizations

Reaction to previous dose
Neurologic
Allergic
Live vaccines
Immunodeficiency
Malignancy
Immunosuppressive therapy
Plasma, or blood transfusion within 2 mo or intravenous immunoglobulin
(IVIG) within 2–10 mo, depending on dosage (for measles only)
Pregnancy

TABLE 4   Consider Discontinuation of Acellular Pertussis Vaccine

Contraindications
   Immediate anaphylactic reaction
   Encephalopathy within 7 days
Precautions
   Seizure, with or without fever, within 3 days of immunization
   Persistent crying or screaming of 3-hr duration within 48 hrs of
      immunization
   Hypotonic-hyporesponsive episode (shock-like state) within 48 hrs of
      immunization
   Temperature more than 104.8°F (40.5°C), unexplained by another cause,
      within 48 hrs of immunization

48 hours) following a previous dose are definitive contraindications to the receipt of pertussis vaccine. Some authorities recommend discontinuing pertussis vaccine for other severe reactions (Table 4).

Premature Infants

Premature infants are generally immunized at the usual chronologic age using routine vaccine dosages. At 2 months DTaP, Hib, and inactivated polio vaccines can be given, even if the infant weighs <1500 g at birth. Rotavirus vaccine has been evaluated in prematurely born infants and shown to be safe and effective in those born as young as 26 weeks gestation.

Preterm neonates born to hepatitis B surface antigen (HBsAg)-positive mothers should be managed identically to full-term neonates (Table 5), receiving hepatitis B immunoglobulin (HBIG) and the first dose of hepatitis B vaccine (at a different site) within 12 hours of life.

In premature neonates with birth weights less than 2000 g whose mothers are HBsAg-negative, hepatitis B vaccine should be delayed until the weight is more than 2000 g or until 1 month of age, whichever comes first. There is no urgency in administering this vaccine early in life so the first dose can be given at hospital discharge if the weight is adequate.

If the birth weight is less than 2000 g and the mother's hepatitis B status cannot be determined within the initial 12 hours of life, both HBIG and hepatitis B vaccine should be given at birth (Table 6).

Immunosuppressed Patients

Immunization of immuncompromised patients may not elicit a protective immune response and in the case of live vaccines, may cause severe disease. Risks must therefore be carefully balanced against potential benefits. However, it should be emphasized that data are quite limited concerning adverse reactions of live vaccine products in immunosuppressed individuals. Inadvertent immunization of HIV-infected infants with live vaccines have rarely resulted in disease, offering reassurance that even these vaccines are relatively safe. Children with congenital disorders of immune function appear most vulnerable to dissemination of live bacterial and virus vaccine microorganisms, particularly BCG and measles, so these should not be given when host immune responses are severely compromised.

TABLE 5   Hepatitis B Prevention for Premature and Full-Term Infants of HBsAg-Positive Mothers

Birth	Hepatitis B immune globulin (HBIG) 0.5 mL IM within 12 hrs of birth
	Hepatitis B vaccine 0.5 mL IM within 12 hrs of birth
1 mo	Hep B vaccine
6 mos	Hep B vaccine

TABLE 6   Hepatitis B Virus Vaccine and HBIG in Neonates

Mother HBsAg-positive (Table 5)
Mother HBsAg-negative
   Full-term and premature >2000 g: vaccine begun birth to 2 mo
   Premature <2000 g: delay vaccine until >2000 g or 1 mo of age
Mother HBsAg-status unknown
   Full-term and premature >2000 g: vaccine at birth (<12 hr) determine
     mothers HBsAg status HBIG within 7 days if mother positive
   Premature <2000 g: HBIG and vaccine within 12 hr of birth

Live virus vaccines, including MMR, varicella, and rotavirus can be given to normal children living in households with a family member who is immunodeficient, and the former two vaccine products are even more important under these circumstances since wild measles and varicella have caused significant disease in immunosuppressed children and adults (Table 7).

Influenza Vaccine

Annual vaccination beginning at 6 months of age is recommended for all children younger than 6 years, those with medical problems that would result in more extensive infection once they developed influenza and for all individuals with increased exposure to potential outbreaks (Table 8).

    The type of vaccine and dosage recommended for various age groups vary with the vaccine prepared each year. Therefore, the physician should consult the package insert or the state health department for specific information.

    Field trials of influenza vaccines in the past have usually shown vaccine efficacy in the range of 70% to 80%. The greatest success is achieved when the antigenic drift of viral strains is anticipated so that the vaccines would include appropriate components. Vaccines now provide protection for both influenza A and influenza B. If an individual receives vaccine each year, only one dose is needed. If vaccine is given for the first time, however, often two doses are required for adequate immunization.

    Outbreaks of influenza occur between October and the end of March. Therefore, the vaccine should be administered before or during the month of October and discontinued by April 1. Often, an outbreak that occurs in December or January, is not documented until February when it receives national attention. This is too late to begin an immunization

TABLE 7   Vaccines for Immunodeficient and Immunosuppressed Children

Definition of immunosuppression
   Immunosuppressive chemotherapeutic agents for malignancy or
     management of transplant rejection
   Congenital or acquired (AIDS) immunodeficiency conditions
   Corticosteroids
     2 mg/kg/day of prednisone or equivalent or 20 mg/day total
      dose given >14 days
   Live vaccines are generally contraindicated in immunodeficient children
     and adults
   Rotavirus vaccine has not been studied in immunodeficient infants so
     is not recommended
   MMR and VZ may be given to AIDS patients who are not severely
     immunosuppressed
   MMR, varicella, and rotavirus vaccines can be given to children when
     there is an immunosuppressed individual in the household

TABLE 8   Influenza Vaccine

Chronic diseases	Immunosuppressive
Pulmonary	therapy
Cardiac	Age >65 yrs
Renal	Hospital personnel
Diabetes mellitus	School teachers
Metabolic	
disorders	
Anemia	
Malignancies	

program since, historically, cases rarely appear after March 1. The best and most efficient system is for the primary care physician to maintain a list of patients who should receive vaccine and, during the month of September, notify these patients so that they may plan for a brief office appointment. The most important aspect in assuring success for vaccination practices is a compulsive and methodical attitude on the part of primary care physicians. The individual patient cannot be expected to remember this aspect of health care.

Rabies Vaccine

Rabies vaccine is currently recommended for animal handlers and anyone traveling to regions of the world where rabies is endemic in domestic animals. It is also used for post-exposure prophylaxis in conjunction with rabies immunoglobulin. For pre-exposure prevention a three dose regimen is required. If pre-immunized individuals are bitten by potentially rabid animals they will still require two post-exposure doses of rabies vaccine, but rabies immunoglobulin is not required. For post-exposure treatment, five doses of vaccine along with rabies immune globulin (RIG) should be administered. The Centers for Disease Control (CDC) now recommends that the full dose of RIG be infiltrated in the area around and into the wound if possible. If the volume is too large, any remaining volume should be injected by the intramuscular route at a site distance from rabies vaccine administration.

PASSIVE IMMUNIZATION

Immunoglobulin

Passive immunization may be accomplished by administering immunoglobulin (previously called immune serum globulin) to individuals exposed to hepatitis A or those traveling into endemic regions of the world where probability of exposure is significant and to non-immune children exposed to measles, and non-immune pregnant women exposed to rubella. The other indication for immunoglobulin is hypogammaglobulinemia. However, this product has been in greatly limited supply for quite a few years and has been largely replaced by intravenous immunoglobulin preparations.

Hyperimmune Human Immunoglobulin

Gammaglobulin prepared from selected hyperimmune donors is particularly useful as passive immunotherapy in modifying or preventing clinical illness from a number of infectious agents (Table 9).

The need for consultation concerning the indications for Varicella-Zoster hyperimmune globulin (VariZIG^{TM}) is more frequent than for any of the other globulin products. This is the result of both the ubiquitous nature of the virus and the large number of patients who benefit from its administration. The most common circumstance is a child with malignancy, usually leukemia, who is exposed to chickenpox. Table 10 outlines the guidelines for using VariZIG.

TABLE 9 Hyperimmune Immunoglobulin

Immune globulin	Trade name	Manufacturer
Human		
Botulism	BabyBIG®	California Department of Health Services—510-540-2646
Cytomegalovirus	Cytogam®	Connaught Laboratories
Hepatitis B	HBIG	Cutter Biological, Abbott, Merck
Rabies	R.I.G.	Cutter Biological
Tetanus	T.I.G.	Cutter Biological, Savage, Hyland, Parke-Davis, Wyeth, Elkins-Sinn, Merck Sharp and Dohme, Hyland Therapeutics
Varicella-Zoster	VariZIG™	FFF Enterprises—800-843-7477
Animal		
Botulism antitoxin (Equine)		Available from CDC
Diphtheria antitoxin (Equine)		Available from CDC
RSV (Palivizumab) humanized mouse monoclonal antibody		MedImmune

TABLE 10 Guidelines for the Use of VariZIG[a]

Time elapsed after exposure is such that VariZIG can be administered within 96 hrs

One of the following underlying illnesses or conditions
Immunocompromised children including HIV infection, without a history of varicella or varicella immunization
Susceptible pregnant women
Newborn of mother who had onset of chickenpox <5 days before delivery or within 48 hr after delivery
Exposed hospitalized preterm infant >28 wk gestation whose mother's history is negative for chickenpox or is seronegative
Exposed preterm infant <28 wk

One of the following types of exposure to chickenpox or zoster patient(s):
Household contact
Playmate contact: face-to-face indoor play
Hospital contact: in same 2–4-bed room or adjacent beds in a large ward; face-to-face contact with an infectious staff member or patient; visit by a person deemed contagious
Newborn contact (newborn of mother who had onset of chickenpox <5 days before delivery or within 48 hr after delivery)

[a] If VariZIG is not available, iVIG may be used.

It is now more readily available through regional distribution centers around the country, which can be located through a central service FFF Enterprises (1-800-843-7477).

Hyperimmune Animal Immunoglobulin

In addition to human hyperimmune globulin preparations, antisera of animal origin are also available for clinical use. These products carry with them a high probability of serum reactions, particularly if the recipient has been exposed to similar animal products previously. Information for these and other products can be obtained through the Centers for Disease Control, Tel.: +404 329 3311 or 329 3644. Materials include: black widow spider equine antivenin, equine western equine encephalitis, botulism ABE polyvalent equine antitoxin, diphtheria equine antitoxin, antirabies serum, polyvalent gas gangrene equine antitoxin, coral snake equine antivenin, and crotalid polyvalent antivenin.

5 | Travel Medicine

INTRODUCTION

Immigrants and naturalized citizens residing in the United States constitute the population most likely to travel with young children to developing countries. These periodic trips are often the only way relatives can maintain family relationships. Clinicians' assessment of priorities and approaches to counseling are therefore very different from those for adults who are simply planning business or exotic leisure travel. The usual conservative approach must be tempered by consideration of more personal issues, otherwise parents would be strongly encouraged to delay exposing young children to serious health problems more prevalent in their (or their parents') native countries.

It should also be kept in mind that many diseases in other regions of the world are not seen in the countries of residence for travelers. Therefore, their illness on returning may not be recognized by primary care physicins. Infectious disease consultants are important for their management. In some cases, infections caused by organisms related to similar pathogens of the country of origin may be more severe, e.g., typhoid fever caused by *Salmonella typhi* versus non-typhoidal *Salmonella* organisms seen in most developed countries. In other cases, disease is less severe, e.g., Mediterranean-spotted fever (Fig. 1) in Europe caused by *Rickettsia conorii* versus Rocky Mountain–spotted fever caused by *R. rickettsii* in the Americas.

RESTRICTIONS FOR FAMILY TRAVEL

As a general recommendation, families should be advised to avoid traveling with infants less than 6 months of age because in this age group diarrheal diseases are more severe and insect-borne illnesses are extremely difficult to prevent and treat. In fact, very few medications for diseases such as malaria, leishmaniasis, or filariasis have been adequately studied in young infants. Perhaps more importantly, immunizations for polio, rotavirus, hepatitis B,

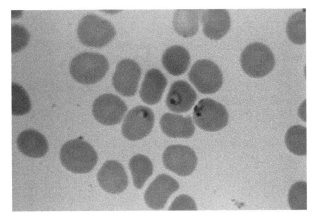

FIGURE 1 Ring stage of *Plasmodium falciparum.* Infection with this species is usually a medical emergency as very high parasitemias causing death may occur as a consequence of severe anemia, renal failure, and cerebritis.

Haemophilus influenzae type b, tetanus, diphtheria, and pertussis are not completed until 6 months and measles, mumps, rubella (MMR), and varicella not routinely before 12 months. As discussed later, consideration can be given to administering MMR and perhaps varicella vaccines as early as 6 months of age.

It is obvious that most children born in developing countries do well without any unique medical intervention. They do not routinely receive special vaccines nor malaria prophylaxis. Also, any infant being breast fed is afforded maximal protection from most infectious agents and is unlikely to develop difficulty following exposure to gastrointestinal pathogens such as *Salmonella* and *Shigella*. However, because special steps can reduce disease in infants and young children, potential preventive measures should be carefully explained to parents.

For infants not being breast fed, bottled water and canned fruits and vegetables must be provided, or at the very least, meticulously boiled water and freshly cooked food should be prepared. These same recommendations pertain to older children and adults as well, but there is greater emphasis on this advice for infants because food-borne disease is more serious in this age group.

MISSIONARY FAMILIES

Missionaries and their families represent a very unique, high-risk group for tropical diseases, a consequence of long duration exposure in rural communities much different from the usual vacation or business traveler. Recommendations for preventive medical interventions are quite varied since there is disagreement as to whether these individuals should be managed as all other residents of the host country or whether they should receive special care similar to that offered transient travelers. There is not a single publication in the medical literature which specifically addresses their needs yet missionaries routinely seek medical advise from their physicians. A survey of the missionary offices of various religious denominations also failed to identify consistent guidelines for medical management of these families.

Anticipated length of stay in a particular region often plays a major role in decisions made by travel medicine clinics. This variable particularly pertains to chemoprophylaxis for malaria. Clinicians' assessment of priorities and approaches to counseling are therefore very different from those for adults who are simply planning business or exotic leisure travel. The usual conservative approach must be tempered by consideration of more personal issues, otherwise missionaries would be strongly encouraged to delay exposing young children to serious health problems more prevalent in developing countries.

ROUTINE IMMUNIZATIONS

All family members should complete the recommended basic series of immunizations that prevent common childhood diseases (Table 1). In the case of *H. influenzae* type b–conjugate vaccine, adequate protection is actually achieved after 2 doses in the primary series. A minimum of 3 immunizations is necessary for hepatitis B, pneumococcus, DTP, polio, and rotavirus. Booster doses of some vaccines may be given earlier than generally recommended to maximize protection prior to travel.

Measles, mumps, and rubella combined vaccine, hepatitis A, meningococcus, and varicella may be given as early as 6 months of age rather than the usual times, if the family will be traveling to or residing in any region where these diseases are highly endemic.

TRAVEL VACCINES

Limitations for Young Children

There are major limitations in making recommendations for children traveling to foreign countries. For example, many vaccines and prophylactic chemotherapeutic agents used against pathogens that are relatively rare in the United States have simply not been thoroughly

TABLE 1 Routine Immunizations and the Age When Protection is Provided

Disease	Recommended vaccine schedule	Age when protection adequate for travel
Hepatitis B	0, 1, 6 mos	6 mos
Diphtheria	2, 4, 6, 15 mos, 5 yrs	6 mos
Tetanus	2, 4, 6, 15 mos, 5 yrs	6 mos
Pertussis	2, 4, 6, 15 mos, 5 yrs	6 mos
Polio	2, 4, 6 mos, 5 yrs	6 mos
Rotavirus	2, 3, 3 mos	4 mos
H. influenzae b	2, 4, 6, 12 mos	4 mos
Measles	12 mos	12 mos
Mumps	12 mos	12 mos
Rubella	12 mos	12 mos
Varicella	12 mos	12 mos
Hepatitis A	12, 18 mos	12 mos
Meningococcus	11–12 yrs	11–12 yrs
Human papilloma virus	11–12 yrs (3 doses)	11–12 yrs

studied in this population (e.g., mefloquine for malaria prophylaxis) or have been shown to be inadequate (e.g., some components of the meningococcal vaccine in children less than 2 years of age). Yellow fever vaccine is associated with a higher incidence of vaccine-related encephalitis in young infants as compared with adults, so it should only be given if benefits clearly outweigh the risks. The yellow fever vaccine is never recommended for infants less than 4 months of age.

There is actually considerable unpublished information concerning the use of most vaccines and medications in young children, because this age group has received many of these agents for years in developing countries in spite of non-approval. In most cases, few adverse reactions have been reported. Table 2 includes information currently available from suppliers concerning reported side effects as well as identified limitations.

Reviews of travel medicine issues have been remarkably conservative in recommendations for infants and young children. Conclusions likely reflect gaps in published management data, as discussed.

TABLE 2 Age Limitations for Vaccines and Chemoprophylaxis

Agent	Limitation and reason
Meningococcal polysaccharide vaccine	<2 yrs Poor antibody response to groups C, Y, and W-135
Meningococcal conjugate vaccine	Not studied <2 yrs of age
Oral typhoid vaccine	Not approved <6 yrs Limited data and no suspension formulation but safe and effective
Yellow fever vaccine	Contraindicated <4 mos Vaccine-associated encephalitis
Mefloquine	<15 kg (approx. 30 mos of age) Limited pharmacologic data but safe and effective
Loperamide	≤2 yrs Not approved as data are limited
Bismuth subsalicylate	≤3 yrs Not approved as data are limited

Active immunizations for other infectious diseases varies according to the country of residence. The necessity for active immunization in children is no different from that in adults and schedules are generally identical (Table 3).

Hyperimmune human immunoglobulin for rabies and hepatitis B is necessary for unimmunized individuals of all ages immediately following direct exposure to these diseases. This would have to be given in the host country and may not be readily available. Families should be apprised of this limitation, which further supports routine vaccination for rabies and hepatitis B.

Hepatitis A

One of the greatest risks during residence in developing countries is exposure to hepatitis A from contaminated food and water. The disease is usually anicteric and quite mild in young children. However, these young family members could subsequently become the contact source of infection for their parents and adult relatives, in whom disease can be more severe. Reported mortality among the older age groups is 3 per 1000 cases.

Hepatitis A vaccine has been licensed and recommended for children as young as 1 year of age who travel or reside in regions of the world where disease is endemic. Limited

TABLE 3 Recommended Preventive Measures for Travel to Countries Where Specific Diseases Are Endemic

Vaccine	Schedule

Hepatitis A vaccine
  Vaqta (Merck)
	2 wks prior to travel and 6–18 mos later
	1–17 yrs of age 0.5 mL (25 U) IM >18 yrs
	  1.0 mL (50 U) IM

Typhoid vaccine, live oral
  Ty21a
  Vivotif Berna (Berna
    Products Corp.) or
	1 cap q.o.d. × 4

Typhoid Vi polysaccharide
  vaccine
  Typhim Vi (Pasteur Meriux
    Connaught)
	0.5 mL IM
	Repeat q 2 yrs if high risk

Meningococcal polysaccharide
  vaccine
  Menomune—A/C/Y/W-135
    (Connaught)
	0.5 mL SQ
	Single dose q 2 yrs

Meningococcal conjugate vaccine (Sanofi Pasteur)	0.5 mL IM

Yellow fever, 17D	Single dose SQ
	Recommended for age >9 mos 4–9 mos
	  individualized based on estimates of risk
	<4 mos contraindicated booster every
	  10 yrs

Rabies
  Rabies vaccine adsorbed
    (RVA) (Smith Kline
    Beecham)
	1 mL IM 0, 7, and 21 or 28 days

Imovax Rabies Imovax Rabies ID	1 mL IM 0, 7, and 21 or 28 days 0.1 mL ID 0, 7, and 21 or 28 days
Japanese encephalitis	SQ doses 0, 7, 30 days or 0, 7, 14 days >3 yrs of age: 1.0 mL 6 mos–3 yrs, 0.5 mL <6 mos: no data but 0.5 mL appropriate

data indicate good antibody conversion in infants younger than 1 year of age. For this reason, it seems prudent to immunize children who are as young as 6 months of age. One dose is required with a booster administration 6 to 12 months later. Another dose might be considered for infants immunized prior to 2 years of age, given sometime after the second birthday.

Typhoid Fever

A common infection in developing countries is typhoid fever, accounting for significant morbidity and mortality in residents of all ages. Although 2 killed vaccines are available, the live oral vaccine is as efficacious as the killed vaccines and preferred for all ages. However, at this time it is not approved in the United States for children younger than 6 years of age. The primary reason for this limitation is that children younger than 6 years are usually unwilling to swallow capsules. Vaccine trials using a suspension formulation actually demonstrated higher efficacy and safety in children than that observed for the capsule when employed in adult studies. Unfortunately, this oral suspension is not commercially available.

A parenteral vaccine, Typhoid Vi, the capsular polysaccharide (ViCPS) of *Salmonella typhi*, is approved for administration to children 2 years of age and older. It requires only a single injection for immunization, but local reactions occur in 7% of recipients. Protective efficacy for the oral vaccine lasts for 5 to 6 years, compared with the ViCPS vaccine which requires a booster every 2 years. Of the 3 typhoid vaccines currently licensed in the United States, only the older parenteral heat-phenol–inactivated product is licensed for children as young as 6 months of age.

A reasonable approach for young children is to open the capsule and place the contents into a gelatin dessert, banana, or other preferred food of infants using the same schedule recommended for older children. It is important to keep in mind that this is a live bacterial vaccine, quite safe, but not recommended for patients who are immunosuppressed or for young children in a household where any adult is immunosuppressed. For reasons not completely understood, mefloquine may reduce the immunogenicity of typhoid vaccine, so this drug should be given more than 24 hours before or after a vaccine dose.

Meningococcus

The meningococcal polysaccharide vaccine contains antigens that elicit a T cell–independent immune response markedly limited in infants. It is therefore not generally recommended until 2 years of age. However, the group A component is immunogenic as early as 3 months of age and this is the serogroup most likely to cause outbreaks in developing countries. Immunization is therefore appropriate for any infant older than 90 days. The risk of invasive meningococcal disease from other serogroups, even in countries which report a high incidence of group A infection, is low enough that immunization for groups C, W135, and Y is rarely essential.

The conjugate meningococcal vaccine has not been studied in young infants, but is likely to affort greater protection than the polysaccharide vaccine in this young age group. It therefore appears reasonable to give this vaccine to infants 3 months of age or older if they will be traveling to countries where meningococcal disease is endemic.

Parents also can be counseled to prevent their children from having close contact with adults during reported outbreaks of meningicoccal disease in local communities; early rifampin prophylaxis is advised following potential exposure. Direct household exposure to infected patients still represents the only well–documented risk factor for secondary cases.

Yellow Fever

Prevention of yellow fever in infants is problematic because immunization is associated with a relatively high incidence of vaccine-induced encephalitis. This reaction can be severe in children less than 4 months of age. Most authorities believe that yellow fever vaccine should never be given to young infants, but this contraindication must be balanced against disease prevalence and the likelihood of exposure for children older than 4 months. The vaccine is considered safe in children over 9 months of age. Yellow fever is endemic in tropical South America (particularly Peru), sub-Saharan Africa, and, periodically in Central America.

Rabies

Few Americans realize that rabies is endemic among domestic animals in most developing countries. It is therefore prudent to consider immunization if living circumstances are likely to create unpreventable exposure. This is usually defined as residence in rural regions for more than 6 months. Because they are less cautious, children are more likely to be bitten by potentially rabid animals and thus are higher priority candidates for vaccine. Two vaccines may be administered by the intramuscular (IM) and one by the intradermal route. Both methods have been shown to be equally efficacious. Most patients prefer the intradermal route because of reduced cost of the 0.1 mL dose used. Only the human diploid cell vaccine (HDCV) is approved for intradermal injection, while both HDCV and rabies absorbed (RVA) may be administered IM using a 1.0 mL dose. A special syringe must be used for the intradermal injection. Both routes require 3 doses given at 0, 7, and 21 or 28 days. Immunization does not mean that additional treatment is unnecessary following an animal bite, but it does offer adequate protection so that only two intramuscular booster doses of vaccine at 0 and 3 days following exposure would be required; rabies immunoglobulin does not have to be given to immunized individuals bitten by potentially rabid animals.

Japanese Encephalitis

Japanese encephalitis is an arthropod-borne disease seen in rural regions of Japan, China, Southeast Asia, and India, primarily during wet summer months. Risk for disease in urban areas is low, and even in endemic regions few cases are reported during the fall, winter, and spring. If risk of exposure is considered high, vaccine (JE-VAX; Connaught, Swiftwater, Pennsylvania, U.S.) may be administered to children at any age. Specific information pertaining to reported infection and availability of vaccine may be obtained from the Division of Vector-Borne Infectious Diseases, Centers for Disease Control and Prevention (970/221-6400).

Infant cribs should be covered with mosquito nets, and aerosol insecticidal sprays should be applied to exposed skin during daytime activity when there is increased risk of exposure to biting mosquitoes. Incidence of disease is highest in children 2 to 7 years of age. The relatively lower rates in infants may be the consequence of protective maternal antibody or reduced exposure to mosquitoes, which are more likely to bite in outside environments. Reported mortality is between 5% and 35%, a difference largely reflecting availability of intensive medical care for various study locations. These high figures support routine immunization for any missionary families at risk. The preferred dosing schedule is 0, 7, and 30 days, if time allows. The 0, 7, and 14 day schedule is also highly protective, but final antibody titers are somewhat lower.

Cholera

Cholera immunization is mentioned only to emphasize that the World Health Organization no longer recommends vaccination for travel to or from cholera-endemic regions, and currently no country requires immunization for entry or re-entry. Although quite safe, this vaccine offers only 50% protective efficacy of very short duration, 3 to 6 months, for selected epidemic serotypes. Risk remains minimal for families residing in homes where proper hygienic precautions are employed.

TUBERCULOSIS SCREENING AND BCG

All long-term emigrants to virtually any country outside of the United States should have a Mantoux tuberculosis skin test (TST). This test serves as important baseline information if exposure occurs during residence. Some countries require documentation of TST responses prior to entry. For U.S. children younger than 12 months of age, such testing is probably unnecessary because the likelihood of prior exposure in this country is so low. On the other hand, if the infant has received Bacille Calmette-Guerin (BCG) vaccine, recording of the TST response is very useful for interpretation of later skin testing. Testing can be done simultaneously with measles vaccination, but testing should be delayed for 4 to 6 weeks if MMR was previously given (1).

Bacille Calmette-Guerin vaccine should be given prior to residence in almost all developing countries, concordant with local recommendations for universal immunization. Methods for BCG administration using a scarification technique are well understood in travel medicine clinics so vaccination is best accomplished in this setting. The Tice strain of BCG is administered percutaneously; 0.3 mL of the reconstituted vaccine is usually placed on the skin in the lower deltoid area (i.e., the upper arm) and delivered through a multiple-puncture disc. Infants <30 days of age should receive one-half the usual dose, prepared by increasing the amount of diluent added to the lyophilized vaccine. If the indications for vaccination persist, these children should receive a full dose of the vaccine after they are 1 year of age if they have an induration of <5 mm when tested with 5 tuberculin units (TU) of purified protein derivative (PPD) tuberculin. If time allows, a tuberculosis skin test (IPPD) should be placed and read to document adequacy of BCG vaccination.

TRAVELER'S DIARRHEA

Traveler's diarrhea usually occurs during the first week of travel and is generally a mild self-limited disease. The incidence is highest among persons visiting Latin America, Africa, Asia, and the Middle East. Numerous organisms are responsible, with the vast majority being due to enterotoxigenic *E. coli* in Americans who travel to Mexico or South America.

If meticulous attention is paid to avoiding potentially contaminated food and water, the incidence of infection is extremely low. Prophylactic antibiotics are no longer routinely recommended because their use leads to the rapid development of bacterial resistance. Antimicrobial therapy should be reserved for symptomatic cases or for individuals entering an extremely high-risk area (poor sanitation) and who will be remaining there for more than 5 days. Recommended antibiotics are trimethoprim/sulfamethoxazole (TMP/SMX), trimethoprim alone, and the quinolones—ciprofloxacin or norfloxacin (for patients older than 18 years). It is most practical to allow travelers to bring appropriate medication with them if they are staying for more than 5 days, but with instructions to begin therapy only if symptoms occur. Loperamide (Immodium®), an antimotility medication is safe, available over the counter, and can be combined with antibiotics for more effective symptomatic care. Bismuth subsalicylate has also been shown to be a useful adjunct to antimicrobial therapy in adults.

For infants and children less than 2 years of age, prophylaxis is not recommended. Once symptomatic, these young patients should be given fluids with a higher electrolyte content such as that contained in oral rehydration solutions (Table 4).

TABLE 4   Traveler's Diarrhea

Prophylaxis not recommended
Early treatment × 5 days
Ciprofloxacin
20–30 mg/kg div. q 12 hrs
TMP/SMX
6–20 mg TMP/30–100 SMX/kg
div. q 12 hrs
Doxycylcine
5 mg/kg div. q 12 hrs

PREVENTIVE INTERVENTIONS FOR DEVELOPING COUNTRIES

Malaria

The most common cause of recurrent fever in travelers returning from malaria endemic countries is malaria. Diagnosis is readily made with thick and thin blood smears during febrile episodes (Fig. 2). The only species that commonly causes life threatening episodes of hemolysis and cerebral disease is *Plasmodium falciparum*, which is endemic in Africa, Haiti, New Guinea and present along with *P. vivax* in some regions of the Pacific Islands, South America, and Southeast Asia.

Primary prevention of malaria relies on a combination of personal protective measures and antimicrobial prophylaxis. International travelers visiting malaria endemic areas should be encouraged to avoid exposure to mosquitoes, use insect repellents and pesticides, and wear long pants and long-sleeved shirts. For a minority of malarious areas, oral chloroquine is the drug of choice for primary prophylaxis. For travel to regions reporting chloroquine-resistant *Plasmodium falciparum*, other drugs should be used (Table 5).

All individuals residing in malaria-endemic regions for short periods of time (< 6 months) should receive chemoprophylaxis beginning before arrival and continued for 4 weeks after returning to the United States or other developed countries. This recommendation applies to family members of all ages, although data concerning the safety and efficacy of appropriate chemoprophylactic regimens are limited in very young children. For regions where chloroquine-resistant *Plasmodium falciparum* has not been identified, chloroquine remains the drug of choice. Such regions include Haiti, the Dominican Republic, Central America west of the Panama Canal, and the Middle East, including Egypt. Atovaquone/proguanil is the drug of choice for travel into chloroquine-resistant malaria regions.

Doxycycline can be used as prophylaxis for short-term travelers, but at the daily dosages recommended are likely to stain teeth in children younger than 8 years of age. The only other alternative is to bring medication appropriate for treatment of young infants and begin therapy once a physician diagnoses malaria. Although anti-malaria agents should be available locally, there may be exceptions in medically underserved areas.

Scheduling

Table 6 summarizes required vaccines, chemoprophylaxis and other recommended intervention prior to travel. Planning should begin far in advance, which in many cases will necessitate multiple visits. A calendar should be prepared for each traveler and printed sheets that detail medical problems unique to specific host countries should be provided. This latter

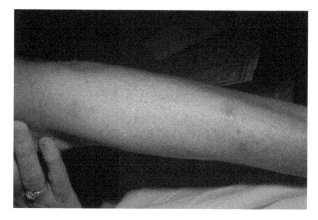

FIGURE 2 (*See color insert.*) Rash of Mediterranean spotted fever caused by *Richettsia conorii* This illness is usually brief and self-limited although the organism is closely related to the bacterium causing Rocky Mountain spotted fever.

TABLE 5 Recommended Antibiotic Regimens and Dosage for Malaria Prevention

Category	Antibiotic regimen
Nonchloroquine-resistant malaria strains (*Plasmodium vivax, P. ovale, P. malariae,* and chloroquine-sensitive *P. falciparum*)	Chloroquine phosphate, 5 mg/kg (max. 300 mg) base (equivalent to 8.3 mg/kg; max. 500 mg salt) once/wk starting 1 wk before travel to a malarious area and continuing during travel until 4 wk after leaving the area
P. vivax and *P. ovale* endemic areas (relapse prevention)	Chloroquine phosphate same dose and regimen as above plus Primaquine, 0.3 mg/kg/day (max, 15 mg/day) for 14 days after leaving the malarious area
Chloroquine-resistant malaria strain (*P. falciparum*)	Atovaquone/proguanil 11–20 kg – 1 peds tab/day 21–30 kg – 2 peds tab/day 31–40 kg – 3 peds tab/day >40 kg – 1 adult tab/day or Mefloquine hydrochloride (tablet, 250 mg) 5–10 kg: 1/8 tab once/wk 11–20 kg: 1/4 tab/wk 21–30 kg: 1/2 tab/wk 31–45 kg: 3/4 tab/wk >45 kg: 1 tab/wk Starting 1 wk before travel and continuing during travel until 4 wk after leaving the malarious area or Doxycycline (alone) ≤8 yr: contraindicated >8 yr: 2 mg/kg (max. 100 mg/day) once/day Starting 1–2 days before travel and continuing during travel until 4 wk after leaving the malarious area or Primaquine 0.6 mg/kg base daily Chloroquine phosphate, same dose and regimen as above plus Proguanil <2 yr: 50 mg once/day 2–6 yr: 100 mg once/day 7–10 yr: 150 mg once/day >10 yr: 200 mg once/day

TABLE 6 Schedule for Immunization and Chemoprophylaxis

Time prior to travel	Vaccine or chemoprophylaxis
6 mos	Hepatitis B
5 mos	Hepatitis B
1 mos	Measles, Mumps, Rubella (MMR) TB Mantoux skin test Hepatitits A Typhoid oral or IM Japanese encephalitis Rabies
1 wk–1 mo	DTP Polio Meningococcal Rabies × 2 Yellow fever Japanese encephalitis
1 wk	Hepatitis B Chloroquine or mefloquine Japanese encephalitis

TABLE 7   Suggested Travel Supplies

Recommended
  Routine medications
  Aspirin or acetaminophen
  Disinfectant for skin cuts and wounds
  Bandages, gauze, Band-aids, tweezers
  Antibiotic ointment
  Sunblock
  Sunhat
  DEET-based insect repellent
  Heating coil (to boil water)
  Iodine tablets or hand-filter (to treat water if no electricity)
  Antihistamine
  Plastic water bottle or flask

Necessary if applicable
  Over-supply of regular prescription drugs
  Copy of important prescriptions using generic names
  Nasal decongestant spray
  Oil of wintergreen (for toothache) ± emergency dental kit
  Antifungal skin cream and foot powder
  Oral rehydration packets (for travel to remote areas)
  Antimotion sickness pills
  Cough syrup
  Thermometer
  Sunburn cream
  Insect sting kit (Epi-pen)
  Ipecac (if traveling with small children)

Items of practical importance that may be necessary or helpful
  Mosquito bed net
  Permethrin insect spray to impregnate clothes
  AIDS-free certificate (for long-term visitors, students, or workers)
  Swiss Army knife
  Sunglasses, spare eyeglasses, copy of eye prescription
  Sewing kit
  Small flashlight
  Knockdown insect spray
  Tissues and toilet paper
  Commercial AIDS prevention kit (needles, syringes, IV infusion tubing)
  Copies of passport front page, airline ticket, important phone numbers (e.g., U.S. embassy, personal physician)
    credit card date
  Supplementary health insurance
  Trip disruption insurance (should include medical evacuation coverage)
  Pre-travel dental checkup
  Pre-signed consent form for medical treatment to minor children left at home

information is available from the Centers for Disease Control and Prevention, Information Service and Traveler's Health Hotline (404) 639-2572.

Travel Supplies

The usual protective measures should be strictly applied to family members. These include providing insecticide-impregnated mosquito nets for cribs and beds, protective clothing, and mosquito repellents. Infants should also spend the majority of time in well-screened areas and have repellents applied every 2 hours. Only products containing low concentrations of meta-N, N-diethyl toluamide (DEET) should be used and applied to exposed skin (excluding the face, hands, or abraded areas). DEET should be removed by washing after the infant returns to indoor screened environments.

Families should also consider bringing with them some other materials which may be helpful in preventing or treating tropical diseases. Suggestions are provided in Table 7.

6 | Procedures

INTRODUCTION

This chapter describes those procedures used to diagnose infectious diseases that are normally performed by pediatricians, emergency medicine staff, family medicine specialists, and primary care physicians. In addition, two procedures, pericardiocentesis and ventricular taps, are included because they may have to be done on an emergency basis by primary care physicians when specialists are not readily available.

ASPIRATE OF CELLULITIS

Needle aspiration of an area of cellulitis should be obtained for culture. The area should be cleansed with an iodine solution and washed with alcohol. A 22- or 23-G needle is attached to a syringe containing 0.5 mL of normal saline *without* bacteriostatic preservative. The needle is advanced 1 cm into superficial subcutaneous tissue, the saline injected and aspirated back into the syringe. The syringe and its contents should be transported to the laboratory for direct plating on appropriate media. Blood culture bottles should not be used because these do not contain adequate growth nutrients for *H. influenzae* and some other organisms.

BLADDER TAP

The procedure is carried out with the patient lying supine and the lower extremities held in the frog leg position. The suprapubic area is cleansed with iodine and alcohol, and the symphysis pubis is located with the index finger. Using a 20-mL syringe and a 22-G, 1/2-in. needle or 2-in. spinal needle in older children, the abdominal wall and bladder is pierced in the midline about 1/2 to 2 cm above the symphysis pubis. The needle is then angled 30° toward the fundus of the bladder. Urine is gently aspirated and the needle withdrawn. No dressing is necessary. As with the venipuncture, local anesthesia is not required in doing vesicopuncture.

BLOOD CULTURE

For those infectious processes where bacteremia is associated, blood cultures represent an important source for etiologic diagnosis. These specimens are essential, particularly, during the initial workup of sepsis, meningitis, endocarditis, pneumonia, cellulitis, osteomyelitis, and septic arthritis. It is prudent to routinely obtain two blood cultures, even from neonates and young infants, because bacteremia is usually not continuous. In addition, two samples will allow easier identification of contaminants present in just one of the cultures. For endocarditis, 3 to 6 are recommended (Table 1).

CENTRAL LINE QUANTITATIVE CULTURES

Often it is difficult to determine whether a catheter is the source of septicemia, particularly if there are other potentially infected sites. Although removal of an indwelling catheter is usually simple and provides a definitive diagnosis in catheter-related sepsis, it may be undesirable to remove permanent catheters from patients who have a limited number of sites for infusion or

TABLE 1 Blood Culture Technique

Wash hands Clean rubber stopper of culture bottle with alcohol Clean skin with 2% iodine or betadine Wipe skin with alcohol Perform venipuncture without touching puncture site Obtain 1–5 mL of blood Change needles aseptically Transfer blood to bottles (aerobic and anaerobic) Volume of sample: a 1:10 to 1:30 dilution (1.0 to 3 mL for 30-mL culture bottles) for routine cultures; 1:50 (1 mL in a 50-mL bottle) is adequate for Bactec methodology

whose parenteral hyperalimentation central lines are the only source of nutrition. Quantitative blood cultures performed with the catheter in place can be compared to quantitative cultures of peripheral blood, thereby establishing whether the catheter is the source of infection and therefore must be removed (Table 2).

LUMBAR PUNCTURE

Cerebrospinal fluid (CSF) should be examined in any child where meningitis is suspected. The only absolute contraindications to lumbar puncture are increased intracranial pressure or a mass lesion of the central nervous system (CNS). In such cases, a computed tomography (CT) scan should first be obtained. Other relative contraindications are anticoagulation, platelet count of less than 20,000, meningomyelocele, severe scoliosis, suspected abscess in the lumbar area, and instability of the patient. Always perform a fundoscopic examination, obtaining a clear view of the optic disc prior to performing a lumbar puncture (Table 3).

LUNG ASPIRATION

Needle aspiration of the lung is the most useful direct method for establishing the etiology of pneumonia in children. Because this procedure is associated with a 1% to 5% incidence of pneumothorax, it should not be undertaken unless determining the causative pathogen would alter therapeutic approaches. Such circumstances are most commonly a severely ill or immune compromised host, suspicion of an unusual organism, or failure of response to initial empiric therapy (Table 4).

TABLE 2 Procedure for Quantitative Blood Cultures

Notify laboratory to provide 2 empty sterile petri dishes and 2 melted TSA deeps (in a beaker of hot water) Flush catheter with 10–20 mL of saline Aseptically draw 2–6 mL of blood from the catheter and from a peripheral vein Using a tuberculin syringe, place 0.1 mL of blood from each site in a separate petri dish Pour TSA over the blood and swirl the dish to evenly suspend the blood Allow agar to harden and transport to laboratory Process the remaining blood as for routine blood cultures Interpretation: quantitative counts from the catheter that are >10-fold those of peripheral blood indicate catheter infection

Abbreviation: TSA, trypticase soy agar.

TABLE 3   Technique for Lumbar Puncture

Restrain patient in recumbent or upright position (upright preferred for
  neonates who may have very low CSF pressure)
Scrub hands, wear surgical gloves and mask
Locate L3–L4 interspace at the level of the iliac crest
Clean with alcohol and apply or inject local anesthetic
Clean the back thoroughly with an iodine solution, wash with alcohol or wipe
  dry
Drape with sterile towels
Insert a 22-G spinal needle (B bevel) in the L3–L4 interspace, directed toward
  the umbilicus
Remove the stylet periodically or when the "pop" of the dura is felt
If blood returns, the procedure may be repeated in the L2–L3 interspace

OSTEOMYELITIS SUBPERIOSTEAL ASPIRATION

Needle aspiration of suspected osteomyelitis should be a routine initial procedure for etiologic
diagnosis. This will not alter interpretation of subsequent bone scans and there is no risk of
introducing disease into bone if there is an overlying area of cellulites (Table 5).

PERICARDIOCENTESIS

Though pericardiocentesis may be done in most any setting as an emergency, under ideal
conditions it is best done in an intensive care unit or cardiac catheterization laboratory (where
fluoroscopic control is possible). Constant ECG monitoring is essential and constant or
frequent BP monitoring is also important.

The patient is placed in a supine position with the head and chest elevated slightly. The
area of the xiphoid is properly prepped and draped. Using sterile technique, the skin and
subcutaneous tissue at and just to the left of the xiphoid are infiltrated with a local anesthetic.
With a syringe attached, an 18- or 20-G needle of 5 to 10 cm length is inserted adjacent to the
xiphoid (in the notch between the xiphoid process and the 7th costal cartilage) and advanced
slowly toward the middle of the left clavicle. The needle is kept at an angle of 20° off the skin.
The needle is passed immediately posterior to the costal cartilage and as it passes through the
pericardium a "pop" may sometimes be felt.

An exploring electrode (V lead) may be attached to the metal hub of the needle with a
sterile alligator clamp and the ECG so monitored. A "current of injury" pattern is noted as the
pericardial space is entered and the epicardium encountered.

Constant negative pressure is kept on the syringe as the needle is advanced and
pericardial fluid is aspirated as soon as the needle perforated the pericardium. As much fluid

TABLE 4   Needle Aspiration of the Lung

Determine with X ray the major site of involvement
Clean skin with an iodine solution, wash with alcohol
Use sterile gloves; sterile towels are rarely necessary
Anesthetize skin and soft tissue down to pleura (2% procaine) above a rib
Attach a 22-G spinal needle (B bevel) to a 10-mL syringe containing 1 mL of
  normal saline without bacteriostatic preservative
Time puncture to maximum inspiration; if possible have patient pause in
  inspiration for 3–4 sec
Rapidly advance needle into lung 3 cm, directed toward the hilum, maintaining
  negative pressure with the syringe; the aspiration should take only 2 sec
Transport needle, syringe, and their contents to the laboratory for inoculation
  into enrichment broth or direct plating

TABLE 5   Technique for Subperiosteal Aspiration

Clean skin with an iodine solution; wash with alcohol
Drape area with sterile towels; use sterile gloves
Anesthetize skin only
Using a syringe containing 0.5 mL of normal saline, aspirate subcutaneous
  tissue as for cellulitis
Using a second 2.5-mL syringe and 20-G needle, advance the needle until the
  bone is touched and aspirate (saline is not needed)
Transport the needle and syringe to the laboratory for direct plating

as possible should be removed, but in the presence of suppurative pericarditis, the purulent material may be difficult to aspirate or may be loculated.

If bloody fluid is obtained, set aside a small sample in a glass tube to observe. Blood that has been in the pericardial space for any significant time will not clot. Blood aspirated from the cardiac chamber will clot normally. Check the hemoglobin content and hematocrit of the fluid aspirated to compare with the patient's peripheral blood values. If the heart has been perforated, remove the needle slowly and observe the patient's vital signs frequently. Perforation of the inferior surface of the right ventricle has rarely resulted in persistent bleeding into the pericardial space.

Some physicians prefer to use a needle-plastic cannula set so that once the pericardial space is entered, the needle can be slipped out of the plastic cannula covering it and fluid can more easily be aspirated via the cannula. This technique may be safer if a large quantity of fluid is to be removed and considerable time is required to remove it. These plastic cannulas, however, may be stiff enough to perforate the heart of a small child, so great care must still be exercised in manipulating the cannula in the pericardial space.

PERITONEAL TAP

An abdominal paracentesis should be accomplished when primary peritonitis is suspected. Most cases of peritonitis secondary to a perforated viscus require surgery at which time appropriate cultures can be obtained (Table 6).

SUBDURAL TAPS

Subdural effusions occurring during or after therapy for bacterial meningitis can be detected clinically by enlarging head circumference, split sutures or fontanels, and lateralizing findings on neurologic examination. Effusions can be evaluated by skull roentgenograms, transillumination of the skull and CT scan. Subdural fluid aspiration, when indicated, is easily done

TABLE 6   Procedure for Peritoneal Tap

Empty urinary bladder
Sedate patient
Place patient in supine position
Clean skin over rectus muscle with iodine from symphysis pubis to umbilicus
Anesthetize skin, soft issue, and peritoneum just lateral to midline in the lower
  third between symphysis pubis and umbilicus
Make 5 mm incision in skin
Assure aseptic technique
Using #14F abdominal trocar, insert through incision directed obliquely up and
  back; continue advancing until release through the peritoneum is felt
Remove stylet and collect fluid for culture, Gram stain, and cell count
Suture incision and apply sterile pressure dressing

on infants with open fontanels. Adequate immobilization of the child is necessary. After shaving the scalp widely around the anterior fontanel, sterile prepping and draping of the scalp, and surgical gloving, an 18- to 20-G subdural needle with stylet is introduced into the lateral recess of the anterior fontanel at the coronal suture. Anesthetic agents are generally not required in infants. The subdural needle is introduced 3 to 5 mm through the dura and the stylet removed. Subdural fluid may well from the needle. If no subdural fluid is encountered, suctioning and probing of the subdural space generally is not recommended. Occasionally by rotating or withdrawing the needle and reintroducing it at a slight angle under the convexity of the skull, flow may be established. A thick exudate of purulent empyema or markedly elevated subdural fluid protein may account for lack of flow. Similarly, loculated fluid beyond the reach of the subdural needle may be present. In these cases, a CT scan may be necessary to exclude the possibility of loculated subdural empyema or ventricular enlargement clinically suggesting subdural effusions. If subdural fluid flow is established, 20 to 30 mL of fluid may be removed and routine studies including cell count, glucose, protein determination, and Gram stain are done. Bilateral subdural taps are indicated in some cases. In general, subdural taps, if done without probing, are innocuous; however, occasionally trauma to the cerebral cortex, bleeding into the subdural space, and prolonged leakage of subdural or subarachnoid fluid following subdural tap may occur. Proper antiseptic preparation precludes infection. Indications for repeated subdural taps are controversial and these increase the risk of fistula formation and iatrogenic infection. The ready availability of CT scans has decreased the indications for subdural fluid aspirations and permitted a more accurate evaluation of effusion size and localization.

THORACENTESIS

Thoracentesis is performed both for diagnosis and therapeutic purposes. For empyema caused by *H. influenzae*, pneumococcus, or group A streptococci, 1 or 2 thoracenteses will often provide adequate drainage, thus avoiding placement of a chest tube. Empyema, as a result of *Staphylococcus aureus*, almost always necessitates chest tube drainage (Table 7).

TYMPANOCENTESIS

This procedure should be considered for any neonate with otitis media where gram-negative coliform bacteria are commonly recovered, and for older patients who have persistent signs and symptoms of middle ear disease after standard therapy (Table 8).

VENTRICULAR TAP

Ventricular taps are generally performed by neurosurgeons; however, the procedure may be useful or mandatory in some emergency situations or in cases where CSF must be obtained

TABLE 7   Procedure for Thoracentesis

Place patient in sitting position
Clean skin with iodine solution; wash with alcohol
Anesthetize skin, soft tissue, and pleura in 7th or 8th interspace (level of the tip of the scapula), posterior axillary line
Drape with sterile towels; use surgical gloves
Use 18-G needle attached to a 3-way stopcock and syringe; enter pleural cavity above a rib
Remove fluid for culture, Gram stain, and chemistries
Obtain post-thoracentesis chest X ray
If patient begins coughing, remove needle immediately
If no fluid is obtained, consider repeating under fluoroscopic direction

TABLE 8   Aspiration of Middle Ear Fluid

Remove cerumen
Clean canal with alcohol
Culture external ear canal to monitor contaminants
Restrain patient
Use an 18-G, 3 1/2-in. spinal needle bent at a double angel (as a fork) attached
    to a 2.5-mL syringe
Use an otoscope with an operating head
Advance needle through a speculum that has been sterilized in alcohol
Penetrate the posterior-inferior aspect of the tympanic membrane
Aspirate middle ear exudate and transport to laboratory for culture and
    gram stain

without lumbar puncture prior to beginning antibiotic therapy. Sterile surgical technique is used in all cases. In infants, the ventricular system can be entered by inserting a spinal or ventricular needle through the lateral aspect of the anterior fontanel at the coronal suture, directing the needle toward the midpoint of the orbit on that side. In older children, a burr hole can be drilled in the midpupillary line at the hairline and the needle introduced. Obviously, these facial landmarks vary and experience and a clear mental image of the ventricular system are needed prior to attempting a ventricular tap. The return of clear or blood-tinged CSF documents correct needle aspiration. Pressure measurements are obtained and sufficient fluid drained both for diagnostic purposes and at times, therapeutic effect. CT and cranial ultrasound are useful in accurately judging the need for and the effects of ventricular tap and should be routinely performed.

VENTRICULOPERITONEAL SHUNT ASPIRATION

Because of the wide variety of shunts currently used in neurosurgery, the surgeon responsible for following the patient's shunt should generally be contacted before aspiration is attempted. Some shunt systems have sites designed for safe aspiration. In other cases, skull radiographs reveal shunt characteristics that help identify the model and specific mechanics. In cases where shunt patency or possible infection is questioned, shunt aspiration is an uncomplicated and safe procedure if sterile technique is used. The goal of the procedure should be not only to obtain CSF, but also to document proximal and distal patency. By elevating the catheter and using a manometer, if necessary, ventricular pressure can be measured. Elevating the catheter and noting drainage of CSF suggests distal patency. Rarely is the quantity of fluid obtained critical. Sufficient fluid should be obtained liberally to carefully and thoroughly perform all cytologic, chemical, and microbiologic cultures and smears (including large amounts of fluid if fungal studies are indicated). Following removal of the needle, CSF may leak and the site should have a sterile dressing and be observed for infection. In general, if the bulb site itself appears infected, no aspiration should be attempted.

7 | Laboratory Diagnosis

INTRODUCTION

The clinical laboratory is continually striving to meet the needs of both the attending physician and the patient by providing prompt and accurate results. Accomplishing this goal in the most proficient manner necessitates good communication and cooperation between the physician and the laboratory technologist. This chapter attempts to provide the clinician with a simplified review of the available laboratory tests to provide information from which to base clinical decisions. Also, there may be times when physicians will have to perform these laboratory studies on an emergency basis or when laboratory technicians are not available.

It is the responsibility of the physician to ensure that an appropriate and properly collected specimen is obtained from the patient and promptly delivered to the laboratory. Upon receipt, the submitted specimen will be inspected to determine if it is of sufficient quality and quantity for adequate evaluation.

STAINS

Microscopic examination of unstained and stained smears of specimens from an infected site is the most direct, rapid, and least technical of procedures. A Wright's stain of a buffy-coat or peripheral blood smear can make the diagnosis of human monocytotrophic ehrlichiosis (Fig. 1). The diagnosis of relapsing fever, caused by spirochetes of the genus, *Borrelia,* is usually made by identifying the corkscrew-shaped organisms on a Wright-stained peripheral blood smear (Fig. 2).

Gram Stain

Gram-positive and gram-negative organisms are differentiated on the basis of the cell wall and cell membrane permeability characteristics to organic solvents. These characteristics are

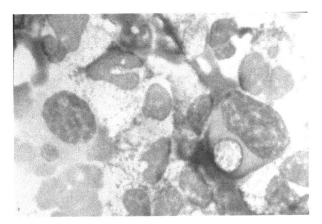

FIGURE 1 A Wright's stain of a buffy-coat peripheral blood smear in a patient with profound leukopenia, thrombocytopenia, and hyponatremia reveals the morulae or mulberry-like clusters of *Ehrlichia chaffeensis* in mononuclear cells, confirming the diagnosis of human monocytotrophic ehrlichiosis.

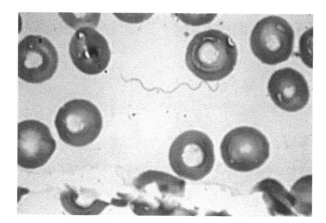

FIGURE 2 Corkscrew-shaped organisms on a Wright's-stained peripheral blood smear of a patient with a third febrile episode in three weeks, confirms the diagnosis of relapsing fever.

probably due to the glycosaminopeptide and lipoprotein composition of the bacterial cell wall. Gram-positive organisms, which do not have significant amounts of lipid as an integral part of their cell wall, retain the crystal violet-iodine complex and stain purple, whereas gram-negative organisms do not retain this complex and stain red from the counterstain (Table 1).

Acid-Fast Stain

This stain should be performed if pulmonary tuberculosis or tuberculous meningitis is suspected. It is based on the observation that the staining of mycobacteria with carbol fuchsin resists decolorization with acid alcohol. Other acid-fast organisms such as *Nocardia* sp. may also be detected using this procedure, but must be identified further with special stains and cultures. A technique using auramine and rhodamine fluorescent dyes is easier to read although it is more time consuming compared to the acid-fast stain (Table 2).

Methylene Blue Stain

Methylene blue is a useful stain to establish the morphology of organisms and to differentiate cells found in the specimen (neutrophils, lymphocytes, monocytes, RBCs, and epithelial cells). Intracellular bacteria, such as *Neisseriae*, are often more evident with this stain as are other bacterial characteristics as demonstrated by the capsules surrounding pneumococci and the metachromatic granules of *Corynebacterium diphtheriae*.

TABLE 1 Gram Stain

Specimen source: most clinical specimens technique
   Air dry smear and fix with methanol (allow to evaporate)
   Flood slide with crystal violet (60 sec)
   Wash, add Gram's iodine (60 sec)
   Decolorize with acetone alcohol (5 sec) and wash immediately
   Counterstain with safranin (15 sec)
Staining identification
   Gram-positive organisms stain purple
   Gram-negative organisms stain red

TABLE 2   Acid-Fast Stain

Specimen source
Sputum
CSF
Technique
Air dry and fix with methanol (allow to evaporate)
Flood slide with Kinyoun carbol–fuchsin (4 min)
Wash with water and decolorize with acid alcohol until faint pink
Wash, counterstain with methylene blue (30 sec)
Identifying organisms
Acid-fast (stain red)
Mycobacteria sp.
Nocardia sp.
Nonacid-fast bacteria and cellular elements stain blue

Abbreviation: CSF, cerebrospinal fluid.

Wright's and Giemsa Stains

Both Wright's and Giemsa stains are extremely helpful in demonstrating organisms, inclusion bodies, or cellular differentiation in various specimens (Table 3).

WET MOUNTS

Unfixed samples can be examined microscopically as wet mounts for bacterial, fungal, parasitic, and other pathogens (Table 4). These commonly used wet mounts are: normal saline, used to detect trichomonads and protozoa; potassium hydroxide (KOH), used primarily for identification of fungal forms; and India ink mounts for identifying encapsulated *Cryptococcus*.

SPECIMEN EXAMINATION AND ANALYSIS

Cerebrospinal Fluid

Collection of Cerebrospinal Fluid (CSF) is performed under sterile conditions and divided into three 1-mL aliquots for microbiologic cultures, chemistry determinations, and cell counts. A 4th sample may be obtained for viral cultures (Table 5).

TABLE 3   Uses of Wright's and Giemsa Stains

Used to stain
Intracellular organisms in blood (buffy coat)
Conjunctival scrapings
Impression smears
Tissue sections
Used to differentiate
Multinucleated giant cells in vesicle fluid of herpes virus skin or mucosal
infections (see "Tzanck Preparation")
Cell types (PMNs, lymphocytes and trachomatis inclusions, eosinophils,
epithelial cells, monocytes)
Used to detect
Rickettsiae
Chlamydiae
Protozoa (malaria)
Selected yeast and fungi

TABLE 4   Three Commonly Used Wet Mounts

Normal saline	KOH	India ink
Specimen source Cervical secretions Vaginal secretions Urethral discharge Urine sediment Feces	*Specimen source* Cervical discharge Skin scrapings Sputum Tissue scrapings	*Specimen source* Cerebrospinal fluid Urine Exudates Sputum
Technique Mix 1–2 drops of 0.9% NaCl and examine microscopically	*Technique* Mix 1 drop 10% KOH, allow to stand 10–15 min and examine microscopically	*Technique* Mix 1 drop of India ink and examine microscopically
Identifiable organisms *Trichomonas* *vaginalis* Protozoa (trophozoites, cysts of *Entamoeba* *histolytica*) Pinworm eggs	*Identifiable organisms* Fungal forms	*Identifiable organisms* Capsule of *Cryptococcus* *neoformans* (must see budding yeast)

In the bacteriologic examination of CSF the gram-stained smear is an extremely important rapid identification of meningitis. It normally takes approximately 1 to 10×10^4 bacteria per milliliter before detection by a direct smear is possible. Centrifugation of the CSF at 2000 rpm for 10 minutes increases the percentage of positive smears made from the sediment. Caution must be taken because of artifacts staining similarly to organisms (Table 6).

Dark-field examination for spirochetes, if syphilitic or leptospiral meningitis is suspected, is available in some laboratories as well a variety of rapid immunologic assays that are capable of demonstrating the type-specific polysaccharide capsule antigens of group B streptococcus, pneumococcus, meningococcus, and *H. influenzae.*

TABLE 5   Processing CSF from Meningitis Patients

Aliquot	Diagnostic tests	Volume of CSF required (mL)
1	Culture [bacteria (and fungi)]	1.0–2.0
2	Protein and glucose (compare with simultaneous blood glucose)	1.0 1.0

3	Total WBC and RBC count
	Sediment for staining
	  Wright's stain cell differential
	  Gram stain (80% positive in meningitis)
	  Acridine orange for rapid detection of
	    bacteria
	  Acid-fast stain
	  India ink (other fungal stains)
	Antigen detection (Latex agglutination, CoA,
	  etc.)
		1.0

TABLE 6   Common Errors in CSF Staining Interpretation

Gram stain
   Confusing precipitated stain as gram-positive cocci
   Identifying false capsules because of poor stain
   Misreading of *H. influenzae* with bipolar staining as overdecolorized
     pneumococci
India ink preparation
   Cells or artifacts that appear to be *Cryptococcus* sp. causing false-positive
     results

Urine

The laboratory aid to the diagnosis of a UTI is only as valid as the care given to the collection of a urine specimen for culture and examination. Consequently, the method of collection (see Chapter 11) of urine is important and it is necessary to know how collection was accomplished in order to interpret results. The volume of urine recommended for a urinalysis is 15 mL or more but as little as 2 mL will suffice for a screen.

Microscopic examination of formed elements must clearly be identified to determine early diagnosis of urinary tract infection. This can be done with wet mounts and staining of urine sediment. Practically all uncentrifuged urine with bacterial colony counts of greater than or equal to 10^5 mL^{-1} will have a positive Gram stain. Several rapid screening methods are available for the identification of bacteriuria. Glucose and nitrite determinations by the dipstick technique to detect bacterial metabolism must be interpreted with caution because dilute urine will result in false-negative results. None of these tests have yet replace bacterial cultures in the detection of UTIs (Table 7).

An important aspect of evaluating a patient with suspected UTI is to identify the organism with routine and quantitative cultures (Table 8).

Quantitative urine cultures may be obtained by using bacteriologic loops that deliver approximately 0.01 mL of a sample of urine. A sterile loop is dipped into urine from a properly collected specimen and streaked on a blood agar plate. After incubation 18 to 24 hours at 37°C the number of colonies of bacteria on the blood agar plate is multiplied by 1000, giving a reasonable approximation of the bacteria per milliliter in the urine specimen. Thus more than 100 colonies on a plate is evidence of significant bacteriuria and a quantitative colony count of 10^5 colonies per milliliter (3).

TABLE 7   Routine Screening Urinalysis

Test	Volume
Screening for bacteriuria	2–3 drops
Gram stain of uncentrifuged specimen	
Quantitative loop culture	
Specific gravity (performed using a refractometer)	1 drop
Microscopic examination of sediment	1 drop of
RBCs, leukocytes, renal epithelial cells, hyaline casts,	concentrated
mucous and excess crystals, microorganisms	sediment
Basic chemical screen (tested with a multiple or single	2 mL
reagent strip)	
pH (7.5 in infection)	
Blood	
Protein	
Bilirubin	
Glucose	
Urobilinogen	
Ketone	
Nitrite	

TABLE 8   Bacteriologic Cultures for Urine

Routine cultures
Blood agar
MacConkey agar or EMB for gram-negative bacilli
TSA
Special considerations
Pyuria in the absence of bacterial growth by routine culture might indicate the possible presence of *Mycobacterium tuberculosis*. Sediment from the first morning specimen should be Gram stained and cultured

Abbreviations: EMB, Eosin-methylene blue agar; TSA, trypticase soy agar.

Urine obtained directly by bladder puncture or catheterization is normally sterile and any growth of urinary pathogens should be considered significant.

Fecal Specimens

Fecal specimens should be collected and transported in paper stool cups. Care should be taken not to contaminate the stool with urine or water because of the possibility of killing trophozoites. The guaiac method represents a suitable test for routine screening of blood in stool (Tables 9 to 11).

A predominance of polymorphonuclear leukocytes (PMNs) is seen with any inflammatory enterocolitis (Table 12).

Ova and Parasites

When parasitism is highly suspected, a minimum of three specimens should be submitted. The major parasitic species that infect the intestinal tract are protozoa and helminths. The protozoa (amebiasis and giardiasis) have 2 major forms, trophozoite and cyst. Inspection of the perianal area at night, after the child is asleep, may reveal adult pinworms (thread-like white worms 1/4 to 1/2 in. long) (Table 13).

Synovial Fluid

Synovial fluid (SF) aspiration may provide information to distinguish between the joint inflammation due to infectious, immunologic, or traumatic involvement. The specimen should be collected using sterile technique to avoid contamination from exogenous birefringent

TABLE 9   Evaluation of Fecal Specimens

Gross examination
Consistency, odor, presence of blood, pus, undigested food, mucus, parasites
Microscopic examination
Fecal leukocytes stained with methylene blue or Wright's stain
Ova and parasites (wet mounts and Scotch tape prep)
Routine cultures: fecal specimens are routinely cultured for
E. coli 0157:H7, *Salmonella, Shigella, Campylobacter,* and *Yersinia.* It is worth noting that enteropathic *E. coli, Vibrio* sp. and viruses require special handling and media
Blood agar
MacConkey or other selective media for gram-negative enteric bacilli
HE agar, Selenite, SS agar for *Salmonella* and *Shigella*
GN (gram-negative) broth
PCR (polymerase chain reaction) for *Campylobacter*

TABLE 10   Guaiac Method for Occult Blood

Place about 0.5 g of feces into a test tube
Add 2 mL of water and mix
Add 0.5 mL glacial acetic acid and guaiac solution
Mix 2 mL 3% H_2O_2 with suspension
Observe for 2 min and note maximal blue intensity as
  1^+, 2^+, 3^+, or 4^+
Green denotes a negative test

TABLE 11   Staining Procedure for Fecal Leukocytes

Place small fleck of mucous or stool on glass slide
Add 2 drops of Loeffler's methylene blue and mix
Wait 3 min and examine under low power
Make a rough quantitative count by approximating
  average number of leukocytes and erythrocytes
Differential is performed under high power

material. Ideally, the patient should be fasting for 6 to 12 hours to allow equilibrium of glucose between plasma and SF. Infected SF tends to clot spontaneously or within an hour, therefore specimens to be examined microscopically for cells and bacteria should be placed immediately into a heparinized tube (Tables 14 and 15).

Pleural, Pericardial, and Peritoneal Fluids

It is important to differentiate these fluids as to whether they are transudates, caused by mechanical factors influencing formation, or exudates that may be caused by infection due to damage of the mesothelial linings (Tables 16 and 17).

CULTURES

Care must be emphasized for proper specimen collection to avoid or minimize unnecessary contamination.

Blood Cultures

Whenever there is a reason to suspect clinically significant bacteremia, a blood culture should be ordered. The necessity for strict aseptic technique in the course of obtaining blood for cultures should be stressed. A newer method using the BACTEC 460 system has recently been introduced to the clinical laboratory. The BACTEC 460 is an instrument used to test inoculated BACTEC blood culture vials for the presence of liberated radioactive carbon dioxide ($^{14}CO_2$). Should a high level of $^{14}CO_2$ be present in a vial, it indicates that there are living microorganisms that originated in the initial inoculum. All cultures are read on the BACTEC each day for 7 days. All positive bottles, whether they be aerobic or anaerobic, are subcultured aerobically unless the gram stain shows a possible anaerobe.

The aerobic subculture should include a blood chocolate biplate, and if gram-negative rods are seen on Gram stain, a MacConkey plate should be set up also. The anaerobic subculture, if done, should include a reducible blood plate and a CNA-LKV biplate.

TABLE 12   Fecal Leukocytes Associated with GI Diseases

Disease	Average predominant leukocyte
Salmonellosis (other than S. typhi)	75% PMNs, 25% mononuclear cells
Typhoid fever	95% mononuclear cells
Shigellosis	84% PMNs
E. coli (invasive)	85% PMNs
Ulcerative colitis (active)	88% PMNs, 8% eosinophils
Amebic dysentery (active)	Commonly mononuclear cells, unless secondary bacterial infection
Viral diarrhea, cholera, and healthy controls	

Abbreviation: GI, gastrointestinal.

TABLE 13   Simple Methods for Detecting Parasites

Direct wet mounts
   Place fleck of stool on glass slide
   Add 2 drops of 0.9% NaCl for trophozoites and ova or 2 drops of iodine
     stain for cysts
Scotch tape preparation for pinworm
   Obtain preparation immediately after child awakens
   Cover one end of a tongue depressor with cellophane tape (sticky side out)
   Apply to perianal area with mild pressure
   On a glass slide place one drop of xylol and then transfer tape to slide
   Examine for ova under microscope

Anaerobic Cultures

Many anaerobic bacteria of clinical importance are fastidious and oxygen intolerant. Special anaerobic containers must be used in specimen collection and transport. Rapid processing of samples also is important in avoiding overgrowth by facultative anaerobes.

Fungal Cultures

Scrapings, hairs, or other specimens are planted on Sabouraud agar and incubated for 2 to 4 weeks at room temperature. Positive cultures are examined microscopically by 1 of the 3 common wet mounts described in Table 4.

Viral Cultures

Several innovative methods for the rapid identification of viral infections have been developed because of the renewed interest in useful viral diagnoses. The etiology of a viral syndrome

TABLE 14   Evaluation of Synovial Fluid

Gross examination
   Color, turbidity, viscosity, clotting (observe clot formation after 1 hr),
     organisms, crystals
Cell counts
   Enumerate WBC and RBC
Stains
   Wright's stain, Gram stain (65% positive in bacterial infected SF),
     methylene blue, acid-fast stain
Glucose
   SF glucose level is usually <50% of the blood glucose level in septic
     arthritis. Levels may be normal particularly in gonococcal arthritis
Mucin
   Normal SF forms tight cord-like coagulum clump in 5% acetic acid that is
     stable for 24 hr
   Fluid from infected joints results in poor unstable mucin clot
Cultures
   Routine cultures include blood agar, nutrient both supportive of anaerobes,
     and chocolate agar or Thayer-Martin for gonococcus. Special
     consideration for *M. tuberculosis*, fungi, or viral agents
Immunologic tests
   Latex agglutination is helpful in detecting antigens of *H. influenzae* and
     S. pneumoniae, especially during antibiotic treatment

TABLE 15 Examination of Synovial Fluid

Test	Normal and noninflammatory	Severe inflammatory	Infectious-septic
Color	Clear straw	Yellow to opalescent	Yellow to green
Clarity	Transparent	Opaque[a]	Opaque
Viscosity	High	Low	Variable
WBC/mm^3	<200	5000–20,000	50,000–200,000
Neutrophils	<25%	>50%	75%
Culture	Negative	Negative	Positive[b]
Mucin clot	Firm	Slightly friable to friable	Friable
Glucose (blood-SF difference in mg/dL)	0–10	0–40	20–100

[a] Monosodium urate crystals in gout or calcium pyrophosphate dihydrate crystals in pseudogout may be found.
[b] Positive in about 50% because of low virulent organisms or partially treated.
Abbreviation: SF, synovial fluid.

may often be established by viral culture, serologic tests, or both. Table 19 outlines the type of specimen necessary for the isolation of a virus from various clinical syndromes (Table 18).

Tzanck Preparation

The Tzanck preparation is done to distinguish between pustular pyodermas and vesicular lesions due to herpes group viruses, although in many laboratories a fluorescent stain specific for herpes simplex or Varicella-Zoster has largely replaced this test. Scrapings obtained from the base of a vesicle are air dried onto a glass slide and stained with Wright's stain. Smears demonstrating multinucleated giant cells with central aggregation of nuclei and/or intracytoplasmic inclusions strongly suggest herpes infection (Table 19).

Chlamydia Culture

Presumptive evidence of *Chlamydia* can be obtained by the examination of stained smears (Giemsa) for the presence of inclusions. Most laboratories today employ a rapid ELISA antigen detection assay or cell culture procedures for the isolation of *Chlamydia*. After inoculation and

TABLE 16 Differentiating Transudates and Exudates

Pleural fluids (PFs)
   90% exudates >3 g/dL total protein
   80% transudates <3 g/dL total protein
   >95% of pleural exudates have at least one of the following characteristics
     (>95% PF transudates have none of the findings)
   Protein/serum protein (ratio >0.5)
   LDH >200 U
   Specific gravity >1.016
   pH <7.4
   WBC >1000 mm^{-3}
Peritoneal fluid
   Total protein 2–2.5 g/dL to separate transudates from exudates

TABLE 17   Evaluation of Fluid Exudates

Gross appearance (color, clarity, odor)
Total WBC and RBC counts
Differential (Wright's stain) or cytologic study
Gram stain
Culture (blood agar, medium selective for gram-negative bacilli, EMB
   anaerobic and aerobic growth, and chocolate agar for *H. influenzae*)
Chemistry (total protein, LDH, glucose)

Abbreviations: EMB, Eosin-methylene blue agar; LDH, lactic acid dehydrogenase.

incubation, the cells are stained with iodine (see "STAINS" in this chapter). Antibodies to *C. trachomatis* are usually measured by CF (group specific) or micro-IF (immunotype-specific) methodology (Table 20).

ANTIMICROBIAL SENSITIVITY TESTING

Antimicrobial sensitivity testing should be performed only when pathogens have unpredictable susceptibility patterns to the commonly used antibiotics. Sensitivities are not routinely performed on group A streptococci or *Neisseria* sp. because they have relatively predictable susceptibility patterns to antibiotics.

TABLE 18   General Procedures for Viral Specimen Collection

1. Specimens should be obtained early in the course of illness, when virus shedding is greatest, preferably within 3 days, and generally no later than 7 days after the onset of symptoms
2. The type of specimen and clinical syndrome should be clearly recorded, because different processing steps prior to attempted isolation are necessary for different types of samples, and only isolation are necessary for different types of samples, and only certain viruses are found in some specimen types
3. Samples collected on swabs (conjunctival, pharyngeal, nasopharyngeal, rectal) should be placed quickly in liquid virus transport; medium provided by the laboratory
4. Because many viruses are heat labile, samples should be placed in sterile containers, packed in wet, crushed ice, and transported promptly to the virology laboratory. Many specimens can be held at 4°C for up to 24 hr (on wet ice or in a refrigerator) without significant decrease in recovery. For prolonged storage, specimens should be frozen at −70°C

Specimen guidelines

1. *Nasal secretions.* A calcium alginate swab is introduced through the anterior nares into the nasopharynx and plunged into the transport medium after removal from the nares. Nasal washings are collected by instilling 4–5 mL of infusion broth into each nostril while the patient extends the neck slightly and closes the posterior pharynx (by pushing against "k" sound). The head is tilted forward and a sample collected in a clean container held beneath the nose
2. *Pharynx.* A swab of the posterior pharynx should be taken by touching the swab to both tonsillar areas and to the posterior pharyngeal wall
3. *Blood.* Citrated whole blood, 3–5 mL, can be used to isolate viruses from the buffy coat (e.g., HSV, rubella)
4. *CSF.* Collect 1–3 mL into a sterile container and process immediately. Avoid freezing particularly for cytomegalovirus
5. *Urine.* Collect 5–10 mL of a clean catch, midstream urine into a sterile container and process immediately
6. *Feces.* Place a 2–5 sample into a clean specimen container without transport medium. A rectal swab is less satisfactory but can be obtained by inserting a cotton-tipped swab stick 5 cm into the rectum and gently rotating the swab. In contrast to rectal cultures for gonococcus, some fecal material should be obtained when doing viral studies
7. *Vesicular fluid.* After decontamination of overlying skin, aspirate the lesion with a pasteur pipette, or a small-gauge needle attached to a tuberculin syringe, or open the vesicle and collect fluids and cellular elements from the base into a swab. If a crust is present, the crust should be lifted off; the fluid beneath the crust then can be swabbed (see "Tzanck Preparation")

TABLE 19 Collections from Suspected Viral Infections

Syndrome	Source of specimen for viral isolation	Most common viral agents
Upper respiratory tract infection	Nasal wash or nasopharynx	Rhinovirus Parainfluenza 1, 3 RSV Adenovirus 1, 2, 3, 5, 14, 21
Lower respiratory tract infection		
Child	Nasal wash Nose or throat swab	RSV Parainfluenza 3, 1, 2 Influenza A
Adult	Sputum	Influenza A
Pleurodynia	Throat swab Stool	Coxsackie A, B
CNS infection		
Meningitis	CSF Throat swab Stool	Mumps Coxsackie A, B ECHO
Encephalitis	Blood	Mumps Herpes simplex 1
Myocarditis and pericarditis	Throat swab Stool	Coxsackie B
Gastroenteritis Stool		Nora virus, Hawaii agents Reovirus
UTI		
Acute hemorrhagic cystitis	Urine	Adenovirus 2, 7, 11 and ECHO 9
Orchitis and epididymitis	Throat swab Stool	Mumps
Parotitis	Throat swab Stool	Mumps
Exanthemata (nonspecific, with fever)	Skin vesicle fluid Throat swab Stool	Coxsackie A9, A16 ECHO 9, 16, 11
Herpangina	Skin vesicle fluid Throat swab Stool	Coxsackie A (1–6, 8, 10, 16, 22) Coxsackie B
Hand-foot-and-mouth disease	Skin vesicle fluid Throat swab Stool	Coxsackie A
Nonspecific febrile illness	Nose and throat swab Stool Blood	Coxsackie A, B ECHO Influenza A, B

The methods available for sensitivity testing include disc diffusion (agar diffusion), agar dilution (plate dilution), and broth dilution (tube or microtiter plate dilution).

Disc Diffusion Testing

The Kirby-Bauer disc diffusion method is the most commonly used antimicrobial susceptibility test. The technique requires the inoculation of an agar plate with a standard inoculum, addition of disc containing a standardized quantity of antimicrobial agent, incubation for 18 hours, and measurement of the zones of inhibition. A 3-category system of reporting results of disc diffusion testing is often used: sensitive, intermediate, and resistant.

Dilution Susceptibility Testing

Dilution susceptibility tests are used to determine the minimal inhibitory concentration (MIC) and minimum bactericidal concentration (MBC) of an antibiotic for an infecting organism.

TABLE 20 Specimens and Tests Used for *Chlamydia* Identification

Organisms	Specimen	Tests

C. trachomatis	Urethral swabs
	Cervical scrapings
	Posterior
	  nasopharyngeal
	Tracheal
	  secretions
	Conjunctival
	  scrapings
		Giemsa stain, cell
		  cultures,
		  serology
		ELISA, CIE, IHA
		  (IgM is
		  diagnostic in
		  infants)

C. psittaci	Respiratory
	  secretions
	Conjunctival
	  scrapings
	Biopsy of lung
	  (postmortem)	

The MIC of the drug is defined as the lowest concentration that prevents visible growth of the test organism under a standardized set of conditions. The MBC of the drug is the lowest concentration that results in complete killing (99.9%) of the test organism. The MIC and MBC are expressed quantitatively in micrograms, international units, or nicromoles of antibiotic per milliliter. Dilution susceptibility testing can be done by a broth dilution or agar dilution method.

β-Lactamase Test

The development of raid assays for β-lactamase permits an assessment of sensitivity to penicillin or ampicillin before standard disc diffusion of broth dilution susceptibility testing results are available. Rapid acidometric, iodometric, and chromogenic cephalosporin methods

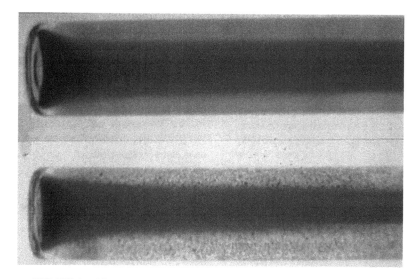

FIGURE 3 (*See color insert.*) Agglutinated red blood cells in a sodium citrate anticoagulation test tube that has been chilled in an ice bath are highly specific for *Mycoplasma pneumoniae* as the cause of pneumonia or other *Mycoplasma* infections.

currently are used to detect β-lactamase production. Bacteria can be tested after overnight growth in media and results are usually available within 30 minutes to an hour.

Successful therapy of infections caused by *Haemophilus influenzae, Staphylococcus aureus,* and *N. gonorrhoeae* may be facilitated by knowing whether the infecting agent is sensitive or resistant to penicilli nor ampicillin. Resistance is correlated with the production of the enzyme, β-lactamase.

SEROLOGIC AND IMMUNOLOGIC TESTING

Serologic methods are employed to detect microbial antigen as rapid diagnostic tests or to determine host antibody responses to suspected pathogens. Because of the nature of the immune response patients generally are 10 to 12 days into their clinical illness before most serologic tests are able to measure tests are able to measure a response. For conclusive evidence of infection, usually either a conversion from negative to positive or a 4-fold rise in titer must be demonstrated. In some cases, the titer will decrease. An acute phase serum and a convalescent serum (2 to 4 weeks after the onset of the infection) should be submitted to the laboratory.

A simple and highly specific test is "bedside cold agglutinins" to identify *Mycoplasma pneumoniae* as the cause of pneumonia. This test can be done by the clinician in just 30 seconds at the bedside. Two to 5 drops of blood are placed in a small blue-top sodium citrate tube, shaken to anticoagulate the blood, and the tube submerged in a cup containing an ice slurry. A control blood sample should undergo the same processing. After 30 seconds, the tube is held up to light and slowly rolled to thin the layer of blood. Agglutination of the red blood cells (Fig. 3) indicates a positive test.

8 | Respiratory Infections

INTRODUCTION

Respiratory tract infections constitute the major complaint for acute care visits to the pediatrician, accounting for an estimated 30% to 40% of all office consultations. The manifestations of the majority of infections are limited to the upper respiratory tract (i.e., ears, nose, and throat), but as many as 5% may involve the lower respiratory tract. It should be emphasized that although the symptoms of a respiratory tract infection are fairly well localized, pathologic and physiologic changes may be widespread. Examples include acute exacerbation of asthma, diarrhea, and myalgia associated with viral respiratory disease.

Greater than 90% of upper respiratory infections are viral in origin (excluding otitis media and sinusitis), while approximately half of all cases of pneumonia in children are caused by bacteria and half by viruses. Difficulty documenting etiology of infection in young children unfortunately has required liberal antibiotic use. The age of the patient, localization of the symptoms, and the status of the host's defenses help predict the organism and the need for antimicrobial therapy. In most cases of upper respiratory infection, fluids, acetaminophen for fever and bed rest are the only therapies necessary (Table 1).

TABLE 1 Etiology of Common Upper Respiratory Infections

Common cold	Rhinoviruses
	RSV
	Parainfluenza
	Coronaviruses
Pharyngitis	Viruses
	Adenoviruses
	Enteroviruses
	Epstein-Barr virus
	Bacteria
	Group A streptococcus
	Arcanobacterium hemolyticum
	Groups C and G streptococcus
	Neisseria gonorrhoeae
	Francisella tularensis
	Treponema pallidum
	Corynebacterium diphtheriae
Sinusitis	*Haemophilus influenzae*
	S. pneumoniae
	Moraxella catarrhalis
Croup (laryngitis, laryngotracheitis, laryngotracheobronchitis)	Parainfluenzae
	Influenza
	RSV
	Adenovirus
	B. pertussis

Abbreviation: RSV, respiratory syncytial virus.

COMMON COLD

The common cold can often be distinguished from the broader category of upper respiratory infections (URIs) by the absence of pharyngitis. Rhinoviruses are by far the most common etiologies, producing primarily nasal symptoms: congestion, mucoid discharge and sneezing. Mild conjunctivitis, throat irritation and low grade fever are occasionally present. For the vast majority of children with simple rhinovirus infection, no treatment is necessary. Parents should be educated that cold remedies are a waste of money and effort.

PHARYNGITIS

Examination of patients who present with sore throat may reveal tonsillitis, tonsillopharyngitis, or nasopharyngitis. An exudative tonsillar membrane with palatal petechiae strongly suggests group A beta-hemolytic streptococcus (GABHS) as the etiology (Fig. 1) while a white shaggy membrane with palatal petechiae is more characteristic of infectious mononucleosis. The absence of pharyngeal inflammation or the presence of either rhinorrhea or laryngitis is much more likely to be associated with viral infection. However, no physical findings clearly separate GABHS from viral, other bacterial, or non-infectious causes.

The primary concern for pharyngitis in children between 3 and 18 years of age is that untreated GABHS may subsequently cause rheumatic fever. To prevent this sequela, adequate antimicrobial therapy should be instituted within 9 days of infection. Rapid antigen detection assays for GABHS are diagnostic if positive since the specificity of such tests is 98% to 99% (1% to 2% false positives). However, sensitivity is only 70% (30% false negatives) requiring follow-up cultures for negative tests if there is strong clinical suspicion for GABHS tonsillopharyngitis. If the clinical information, i.e., history, physical, and epidemiology do not support GABHS, a culture is not necessary.

The drug of choice for treatment of group A streptococcus remains penicillin V although many experts recommend a higher dosage than what has been used previously. A minimum of 20 mg/kg/day should be prescribed; larger children would generally receive 500 mg div. b.i.d. × 10 days. Many clinicians prefer amoxicillin because of a more pleasing taste and therefore better compliance. Relapses or failure should be treated with an antibiotic active against β-lactamase producing organisms, i.e., macrolides, cephalosporins, clindamycin, or amoxicillin/clavulanate. The hypothesis is that colonizing pharyngeal bacteria that produce penicillinase have inactivated penicillin, resulting in treatment failure.

Other bacteria which can occasionally cause pharyngitis and require antimicrobial therapy are the following: *Arcanobacterium hemolyticum*, streptococci groups C and G,

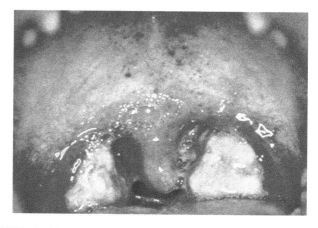

FIGURE 1 (*See color insert.*) Tonsillopharyngitis with an exudative tonsillar membrane and palatal petechiae in an adolescent with a positive strep screen.

N. gonorrhoeae, F. tularensis, and *Treponema pallidum.* In some developing countries, diphtheria is still seen.

No treatment is of any benefit for the usual viral causes of pharyngitis. Throat lozenges, sprays, mouth washes offer only transient benefit. The use of decongestants and anti-histamines should be discouraged as they have not been shown to be efficacious.

SINUSITIS

Acute paranasal sinusitis is a more difficult diagnosis to make in children than in adults because the characteristic symptoms are less likely to be present. Furthermore, there is considerable controversy about sensitivity of laboratory methods for documenting this infection. Maxillary or ethmoidal sinusitis usually follows a viral upper respiratory tract infection. Symptoms may include cough, purulent nasal discharge, facial pain, and fever. Diagnosis is most often considered when a URI with a daytime cough and purulent nasal discharge lasts longer than 10 days. The diagnosis can be supported with sinus X-rays, but the best radiographic study is a limited CT scan; sinus puncture with culture is the most definitive test, but is infrequently performed due to its invasive nature. The organisms commonly recovered are considered pathogens when isolated from the sinuses, even though they are part of the normal flora in other parts of the respiratory tract.

Several antibiotics are effective given orally. The increased resistance to amoxicillin resulting from β-lactamase production by approximately 60% of *H. influenzae* and 90% to 100% of *Moraxella catarrhalis* and an alteration in penicillin binding proteins which occurs in about 50% of *S. pneumoniae* have questioned the reliability of amoxicillin as first line therapy of sinusitis. If amoxicillin is considered a high dosage (75 to 90 mg/kg/day) should be prescribed. Alternatives include cephalosporins, macrolides, and trimethoprim-sulfamethoxazole (Table 2).

EPIGLOTTITIS

Acute epiglottitis is a life-threatening acute inflammation of the supraglottic region predominately caused by *Haemophilus influenzae* type b (Hib). Since the routine administration of Hib vaccine in the early 1990s, the prevalence of disease caused by this pathogen has dramatically decreased. Mostly affecting children under 4 years of age, epiglottitis presents with a rapid onset of toxicity and respiratory distress (Table 3).

A diagnosis is made from the characteristic presentation in most cases. In severe or classic cases, nothing is to be gained by obtaining a lateral neck radiograph to confirm the diagnosis. Hyperextending the neck to obtain a proper radiograph may actually induce laryngospasm. A patent airway must be established as rapidly as possible. However, radiographic examination may provide useful information in the patient with mild symptoms in whom the diagnosis of croup is more likely. With this diagnosis, X-rays demonstrate a

TABLE 2   Acute Sinusitis

Age	Usually >2 years
Symptoms	Cough, nasal discharge, fever, face pain, prolonged URI
Organisms	*Haemophilus influenzae*
	S. pneumoniae
	Moraxella catarrhalis
Complications	Cavernous sinus thrombosis
	Periorbital cellulitis
	Meningitis
	Maxillary osteomyelitis
	Brain abscess

Abbreviation: URI, upper respiratory infection.

TABLE 3 Signs and Symptoms of Epiglottitis
at Time of Hospital Admission

Sign or symptom	Incidence (% of patients)
Respiratory distress	100
Stridor	92
Fever	92
Drooling	63
Delirium	58
Dysphagia	58
Pharyngitis	50
Hoarseness	33
Cough	29

TABLE 4 Differential Diagnosis of Epiglottitis

Croup
Bacterial tracheitis
Peritonsillar abscess
Retropharyngeal abscess
Severe tonsillitis
Foreign body aspiration
Angioedema
Infectious mononucleosis

subglottic "steeple sign" which is representative of viral induced edema. If radiographic examination is elected, the physician should accompany the patient at all times. Acute epiglottitis must be differentiated from other disorders which produce supraglottic and subglottic upper airway obstruction (Table 4).

Once a diagnosis of epiglottitis is seriously suspected, preparations must begin immediately to secure the airway. When treated early and aggressively, the prognosis for epiglottitis is excellent (Table 5).

CROUP (LARYNGOTRACHEOBRONCHITIS)

Laryngotracheobronchitis (LTB) is the most common cause of acute partial upper airway obstruction in children. The terminology describing this disease and those in its differential diagnosis has been confusing. LTB (or croup) refers to partial airway obstruction due to a viral infection with erythema and edema concentrated mostly in the subglottic area (Fig. 2). The organism is usually parainfluenza (in order of frequency types 1, 3, 2), although other organisms can cause croup during periods of increased prevalence [respiratory syncytial virus

TABLE 5 Treatment of Epiglottitis

Secure airway
Keep child calm
Let child assume most comfortable position, preferably in parent's arms
Administer oxygen by face mask without agitating the child
Contact anesthesiologist, otolaryngologist, and operating room supervisor
Transport child as soon as possible to operating room with parent (to calm child), physician, and all equipment needed to secure airway if distress increases
Induce anesthesia by allowing child to breathe spontaneously from mask (halothane and 100% oxygen) while in sitting position; then establish intravenous line
Epiglottis is visualized by direct examination
Nasotracheal tube is inserted and taped securely (if not possible, orotracheal intubation is attempted, followed by bronchoscopic intubation, or tracheostomy as a last resort)
Antibiotics
Ceftriaxone or cefotaxime
Supportive care
Observe in intensive care unit
Keep sedated and restrained
Provide 2–4 cm H_2O continuous positive airway pressure and humidification through endotracheal tube
Assure hydration (intravenous)
Extubation
After approximately 48 hr intubation, the epiglottis is again examined directly
If edema and inflammation have subsided, and a leak is present around the tube, it may be removed
If not, tube is left in place and epiglottis is re-examined in 24 hr

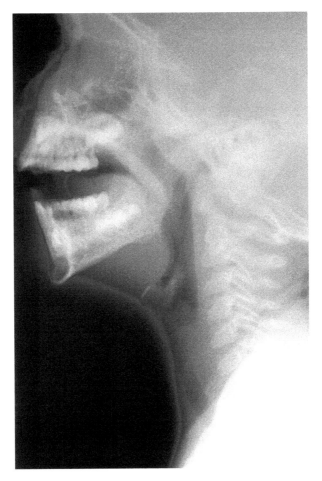

FIGURE 2 Lateral neck radiograph of a child with subglottic viral croup.
The tracheal air column is narrow and less radiolucent in the larynx due to
laryngeal edema, but the epiglottis is normal.

(RSV), human metapneumovirus, influenza, and rhinovirus]. The peak ages are between
6 months and 2 years. The clinical presentation is that of a child with a few days of upper
respiratory tract infection who then develops inspiratory stridor, retractions, and a harsh
barking cough. The degree of fever depends on the organism and is usually mild with
parainfluenza. The severity of the obstruction is variable throughout the day and is often
worse at night. The illness gradually resolves spontaneously over several days. No laboratory
test is needed for confirmation but neck X-rays show characteristic subglottic narrowing
(steeple sign). Therapy at home is symptomatic (i.e., antipyretics for fever) and mist. In-
hospital therapy should include steroids, dexamethasome 0.6 mg/kg given as a single dose;
management of more severe cases might include mist, oxygen, and racemic epinephrine (1:4
concentration of 2.25%, with increasing concentration to 1:1 as needed) by inhalation. Because
of the potential for rebound (i.e., returning to baseline clinical status), the use of racemic
epinephrine commits the patient to further observation. It is uncommon for croup to require
intubation. Because edema and inflammation are in the narrowest portion of the child's
airway, a somewhat narrower endotracheal tube should be selected to decrease the likelihood
of post-intubation subglottic stenosis.

Spasmodic croup occurs in the slightly older child and is probably a variant of reactive
airway disease rather than an infection, although a viral disease may be a predisposing factor.
Characteristically the previously well child awakens suddenly with stridor and coughing, which

TABLE 6   Therapy for Infectious Croup

At home
Mist-humidity
Antipyretics
Observation
In-hospital
Dexamethasone 0.6 mg/kg IM, single dose on
admission
Mist-humidity
Racemic epinephrine
Oxygen
Intubation

lasts 45 to 90 minutes before abating spontaneously. It recurs in an irregular pattern. Steroids, shown to be helpful in infectious LTB, may also be beneficial in spasmodic croup (Table 6).

PERTUSSIS

Despite vigorous immunization programs, pertussis has remained a common disease in infants and young children. The current strategy for improved disease control now includes a booster dose of vaccine for everyone over 10 years of age. This will reduce the human reservoir of the pathogen and prevent spread of disease to young vulnerable infants.

The clinical course is traditionally divided into 3 phases: catarrhal, paroxysmal, and convalescent. During the catarrhal phase, the disease is indistinguishable from the common cold. It is during this phase that the organism, *Bordetella pertussis*, is most likely to be isolated but unfortunately prior to the classic symptoms that suggest the diagnosis of pertussis. The subsequent phase is that of paroxysmal coughing, often interspersed with loud inspiratory "whoops." Coughing may be triggered by feeding, activity, or crying. Unfortunately, this phase can persist for weeks despite appropriate antibiotic therapy. Cultures are negative in 85% of patients during this phase of the illness when the child is most likely to be brought to the physician. Nevertheless, the diagnosis can be made using a PCR assay or fluorescent antibody test on a posterior nasopharyngeal swab. Diagnosis is also strongly suggested by a marked lymphocytosis.

Treatment includes azithromycin 10 mg/kg/day as a single dose × 5 days, clarithromycin 15 mg/kg/day div. b.i.d. × 7 days, or erythromycin 50 mg/kg/day ÷ q 6 hours for 14 days.

BACTERIAL TRACHEITIS

Also termed membranous croup, bacterial tracheitis represents a secondary complication of viral LTB characterized by necrotizing inflammation of the trachea, abundant thick secretions and occasionally sudden airway obstruction. Except for its viral prodrome, the clinical presentation is quite similar to that of *H. influenzae* epiglottitis. Bacterial tracheitis is therefore a more likely diagnosis in a fully immunized child with high fever and rapid onset upper airway obstruction. Presenting symptoms are itemized in Table 7.

A diagnosis of bacterial tracheitis is most likely to be confirmed with airway radiographs showing tracheal irregularities or a membrane. Additional findings include pulmonary infiltrates, atelectasis, hyperinflation, and pulmonary edema.

The viral etiologies of the prodromal LTB include parainfluenza, influenza and adenoviruses. Recovered bacteria have been quite variable (Table 8). Earlier reports indicated that *Staphylococcus aureus* was most common accounting for one-half of cases. Recent outbreaks of disease caused by *Moraxella catarrhalis* and *Corynebacterium pseudodiphteriticum* have been reported associated with less severe illness and a markedly decreased requirement for tracheal intubation.

Management includes empiric broad spectrum antibiotics for coverage of *S. aureus* and β-lactamase producing *M. catarrhalis* and *H. influenzae*. A third generation cephalosporin

TABLE 7 Epidemiology and Presenting Symptoms of Bacterial Tracheitis

Epidemiology
    Peak age 4 years
    Early winter outbreaks
Clinical course
    Prodromal URI
    Cough, stridor
    High fever >39°C
    Toxic appearance

TABLE 8 Etiology of Bacterial Tracheitis

Staphylococcus aureus	35–75%
Haemophilus influenzae	6–40%
a-hemolytic *Streptococcus*	0–40%
Moraxella catarrhalis	0–27%
Group A Streptococcus	0–25%

(ceftriaxone or cefotaxime) plus clindamycin, vancomycin, or linezolid combination are most appropriate. Protection of the airway and prevention of endotracheal occlusion are the priority. Humidification, frequent suctioning of the airway, and intravenous hydration should be started early. Endoscopy to confirm the diagnosis and remove any potentially obstructive membrane or exudative material should be undertaken for patients with significant airway symptoms. Even after endotracheal intubation these patients may develop obstructive plugs or membranes below the tube.

BRONCHITIS

The diagnosis of bronchitis is difficult to make in pediatrics because definition is lacking. If simple inflammation of the trachea and major divisions of the bronchi constitute pathogenesis, bronchitis would be synonymous with the common cold. Chronic or recurrent bronchitis is also difficult to define, but most authors suggest that a productive cough is a prominent feature and that symptoms persist for a period of weeks or recur regularly. As contrasted with adults, bronchitis in children is caused almost exclusively by viral agents (Table 9). *Mycoplasma pneumoniae* is the only common pathogen for which antimicrobial therapy is indicated.

BRONCHIOLITIS

Bronchiolitis is a very common lower respiratory tract infection, affecting perhaps as many as 1% to 2% of all infants. The peak age ranges from 2 to 10 months. RSV is the predominant organism with other viruses being responsible in some reported epidemics. The clinical manifestations are preceding coryza, cough, tachypnea, and wheezing. The chest X-ray shows hyperinflation, peribronchial thickening, and varying amounts of atelectasis. Histologically, there is mononuclear inflammation and sloughing of the bronchiolar epithelium with partial obstruction of the bronchiolar lumen (Table 10).

    Therapy is primarily supportive with maintenance of adequate oxygenation and appropriate hydration and nutrition. One-third to one-half of children will benefit from albuterol bronchodilator therapy; a therapeutic trial either in the emergency room or shortly after

TABLE 9 Viruses Causing Lower Respiratory Tract Infection

Organism	Bronchitis	Bronchiolitis	Pneumonia
RSV	+++	++++	++
Metapneumovirus	++	+++	++
Influenza (A and B)	++	+	++
Parainfluenza	++	++	++
Adenovirus	+++	+	+++
Rhinovirus	+	++	++

++++, most frequent
+, occasional

TABLE 10   Bronchiolitis

Age	2–10 mos
Organism	Respiratory syncytial virus predominates, metapneumovirus, adenovirus, parainfluenza
Symptoms	Wheezing and tachypnea
Therapy	Trial of bronchodilator therapy with aerolized β_2 agonists: albuterol 2.15 mg in 3 mL NS; neonate/infant 0.05–0.15 mg/kg/dose children 1.25–2.5 mg/dose q 4–6 hrs Supportive (O_2, etc.)
Sequelae	Recurrent wheezing Predilection for chronic obstructive pulmonary disease

hospitalization should be offered. Treatment should be discontinued if improvement cannot be documented. A small percentage of infants will require mechanical ventilation. Antibiotics are not indicated as this is exclusively a viral illness. Chest physical therapy may be beneficial to those infants with atelectasis. Steroids have not been beneficial in several large studies.

Although bronchiolitis seems to be a self-limited and a generally benign illness, the long-term sequelae may be significant. Up to 50% of the patients have subsequent wheezing or frank asthma. It is yet unclear what role small airway insults early in life have on chronic obstructive lung disease in adults. Some children appear to have asymptomatic small airways dysfunction years after the episode of bronchiolitis, suggesting a propensity for progressive dysfunction later in life.

Afebrile Pneumonia of Infancy

Afebrile pneumonia in infants less than 3 months of age is caused by a unique group of pathogens which are acquired during the perinatal period from colonized mothers. Mixed infection is common. The clinical presentation is tachypnea, poor weight gain, and inspiratory crackles; wheezing is uncommon. The chest X-ray usually shows interstitial pneumonia, hyperaeration, peribronchial thickening, and scattered areas of atelectasis. The diagnosis should be made by culture. *Chlamydia trachomatis* is suggested by eosinophilia, elevated immunoglobulins, and clinically by the presence of conjunctivitis. Rapid enzyme linked immunosorbent assay (ELISA) or fluorescence assays for chlamydia antigen from posterior nasopharyngeal washings or conjunctival exudate can confirm diagnosis. Other agents require culture for identification (Table 11).

INFLUENZA

Influenza occurs during well-publicized epidemics and is characterized by fever, headache, myalgia, cough, and any combination of upper respiratory tract symptoms. Croup or pneumonia are frequently the primary diagnoses. Because disease is spread by direct person to person contact, hospitalized patients require isolation.

Etiology is best confirmed by viral culture during the first 3 days of illness. Thereafter the low quantity of virus may result in falsely negative cultures. Rapid antigen detection

TABLE 11   Afebrile Pneumonitis of Early Infancy: Etiology and Treatment

Pathogen	Treatment
Chlamydia trachomatis	Azithromycin 20 mg/kg/ day × 3
Cytomegalovirus	Ganciclovir, CMV immunoglobulin
Pneumocystis carinii	TMP/SMX 20:100 mg/kg/day div. b.i.d. × 14 days
Ureaplasma urealyticum	Erythromycin 50 mg/kg/day div. q.i.d. × 14 days

Abbreviation: CMV, cytomegalovirus.

TABLE 12 Antiviral Agents for Influenza A and B

Generic	Trade name	Virus	Treatment age	Prophylaxis age
Oseltamivir	Tamiflu®	A and B	>1 yr	>1 yr
Zanamivir		A and B	>7 yrs	>5 yrs
Rimantadine		A	>13 yrs	>1 yr
Amantidine		A	>1 yr	>1 yr

assays such as immunofluorescence are available but results in the usual office or hospital setting are quite variable.

Two current antiviral agents are effective against influenza A and B (Table 12), most useful when both strains are known to be causing disease or early in epidemics before infecting strains have been identified. The agent of choice for influenza A prophylaxis and treatment had been rimantadine or its parent compound, amantadine. However, in 2005–2006, circulating influenza A strains were resistant. Updated information each year is therefore needed for treatment and prophylaxis recommendations. Influenza vaccine should be mandatory for high-risk children and strongly considered for universal administration, usually given during the month of October (Table 8).

PNEUMONIA

Although the vast majority of acute pneumonias in children are viral in etiology, standard practice dictates empiric administration of antimicrobial agents for most young pediatric patients. Variables for antibiotic therapy and for hospitalization of infants and children include epidemiologic considerations, clinical symptoms, predisposing host factors, age, and radiographic findings. The virtual elimination of Hib as a respiratory pathogen and recent recognition of *Chlamydophila pneumoniae* as a common cause of pneumonia in older children have recently changed our selection of initial empiric antimicrobial therapy for lower respiratory tract infections in pediatric patients. New, rapid diagnostic tests are also useful in making clinical decisions and are particularly important for children who are unable to produce sputum for examination and whose small airways limit utilization of bronchoscopy.

Pneumonia is diagnosed in approximately 20 of 1000 infants younger than 1 year and in 40 of 1000 children aged 1 to 5 years. The practitioner's primary responsibility is to differentiate upper respiratory tract infections from pneumonia. The practitioner must also decide which patients with lower respiratory tract disease warrant more aggressive management.

Etiology

It is estimated that 50% of pediatric pneumonias are caused by viral agents. Approximately 60% of documented viral lower respiratory infections in children are caused by RSV, 20% by human metapneumovirus (hMPV), 10% by parainfluenza types 3 and 1 and a smaller number of pneumonias result from influenza A and B or adenovirus. Rhinovirus is occasionally implicated. Four of these groups of viral agents (RSV, hMPV, parainfluenza, and influenza) are seen almost exclusively during the winter months. Adenovirus is the more common viral pathogen during the remainder of the year. Such specific seasonal clustering implies a greater likelihood of bacterial causes during the spring, summer, and fall.

Chlamydophila pneumoniae is an increasingly recognized pathogen in pediatric community acquired pneumonia as well as otitis media. The reported incidence of this infection varies from 1% to 15%. The symptoms associated with *C. pneumoniae* infection are similar to that seen with *M. pneumoniae*; however, sore throat and hoarseness are reported more frequently. Pleural effusions may be seen in as high as 25% of infections. In most studies, the diagnosis has been made by serology but these assays are still not widely available.

TABLE 13 Bacterial and Fungal Causes of Pneumonia Related to Age of the Pediatric Patient

Age group	Common pathogens
0–48 hrs	Group B streptococci
1–14 days	*E. coli, K. pneumoniae*, other Enterobacteriaceae, *L. monocytogenes, S. aureus*, anaerobes, group B streptococci
2 wks – 2 mos (premature neonates)	Enterobacteriaceae, group B streptococci, *S. aureus, S. epidermidis, C. albicans, H. influenzae, S. pneumoniae*
2 mos – 10 yrs	*S. pneumoniae, Chlamydophila pneumoniae, Mycoplasma pneumoniae*
10–21 yrs	*Mycoplasma pneumoniae, Chlamydophila pneumoniae, S. pneumoniae*

Bacterial and fungal organisms causing pneumonia are primarily related to the age of the pediatric patient (Table 13).

The greatest number of potential pathogens are seen in neonates who require prolonged intensive care, particularly those born prematurely. Group B streptococci (*Streptococcus agalactiae*) and gram-negative enteric bacilli, particularly *Escherichia coli*, are the most common pathogens causing neonatal pneumonia, often in association with generalized sepsis.

Group B streptococcal respiratory infection usually develops during the first few days of life. Rapidly progressive radiographic findings mimic respiratory distress syndrome. Coliform pneumonia in neonates also occurs during the early neonatal period; it is acquired perinatally from a colonized mother. Pulmonary infection in neonates of 3 to 4 weeks of age is more likely nosocomially transmitted during difficult intensive care management. In patients who have been hospitalized for more than 2 weeks, *Staphylococcus epidermidis* is a relatively common cause of sepsis and pneumonia. Infection with *Candida albicans* is a consequence of long-term intravenous catheterization and the administration of broad-spectrum antibiotics.

Other data used to determine probable causes include associated clinical signs and symptoms, chest X-ray findings, and diagnostic laboratory tests (Table 14).

Sputum is rarely produced by children during episodes of pneumonia, so the usual first step in the management of adult pneumonias, Gram's stain examination of sputum is eliminated.

Clinical Appearance

It is not possible to distinguish between viral and bacterial pneumonia on clinical grounds alone. Signs and symptoms together with other assessments, however, allow the practitioner

TABLE 14 Suggested Diagnostic Evaluation for Pneumonia in Children

Chest roentgenograms (PA and lateral decubitus view if there is
  consolidation or evidence of effusion)
Blood culture
Complete blood count
Tuberculin skin test
Bedside cold agglutinins (see text)
Afebrile and <20 weeks of age (in addition to above):
  Chlamydia monoclonal fluorescent antibody or ELISA staining of
    posterior nasopharyngeal swab
  Rapid antigen assay or Wright-Giemsa stain of conjunctival
    scraping (for *Chlamydia*) if there is conjunctivitis

to categorize the correct cause in a majority of cases. Children with bacterial disease have histories suggesting rapid onset, are more likely to appear very sick, and have temperatures above 39°C (102.2°F).

Patients who have viral processes generally have low-grade fever and are usually irritable, although they may not appear toxic. Other important symptoms associated with influenza, parainfluenza, and adenovirus infection are headache, photophobia, myalgia, and gastrointestinal complaints. In addition, there is a prodrome of longer than 2 days associated with these 3 viruses, and even more commonly present when rhinovirus is the responsible pathogen.

In older children who are infected with *Mycoplasma pneumoniae*, onset and disease evolution are more suggestive of viral pneumonia because multiple organ systems may be involved. Mycoplasma infection may be severe and rapidly progressive in children with sickle cell disease.

Chest Roentgenograms

Chest roentgenograms most readily confirm clinical findings that are compatible with pneumonia. In many cases chest X-rays help differentiate viral from bacterial causes. They may even suggest specific pathogens. Viral pneumonias are associated with 4 roentgenographic findings: hyperexpansion, parahilar peribronchial infiltrates, atelectasis, and hilar adenopathy. The latter finding is only commonly associated with adenovirus. Consolidated alveolar or diffuse interstitial infiltrates and large pleural effusions are rarely seen. More severe X-ray changes in young infants suggest respiratory syncytial virus disease.

The chest roentgenogram demonstrating infection with *Chlamydia* classically reveals diffuse interstitial infiltrates with hyperaeration, peribronchial thickening, and scattered areas of atelectasis. The more extensive diffuse interstitial infiltrates that usually accompany *Chlamydia* infection help distinguish this etiology from viral infections.

Alveolar disease, consolidation, the presence of air bronchograms, and pleural effusions are characteristic of bacterial pneumonia. These roentgenographic findings alone dictate institution of antimicrobial therapy. *Staphylococcus aureus* must be suspected if there is evidence of a consolidated infiltrate accompanied by an effusion or a pneumatocele (Fig. 3). This cause is relatively more common in young infants (<12 months of age) and neonates, and warrants hospitalization and daily roentgenographic monitoring. The primary reason for repeating chest X-rays within 24 to 48 hours is to delineate changes compatible with a staphylococcal cause.

Aspiration pneumonia is often suspected on clinical grounds such as a preexisting seizure disorder or severe gastroesophageal reflux. Radiographic findings classically include a consolidating infiltrate in the right lower lobe. Young patients who aspirate while recumbent, however, are more likely to develop disease in the upper lobes.

Extensive destruction of lung tissue may result in the formation of multiple small abscess cavities, termed necrotizing pneumonia. This roentgenographic finding should alert the clinician to the presence of less common pathogens, including *Pseudomonas aeruginosa*, *Klebsiella pneumoniae*, *Proteus mirabilis*, other Enterobacteriaceae, and anaerobes. Predominant organisms are often locally unique, and antibiotic sensitivies for such organisms vary considerably from hospital to hospital. Antibiotic regimens generally include a broad spectrum penicillin (for anaerobic coverage) plus an aminoglycoside (for synergistic activity against *Pseudomonas* and other *Enterobacteriaceae*). Despite early and appropriate antimicrobial therapy, necrotizing pneumonia is often fatal.

Laboratory Diagnosis

The "gold standard" for documenting both bacterial and viral causes of pneumonia is culture. The best source of culture material is a lung aspirate. Published reports have suggested that bacterial pathogens can be isolated in approximately 33% of patients undergoing this

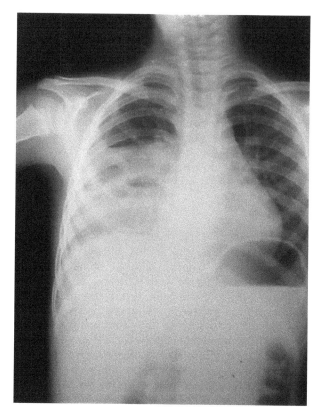

FIGURE 3 Consolidated pneumonia with empyema and pneumatoceles. Thoracentesis fluid grew *Staphylococcus aureus.* A chest tube was required to provide drainage of the abscess.

procedure. Such studies have been biased, however, because severe cases were more likely to be enrolled. The typical viral pneumonia with a centrally located parahilar peribronchial infiltrate does not safely lend itself to needle aspiration. Bacteremia is only documented in 9% to 10% of all febrile children with pneumonia while more than 50% of community acquired cases are bacterial in origin.

In neonates, pneumonia is frequently associated with generalized sepsis. Organisms recovered are similar to those implicated in other serious infections such as meningitis, septic arthritis, and pyelonephritis. A workup for sepsis, including lumbar puncture, is always indicated in neonates who have febrile pneumonia.

Culture is the only reliable method of identifying influenza viruses. Rapid identification of RSV, however, can be achieved with direct fluorescent staining or ELISA techniques. Likewise, fluorescent staining reagents and ELISA that differentiate other potential viral pathogens, such as parainfluenza virus and adenovirus, are also available. Tracheal aspirates or posterior nasopharyngeal secretions are required as specimens for examination.

Respiratory syncytial virus testing is feasible in community hospitals, but other viral cultures are usually performed in reference laboratories. Unfortunately, because of the time required for isolation and identification of viruses, such tests do not generally provide clinically useful information.

P. carinii, U. urealyticum, and CMV, must be cultured from tracheal aspirates. *P. carinii* has been successfully recovered in only a few laboratories where investigations of this organism are in progress. Detection of *Pneumocystis* antigen in serum is also performed only in research laboratories.

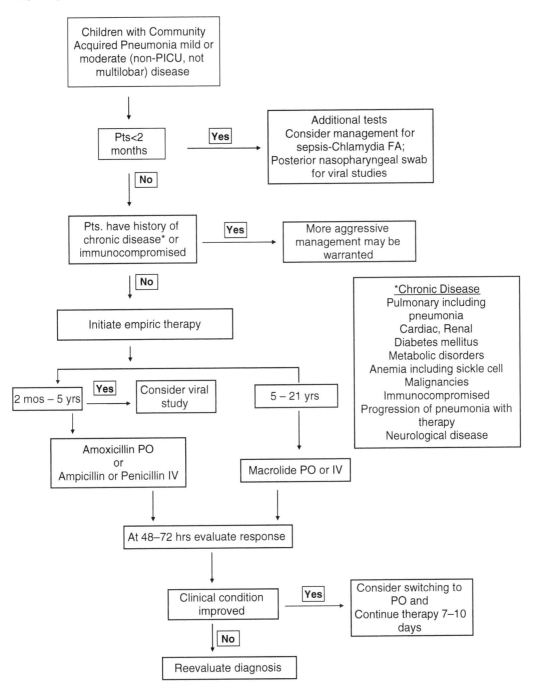

FIGURE 4 Inpatient and outpatient management of children with community acquired pneumonia.

An important rapid diagnostic step for *Mycoplasma* infection is the bedside cold agglutination test. Although only 50% sensitive in identifying this cause, a positive result can guide early specific therapy, because specificity is close to absolute. Most critical is that the test be performed correctly. Two to 5 drops of blood (0.1 to 0.3 mL) are placed in a 64 mm (small blue top) tube containing sodium citrate anticoagulant. An identical tube with control blood is also obtained. These tubes are refrigerated in an ice bath for 1 minute, after which time the tubes are rolled by their ends and blood is observed for agglutination. When the blood is warmed to room temperature, agglutination is no longer apparent. Common mistakes are drawing too much blood, using too large a tube, or using the wrong anticoagulant.

Antimicrobial Therapy

Management of children with community acquired pneumonia is presented as an algorithm in Figure 4. Early empiric treatment for either bacterial or viral disease is imperative for patients whose condition might take a rapidly progressive course if therapy is delayed. Certainly febrile neonates and infants less than 2 months of age belong in this category. Late institution of antibiotics in these patients is associated with higher rates of mortality and morbidity.

Antibiotics are selected primarily on the basis of age and severity of illness (Table 15). Dosages for these agents are listed in Chapter 20. Duration of therapy is 7 to 10 days for uncomplicated pneumonia. Once the causative agent is identified by culture or with 1 of the rapid antigen detection assays, specific therapy may be readily selected.

Azithromycin is the drug of choice for outpatient treatment of pneumonia in the 2-month to 5-year age group, since 25% to 50% of *S. pneumoniae* are resistant to penicillins. However, half of this is intermediate resistance (MIC 0.06 to 1.0 μg/mL) so can be managed with the higher dosages of amoxicillin (75 to 90 mg/kg/day). In areas of the country that report an even higher incidence of highly penicillin resistant (MIC $\geq$2.0 μg/mL) pneumococcus, oral antibiotics active against these organisms may be more appropriate. Such antibiotics include cefdinir (Omnicef) cefprozil (Cefzil), cefpodoxime (Vantin), azithromycin (Zithromax), clarithromycin (Biaxin), or erythromycin. Selection among these may be made on the basis of relative cost, because all are associated with a very low incidence of significant adverse reactions.

Treatment of pneumonia is usually empiric. If *C. pneumoniae* is suspected as the responsible pathogen, azithromycin should be used as primary therapy. When *M. pneumoniae* is likely, particularly in the older teenager, newer quinolones or tetracycline-based antibiotics can be considered when macrolides are not tolerated.

If a child does not respond to initial antibacterial therapy, the most likely explanation is a viral cause. Other bacterial causes might also be considered, such as *S. aureus*, multi-resistant pneumococcus, ampicillin-resistant *H. influenzae*, or anaerobes. If these latter pathogens are likely, hospitalization is warranted. Hospitalization is also based on age, clinical, and roentgenographic factors (Table 16).

Necrotizing Pneumonia

Necrotizing bacterial pneumonias are occasionally seen in patients who are debilitated, immunocompromised, or who have undergone prolonged hospitalization. Responsible

TABLE 15   Empiric Antimicrobial Therapy for Presumed Bacterial Pneumonia

Age group	Antibiotics
Younger than 2 mos	Ampicillin + ceftriaxone or cefotaxime (oral erythromycin if *C. trachomatis* is suspected in infants younger than 20 wk) + Clindamycin (optional) vancomycin (for *S. aureus.* or multi-resistant pneumococcus) if the illness appears life threatening
2 mos – 5 yrs	
Mild	Azithromycin or cefdinir (oral)
Severe	Ceftriaxone or cefotaxime; add clindamycin or vancomycin (for multi-resistant pneumococcus) or if the illness appears life threatening and *S. aureus* is suspected
5–21 years	Azithromycin (oral or intravenous depending on severity)

TABLE 16 Children with Pneumonia Warranting Consideration of Inpatient Management

Toxic appearance
Respiratory distress
Pleural effusion
Age factors
   Less than 2 mos
   Less than 3 yrs with lobar pneumonia
   Less than 5 yrs with involvement of more than 1 lobe
Those with chronic diseases
   Pulmonary (including asthma)
   Cardiac
   Renal
   Diabetes mellitus
   Anemia (including sickle cell disease)
   Malignancies
Immunocompromised host
Progression during outpatient therapy

pathogens are often nosocomial organisms such as *Pseudomonas aeruginosa, Klebsiella pneumoniae, Proteus mirabilis,* and related species. Penicillin or clindamycin are recommended for these pathogens.

Aspiration Pneumonia

Pneumonia due to aspiration of gastric contents or oropharyngeal secretions occurs in patients with impaired neurologic function. A depressed level of consciousness, albeit transient, as in seizure disorders, induction of anesthesia, or diabetic coma, or permanent as in mental retardation, is a fairly constant predisposing factor. Chronic aspiration also occurs in patients with an uncoordinated swallowing mechanism. Careful history and physical examination should uncover the potential for aspiration pneumonitis. The organisms are usually anaerobes, and frequently more than 1 organism is isolated. The infiltrates on chest X-ray are usually in the dependent lobes; effusions and abscesses are common (Table 17).

TABLE 17 Organisms Causing Aspiration Pneumonia

Peptostreptococcus
Peptococcus
Microaerophilic cocci and streptococci
Bacteroides sp.
Fusobacterium sp.
S. aureus
Streptococcus pyogenes
Streptococcus sp.

TABLE 18 Empyema in Children

Stages of infection
   Exudative: allows needle aspiration
   Fibrinopurulent: may be loculated
   Organizing
Treatment options
   Exudative: repeated needle aspiration (1–5 days)
   Exudative or fibrinopurulent: chest tube drainage
   Organizing: limited thoracotomy after 3–5 days of
      drainage
   Organized: decortication >50% limitation of lung
      by CT scan After 2–4 wk of medical
      management
   Tachypnea
   Asymmetry of chest wall expansion
   Fever
   Leukocytosis

PLEURAL EMPYEMA

Collection of exudate within the pleural cavity results from the inflammatory response induced by bacterial pneumonia. This empyema progresses through 3 overlapping stages from initial thin fluid accumulation to organized fibroblast deposition and entrapment of lung (Table 18). Decisions to drain this exudate must be made in a timely manner to prevent pleural thickening and any subsequent need for decortication.

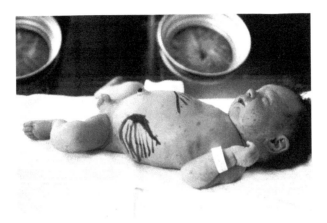

FIGURE 1.1   The classical triad of jaundice, hepatosplenomegaly, and a petechial "blueberry muffin" rash is seen with congenital CMV, rubella, and toxoplasmosis.

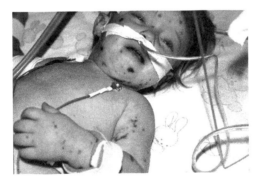

FIGURE 2.3   The rash of meningococcemia is usually a combination of petechiae, ecchymoses, and purpura as seen in this 13-mo-old. Larger purpura have a straked appearance as contrasted with the purpura with Henoch-Schonleion disease which are round. Severe infection with disseminated intravascular coagulation caused by many other bacterial pathogens may look identical to meningococcemia.

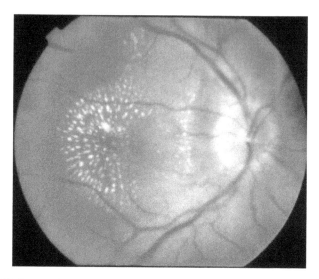

FIGURE 3.1 Cat scratch disease was diagnosed in this adolescent male with a large, tender, axillary node and flu-like illness of three weeks duration. Ophthalmologic examination when he experienced decreased vision in his right eye revealed papilledema and white spots in the macula in a unique configuration, giving this finding the name "macular star."

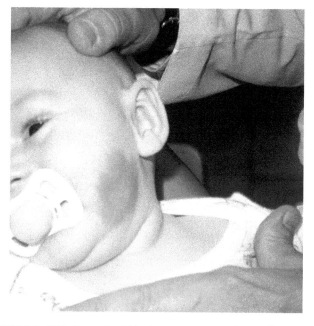

FIGURE 3.2 This 5-month-old had a temperature of 104.5°F and a hot, painful area of cellulitis on the cheek with well-demarcated borders characteristic of erysipelas. A blood culture grew group A β-hemolytic streptococcus.

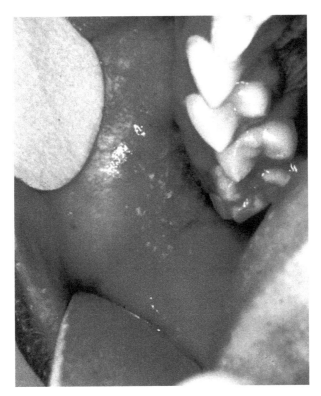

FIGURE 4.1 The Koplik spots with measles allow an early definitive diagnosis. They appear on the buccal mucosa opposite the upper and lower premolar teeth 24 to 48 hours before onset of the rash and may persist for 48 to 72 hours after the rash begins. If the spots are not present 24 hours before and after onset of the rash, the diagnosis of measles is unlikely.

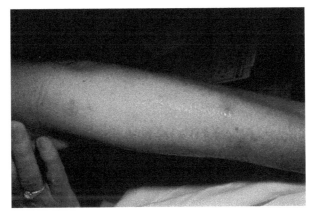

FIGURE 5.2 Rash of Mediterranean spotted fever caused by *Richettsia conorii*. This illness is usually brief and self-limited although the organism is closely related to the bacterium causing Rocky Mountain spotted fever.

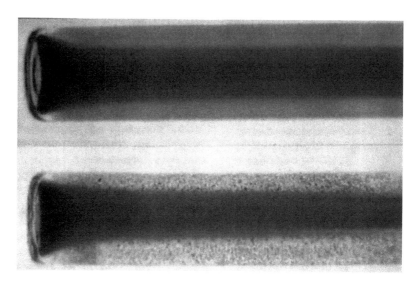

FIGURE 7.3 Agglutinated red blood cells in a sodium citrate anti-coagulation test tube that has been chilled in an ice bath are highly specific for *Mycoplasma pneumoniae* as the cause of pneumonia or other *Mycoplasma* infections.

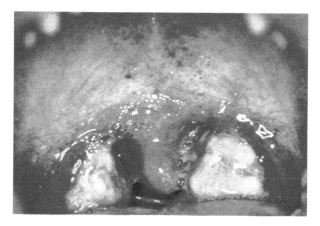

FIGURE 8.1 Tonsillopharyngitis with an exudative tonsillar membrane and palatal petechiae in an adolescent with a positive strep screen.

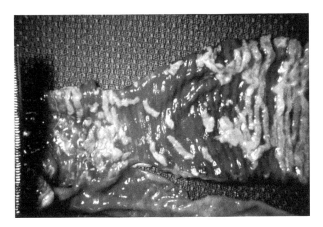

FIGURE 9.3 Pseudomembranous colitis with resulting peritonitis, shock and death in an infant on cephalothin. Autopsy specimen of the colon.

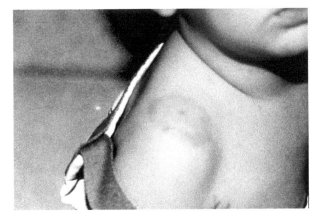

FIGURE 10.3 Erythema migrans rash at the site of a tick bite in an 18-month-old with acute Lyme disease. This lesion with central clearing measured 6×7 cm in diameter.

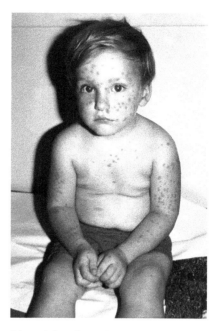

FIGURE 12.2 Gianotti-Crosti syndrome, also known as papular acro-dermatitis of childhood, is characterized by the rapid development of symmetrical flat-topped (lichenoid) skin-colored or erythematous papules in a centrifugal distribution.

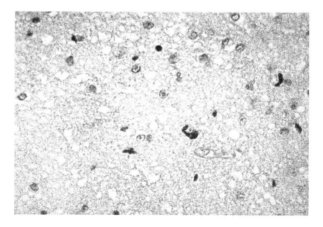

FIGURE 13.2 Brain biopsy in a 6-year-old showing scattered areas of cells containing cytoplasmic viral inclusions characteristic of herpes simplex encephalitis.

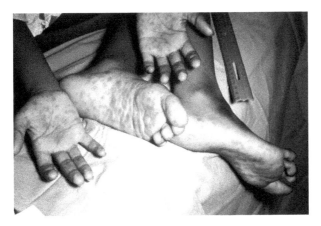

FIGURE 15.1 Secondary syphilis. Copper-colored papulosquamous rash including the palms and soles in this 9-year-old girl following sexual abuse.

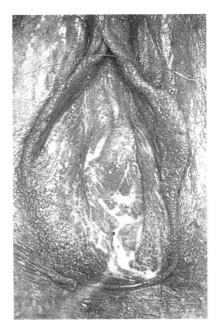

FIGURE 15.3 Bacterial vaginosis, also called nonspecific vaginitis, results from the overgrowth of *Gardnerella vaginalis* and/or anaerobes such as *Mobiluncus* species. The diagnosis is suggested by the presence of this homogenous discharge with a pH >4.5 and a positive amine odor test.

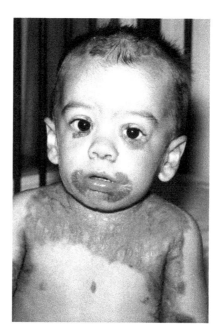

FIGURE 17.2 Chronic mucocutaneous candidiasis, an inherited defect of T cell and mononuclear phagocyte function, presents with persistent candidal infection of the mouth, scalp, skin, and nails.

9 | Gastrointestinal Infections

AMEBIASIS

Amebiasis is primarily an infection of the colon, caused by the protozoan parasite *Entamoeba histolytica*. The organism exists both in trophozoite and cyst forms. Small trophozoites are 10 to 20 µm in diameter and are not associated with invasiveness. Large forms are usually found in the presence of invasive disease and range from 20 to 60 µm in diameter. The presence of ingested red blood cells in the endoplasm of a large trophozoite is the most reliable morphologic feature in identifying the organism as *E. histolytica*. The cyst form measures 10 to 20 µm in diameter and contains between 1 and 4 nuclei (as contrasted with *Entamoeba coli* which contains 4 to 8). Cysts transmit disease and are resistant to drying, cold, and routine chlorination of water.

Entamoeba histolytica is more common in the United States than previously suspected. Its prevalence ranges from 1% in Alaska to 10% in southern states. Worldwide, it is more common in tropical and subtropical climates, and affects 10% of the world's population each year. There are approximately 3500 cases reported each year in the United States; it is estimated that an additional 40% of cases are undetected. Transmission is via the fecal-oral route following ingestion of contaminated water, raw fruit, or vegetables. Insects and flies have also been implicated and there is possible sexual transmission. Poor sanitation and crowding account for reported epidemics. More severe infection is seen in pregnant women, younger children, immunosuppressed patients, patients with AIDS, and patients on corticosteroid medications. The disease is more common in the third to fifth decade of life but occurrences in all ages, including neonates, have been reported.

The pathogenicity of the organism is related to its ability to attach to the colonic mucus layer and disrupt local immune mechanisms. Attachment may be aided by adherence proteins produced by *E. histolytica*. The organism has direct cytotoxic activity toward the intestinal cells as well as toward neutrophils, macrophages, and T cells.

Three forms of amebiasis exist (Table 1). Asymptomatic carriage of *E. histolytica* is most common and accounts for 90% of infections. Occasional vague symptoms such as abdominal

TABLE 1   Clinical Forms of Amebiasis

Asymptomatic carrier
Dysenteric form
Pain
Tenesmus
Diarrhea with blood and mucus
Fever
Abdominal distention
Extraintestinal form
Liver abscess(es)
Thoracic involvement
Cerebral abscess
Cutaneous (perineal)
Heart and pericardium
Larynx
Scapula
Stomach
Aorta

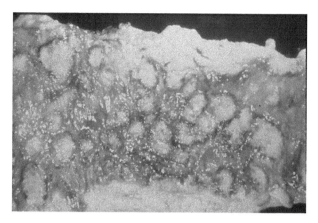

FIGURE 1   Severe colonic lesions of amebiasis with hemorrhagic rings around necrotic areas.

pain, fatigue, headache, or cough are observed but may not be related to the presence of ameba in the bowel. The incubation period is quite variable, 8 to 95 days and precedes invasion of the bowel mucosa to produce a dysenteric form. Progression of symptoms is usually gradual (over 3 to 4 weeks) and dysentery may not occur until later in the course. Abdominal pain and tenesmus are the most common symptoms. Infants may have a much more rapid and fulminant course with severe watery diarrhea and hematochezia. Blood is present in the stools in over 95% of patients. The leukocyte count is usually elevated with a shift to the left, but eosinophilia is absent.

Endoscopic examination of the colon reveals superficial ulcers surrounded by normal mucosa. A characteristic flask-shaped ulcer is seen in some patients. These ulcerations may then deepen and enlarge with the adjacent mucosa becoming hyperemic and friable (Fig. 1). Occasionally, granulation tissue without fibrosis (ameboma) forms. Complications of intestinal disease include necrotizing enterocolitis, toxic megacolon, perforation, abscess formation, stricture, and obstruction by amebomas.

Amebae spread to the liver via the portal circulation. Although less frequent than in adults, liver abscesses are the most common extra-intestinal form of amebiasis in children with invasive disease occurring in 1% to 7% of cases. This process is more fulminating in children. Hepatic involvement is 10 times more common in men than women; there is no difference between genders in prepubescent children. Approximately one-half of patients with amebic abscesses have no history of amebic colitis. The right lobe of the liver is more commonly involved than the left lobe and abscesses are usually solitary. Abscess fluid has been typically described as a reddish "anchovy paste" but can be white or green. Amebae are found in the walls of the abscess but rarely within the fluid. Little inflammatory reaction is evident in the abscess, which explains normal or minimally elevated liver transaminases.

Clinical symptoms of liver abscesses are abdominal pain, fever, and tender hepatomegaly. A non-productive cough, decreased diaphragmatic excursion, and pleural effusions may be found but jaundice is unusual. Intestinal disease is found in the majority of children with amebic liver abscesses. Laboratory values of infected patients include a normal or elevated leukocyte count and an invariably elevated sedimentation rate. Normochromic, normocytic, mild anemia may be present. Other extra-intestinal manifestations of amebiasis are thought to occur via spread from the liver. Extension into the thoracic cavity is the most common and occurs in 10% of patients with liver diseases.

Diagnosis of amebiasis is usually made by stool examination (Table 2). If a specimen cannot be processed within 30 minutes, then it should be put into a preservative (polyvinylalcohol or formalin). Identification of *E. histolytica* in stools can be difficult; a survey of public and private parasitology laboratories revealed that 20% were unable to identify trophozoites and 35% could not identify cysts. The cysts of *E. histolytica* resemble those of both *Entamoeba coli* and other non-pathologic forms of *Entamoeba*. Stained material

TABLE 2   Diagnosis of Amebiasis

Colonic involvement
    Examination of stool or mucus from
        bowel
    Biopsy of colonic ulcer
    Serology
Hepatic involvement
    Scintigraphy
    Computed tomography
    Ultrasound
    Serology

Note: Decisions for therapy and its duration are guided by location and severity of disease.

TABLE 3   Treatment of Amebiasis

Asymptomatic	Paromomycin 30 mg/kg/day PO div. q 8 hr ×
	    7–10 days (max. 1.5 g/day), iodoquinol
	    30–40 mg/kg/day PO div. q 8 hr × 20 days
	    (max. 650 mg q 8 hr), or diloxanide
	    20 mg/kg/day div q 8 hrs × 10 days

Intestinal	Metronidazole 35–50 mg/kg/day PO div. q
	    8 hrs × 10 days (max. 750 mg t.i.d.) or
	    tinidazole 50 mg/kg/day (max. 2 g) q ×
	    3 days followed by iodoquinol or
	    paromomycin (as above)

Extraintestinal	Same as intestinal except tinidazole × 5 days
Failed treatment of invasive disease: dehydroemetine as above	

obtained from mucus or scrapings of the base of an ulcer during endoscopic examination may also reveal the organism. Numerous serologic tests are also available. Most public health facilities use indirect hemagglutination, which is positive in 58% of asymptomatic patients, 61% of those with moderate involvement, and 95% with severe involvement. Almost 100% of patients with extra-intestinal amebiasis have positive antibody titers. Serology is less sensitive in newborns and young infants, even in the presence of severe extra-intestinal amebiasis. An elevated titer does not differentiate between acute or past infection and titers may remain positive from 6 months to 3 years after the acute infection. A high titer (≥1:512) is more suggestive of recent infection. Liver abscesses may be diagnosed by several methods including liver scans, computed tomography (CT), and ultrasound (Tables 2 and 3).

Most liver abscesses do not require needle aspiration. Drainage is indicated for subcapsular hepatic abscesses or abscesses of the left lobe as these can rupture into the pleural cavity or pericardium. If a liver abscess does not respond to medication, closed-needle aspiration under CT or ultrasound guidance may be necessary. If no response is seen, a laparotomy and open drainage should be performed. Other indications for surgery are perforation of the bowel or abscess formation if unresponsive to conservative therapy. Brain abscesses should be treated with early drainage through a burr hole and the abscess residua followed carefully by CT. If a response is not seen, more definitive surgery may be needed. Pericardial abscesses are treated by repeated needle aspirations. Antibiotics are only necessary in patients with secondary infection. Corticosteroids should not be given as this increases the severity of disease.

CAMPYLOBACTER

Campylobacter gastroenteritis has been identified as one of the leading bacterial infections of the gastrointestinal tract in children. The primary organism causing disease in children was formerly termed *Campylobacter fetus* subspecies *jejuni* but is currently referred to as *C. jejuni* (Table 4).

The incidence of intrafamilial spread of infection occurs at a much lower rate than would be expected. This is probably an indication that the organism is not viable for long periods outside of the body. Several instances of spread from animals to humans have also been recorded and include either direct contact and contamination from the animal or ingestion of contaminated meat that has been inadequately cooked.

Fever, diarrhea, and abdominal pain are the primary symptoms of *Campylobacter* infection (Table 5). Fever can be quite high and children may appear toxic. Hematochezia has been found in at least half of infected children and typically appears several days after onset of the illness. Abdominal pain may be so severe as to suggest an acute abdomen. Many patients complain of malaise and fatigue (especially in the recurrent form of the illness) and these may

TABLE 4   Clinical Characteristics of *Campylobacter*

Incubation period	1–10 days (mean 3–5 days)
Peak ages of infection	<1 year old Young adults
Transmission	Contaminated food and water Vertical transmission Person-to-person (family, daycare centers) Via animals (chickens, dogs, pigs, cats)
Duration of symptoms	7 days (mean), can be recurrent or chronic

TABLE 5   Symptoms of *Campylobacter* Infection

Fever
Headache
Diarrhea
Hematochezia
Abdominal pain
Malaise
Vomiting
Toxic appearance

be the only symptoms present between bouts of diarrhea. Vomiting is noted in approximately one-third of patients but is usually mild and does not result in dehydration.

There are several presentations of *Campylobacter* gastroenteritis, (Table 6) the most common being self-limited diarrhea lasting up to 1 week. Recurrent or chronic diarrhea can occur and *Campylobacter* has been implicated as a cause of traveler's diarrhea. *Campylobacter* may cause an exacerbation of symptoms in patients with previously diagnosed inflammatory bowel disease, resembling a relapse of their primary disease. Involvement of the gut can also result in toxic megacolon. Concomitant infection with *Salmonella*, *Shigella*, *Giardia*, and rotavirus has been documented.

The most common extra-intestinal manifestation of *Campylobacter* infection is reactive arthritis, which occurs more frequently in men with the HLA-B27 histocompatibility antigen (Table 7).

Diagnosis of *Campylobacter* by stool culture is relatively easy to perform with selective medium. Direct examination of the stool is usually positive for red blood cells and leukocytes. Dark-field or phase-contrast microscopic examination reveals the characteristic darting motion of the *C. jejuni* organism. A technique for staining stool smears with fuchsin has been shown to correlate well with stool cultures.

Treatment is not necessary for children with mild disease. Many patients are asymptomatic when the diagnosis by stool culture is made. Treatment beginning later than 4 days after onset of symptoms will not change the natural course of the disease. Studies evaluating treatment instituted prior to 4 days duration of illness have shown conflicting results. However, with treatment, stool cultures become negative within 72 hours; without treatment *Campylobacter* can be cultured from stool for up to several weeks. The incidence of intra-familial spread of *Campylobacter* is low, but antibiotics may be useful in a group setting such as a daycare center. If treatment is initiated, erythromycin or azithromycin is the drug of

TABLE 6   Gastrointestinal Manifestations of *Campylobacter* Infection

Recurrent or chronic diarrhea
Traveler's diarrhea
Colitis or enterocolitis
Ulcerative
Nodular (Crohn's-like)
Pseudomembranous
Massive gastrointestinal bleeding
Acute abdomen
Cholecystitis
Pancreatitis
Appendicitis
Mesenteric lymphadenitis
Exacerbation or inflammatory bowel disease
Toxic megacolon

TABLE 7   Extraintestinal Manifestations of *Campylobacter* Infection

Reiter's syndrome	Reactive arthritis
Guillain-Barré syndrome	Meningitis
	Urinary tract infection
Septic arthritis	Hemolytic uremic syndrome
Bacteremia	
Glomerulonephritis	Carditis

TABLE 8 Treatment of *Campylobacter* Infection[a]

Enteritis
PO: erythromycin or azithromycin $\times$ 5–7 days
Systemic
Intravenous aminoglycosides, meropenem, imipenem, and cephalosporins
guided by susceptibility tests
Alternatives
Doxycycline
Ciprofloxacin

[a] For dosage, see Tables 12 and 13.

choice in children and adults. For systemic infection, gentamicin may be added or substituted. Parenteral therapy is probably not needed for asymptomatic bacteremia, except in immunocompromised patients. Table 8 provides a summary of treatment for *Campylobacter* infection.

DIARRHEA AND DEHYDRATION

One of the most common diseases encountered in pediatrics is gastroenteritis, most episodes being mild and self-limited. Young infants are particularly vulnerable to dehydration as a consequence of diarrhea, and this may require hospitalization for rehydration and correction of acid-base or electrolyte disturbances. Acute infectious diarrheal illnesses may be caused by bacteria, viruses, or protozoa. Some of the more common causes of acute infectious diarrhea may be differentiated on clinical grounds (Table 9).

Treatment of diarrhea is predominantly supportive with correction of fluid and electrolyte abnormalities. Antibiotic therapy is recommended in some form of bacterial or protozoan diarrhea (see individual sections). Treatment of dehydration requires recognition of the type of dehydration present, as well as its severity.

ESCHERICHIA COLI

Escherichia coli is the most common coliform bacteria found in the bowel. Several strains are capable of producing enteric disease, and are classified according to their virulence, resulting symptoms, and epidemiology.

Virulence factors are found in plasmids, and each classification group has a characteristic mechanism by which it interacts with the intestinal mucosa. Antigens expressed by these

TABLE 9 Comparison of Clinical Findings in Acute Infectious Diarrhea

Finding	*Shigella*	*Salmonella*	*Campylobacter*	Rotavirus
Vomiting	Rare	Common	$\pm$	Common
Fever	Present	Variable	Present	Variable
Stool				
Volume	Small	Moderate	Moderate	Large
Consistency	Viscous	Slimy	Watery	Watery
Odor	Odorless	Foul	Foul	Odorless
Blood	$+++$	Variable	Common	$\pm$
Mucus	$+++$	Moderate	Variable	Absent
White blood cells	$+++$	$+++$	Present	$\pm$
Bronchitis	Common	Absent	$\pm$	$\pm$

$+++$, very common; $\pm$ uncommon.

bacteria are called O, H, and K antigens. O and H antigens are used to classify bacteria in the O H system of which there are approximately 180 O and 60 H currently identified serotypes.

Enterotoxigenic *E. coli* (ETEC) binds to mucosa in the small bowel and produces an enterotoxin which results in secretory diarrhea. It is a frequent cause of traveler's diarrhea and infant diarrhea in developing nations, but is rare in the United States. ETEC is acquired by ingestion of contaminated food or water, and causes nausea, watery diarrhea, abdominal pain, and mild fever. Traveler's diarrhea usually lasts for 4 to 5 days. Treatment with trimethoprim/sulfamethoxazole or ciprofloxacin for 5 days is usually adequate, but the disease is often mild and self-limited.

Enteropathogenic *E. coli* (EPEC) attaches to the intestinal mucosa and destroys its microvilli, yet it is not invasive and does not produce a toxin. EPEC causes watery diarrhea (chronic and acute), nausea, abdominal pain, vomiting, fever, malaise, and polymorphonuclear leukocytes in the stool. It is more severe in infants and has been implicated in outbreaks of diarrhea in nurseries. Treatment with trimethoprim/sulfamethoxazole may be helpful.

Enterohemorrhagic *E. coli* (EHEC) also attaches to the intestinal mucosa, but then produces cytotoxins. These result in the destruction of microvilli in a manner distinctive from EPEC. The most common serotype found is 0157:H7 which has been associated with several outbreaks in the United States (through contaminated beef which was improperly cooked). Cattle are the normal reservoir for this organism. Initial symptoms of EHEC are diarrhea, progressing to bloody diarrhea, abdominal pain, fever (low grade), and nausea. Severe cases result in hemorrhagic colitis and serotype 0157:H7 is associated with hemolytic syndrome (HUS), thrombotic thrombocytopenic purpura, and intussusception. Children less than 5 years of age are more commonly affected and more likely to develop HUS than older patients. The use of antimotility drugs and antibiotics may pre-dispose patients to developing HUS. The empiric administration of these agents for diarrhea of undetermined etiology should therefore be avoided. A vaccine to prevent *E. coli* 0157:H7 is in the early stages of development.

Enteroinvasive *E. coli* (EIEC) causes a dysenteric profile similar to that of *Shigella*. Colonic mucosal cells are invaded by EIEC, with proliferation of the bacteria and resulting cell death. Clinical findings are diarrhea with blood and mucus, abdominal pain, fever (often high), and a toxic appearance. A stool smear may reveal sheets of polymorphonuclear leukocytes and blood. Treatment recommendations are the same as for *Shigella* (see individual section).

Escherichia coli are grouped as enteroadherent (EAEC) according to their ability to adhere to Hep-2 cells in tissue culture. EAEC do not produce toxins nor invade the mucosa; their exact method of pathogenicity is not defined. They have been identified as a cause of chronic diarrhea in children, especially in developing nations. Treatment with neomycin (100 mg/kg/day for 5 days) may be useful.

The diagnosis of enteric *E. coli* infections can be difficult. Clinical information, such as recent travel to an underdeveloped nation or a dysenteric profile with a negative culture for *Shigella*, is useful. Other more easily identifiable enteropathogens should be looked for, and a stool smear for white blood cells performed. EPEC and EHEC do not ferment sorbitol and this observation is used to help identify these organisms. A sorbitol screen and definitive latex agglutination test for serotype OH:157 are readily available. EIEC does not ferment lactose, a finding that can aid its diagnosis. DNA probes are available for several types of *E. coli*. Serotyping is used primarily for epidemiologic studies (Table 10).

TABLE 10   Classification of Diarrheagenic *Escherichia coli*

Enterotoxigenic *Escherichia coli* (ETEC)
Enteropathogenic *Escherichia coli* (EPEC)
Enterohemorrhagic *Escherichia coli* (EHEC)
Enteroinvasive *Escherichia coli* (EIEC)
Enteroadherent *Escherichia coli* (EAEC)

TABLE 11   Epidemiologic Aspects of Food Poisoning

Organism	Pathogenesis	Source	Prevention
Salmonella	Infection	Meats, poultry, eggs, dairy products	Proper cooking and food handling pasteurization
Staphylococcus	Preformed enterotoxin	Meats, poultry, potato salad, cream-filled pastry, cheese, sausage	Careful food handling, rapid refrigeration
Clostridium perfringens	Enterotoxin	Meats, poultry	Avoid delay in serving foods, avoid cooling and re-warming foods
Clostridium botulinum	Preformed neurotoxin	Home-canned goods, uncooked foods	Proper refrigeration
Vibrio parahaemolyticus	Infection enterotoxin	Sea fish, seawater, shell-fish	Proper refrigeration
Bacillus cereus			
Vomiting type	Preformed toxin	Cooked or fried rice, vegetables, meats, cereal, puddings	Proper refrigeration of cooked rice and other foods
Diarrheal type	Sporulation enterotoxin	Many prepared foods	Proper refrigeration

FOOD POISONING

Bacterial food poisoning may be caused by a variety of organisms, the most common being *Salmonella* and *Staphylococcus aureus* (Table 11). At least 300 outbreaks of food-borne disease are reported each year with this likely to be 1% to 10% of the true figure. The majority of patients experience self-limited disease. Disease may be caused by ingestion of preformed toxin, elaboration of toxin into the gastrointestinal tract, or direct invasion of mucosa by organisms. Ingestion of preformed toxin is associated with a shorter incubation period. Most patients with food poisoning only require supportive therapy (Table 12), the major exception being botulism which represents a medical emergency (see Chapter 2).

GIARDIASIS

Giardia lamblia is second only to *Enterobius vermicularis* (pinworm) as the most common parasite found in the United States, but with the benign nature of pinworm infestation, *Giardia*

TABLE 12   Clinical Aspects of Food Poisoning

Organism	Incubation	Symptoms	Duration	Treatment
Salmonella	8–72 hrs average	Diarrhea (blood) abdominal pain, fever, chills nausea, vomiting	3–5 days	None unless severe or <3 mos of age
Staphylococcus	1–6 hrs	Severe vomiting, abdominal pain, diarrhea	6–8 hrs	None
Clostridium perfringens	8–24 hrs	Watery diarrhea crampy abdominal pain, nausea, vomiting rare	≤24 hrs	None
Clostridium botulinum	12–36 hrs	Nausea, vomiting diarrhea, dysphagia, dysarthria, muscle weakness, respiratory paralysis	Death within several days unless treated	Supportive
Vibrio parahaemolyticus	4–48 hrs	Severe watery diarrhea, abdominal cramps, nausea, vomiting fever, chills, can produce dysentery	2 hrs to 10 days	None
Bacillus cereus				
Vomiting type	1–6 hrs	Vomiting, abdominal pain	8–24 hrs	None
Diarrheal type	6–12 hrs	Diarrhea, abdominal pain, vomiting	20–36 hrs	None

TABLE 13 Clinical Symptoms of Giardiasis

No symptoms
or
Diarrhea (may be episodic)
Weight loss/failure to thrive
Anorexia
Vomiting
Abdominal cramps
Belching
Malodorous stools

is regarded as the most significant parasitic pathogen. Giardiasis is especially prevalent in day-care centers, institutional care facilities, areas with overcrowding, and in the tropics. Children are more often affected than adults with person-to-person transmission being most common. Infants and toddlers may be an important reservoir for infection as up to 50% are asymptomatic. Transmission may also occur through contaminated water and food. Prevalence rates in children attending day-care centers range from 17% to 90% with an average of 20% to 30%.

Clinical symptoms vary with age (Table 13); young children are more likely to be symptomatic.

Diagnosis of giardiasis is most readily achieved by antigen detection in stool using commercially available immunofluorescent and enzyme immunoassay techniques. These assays have a sensitivity of 92% and specificity of 98% for a single stool sample and have largely replaced microscopic identification. Direct examination of three stool samples by a laboratory with expertise in parasitology will establish the diagnosis in 85% of cases. Medications (such as antacids) or concurrent diagnostic testing (such as upper gastrointestinal radiographs with barium) may obscure these organisms. Detection of trophozoites (Fig. 2) requires examination of fresh stools (within 1 hour) or stools preserved in polyvinyl (PVA). Cysts are quite hardy and will survive at room temperature. However, as infection with more than one parasite is frequently encountered, fixatives to preserve both trophozoites and cysts allow for detection of other parasites. These tests also have the convenience of home collection of samples as the bottles containing fixatives can be mailed to the laboratory (Table 14).

Three medications are primarily used for treatment of *Giardia* infection, metronidazole, tinidazole, or nitazoxanide (Table 15). Alternatives include paromomycin, furazolidone, quinacrine, and albendazole. The major advantage of furazolidone is the liquid form. Many of these medications produce an antabuse-like effect, so those containing alcohol should not be

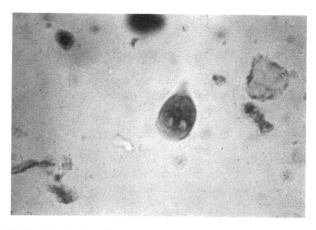

FIGURE 2 *Giardia lamblia* trophozoite in a fresh stool specimen.

TABLE 14 Diagnosis of Giardiasis

Antigen in stool—enzyme immunoassay (EIA)
Stool examination (fresh or with fixatives) with direct fluorescent antibody
Duodenal fluid examination
EnteroTest capsule[a]
Direct aspiration of small bowel
Biopsy of duodenum or jejunum
Serology—antibodies to *Giardia*

[a] Health Development Corporation, Palo Alto, California, U.S.A.

given concomitantly. Quinacrine and metronidazole must be compounded into solution and have a bitter taste. Persistent symptoms after therapy may indicate small bowel overgrowth or incomplete eradication of the pathogen requiring a second course of medication.

HELICOBACTER

Gastric infections with *Helicobacter pylori* has been associated with gastritis, duodenal ulcer disease, and gastric ulcers. The organism is a multiflagellate, unipolar, spiral bacteria. It can assume a dormant coccoid form in unfavorable environments making it more resistant to eradication. *Helicobacter pylori* is more often found in developing countries. However, some areas of the United States have similar prevalence rates. In the United States, prevalence in healthy adults is 20% to 45% and 4% to 31% in children. Many factors influence these rates including age, race, ethnicity, and occupation (Table 16).

Transmission is thought to be via the fecal-oral route (person-to-person and possibly by contaminated food or water). Humans are the only natural host and there is no known animal reservoir.

TABLE 15 Treatment of Giardiasis

Drug	Dosage
Metronidazole	15 mg/kg/day PO div. q 8 hr for 5 days (max. 750 mg/day)
Nitazoxanide	1–3 yr: 100 mg q 12 hr × 3 days
	4–11 yr: 200 mg q 12 hr × 3 days
Tinidazole	50 mg/kg PO single dose (max. 2 g)
Alternatives:	
Paromomycin	25–35 mg/kg/day div. q 8 hr × 7 days
Furazolidone	6–8 mg/kg/day PO div. q 6 hr for 7–10 days (max. 400 mg/ day)
Quinacrine	6 mg/kg/day PO div. q 8 hr for 5 days (max. 300 mg/day)
Albendazole	7–10 mg/kg/day div. qd × 5 day

TABLE 16 Epidemiologic Factors Associated with *Helicobacter pylori*

Increasing age
Lower family income
Family member in home with *Helicobacter pylori*
Patients in institutions for the mentally retarded
Contaminated water supplies
Meat handlers
Doctors and nurses involved in endoscopy
Black races
Hispanic ethnic groups

TABLE 17   Clinical Disease Associated with Helicobacter Infection

Gastritis and gastric erosions (primarily of antrum and fundus)
Atrophic gastritis
Antral nodularity in children
Nonulcerative dyspepsia
Duodenal ulcers and duodenitis
Gastric cancer

TABLE 18   Diagnosis of Helicobacter Infection

Serology by ELISA (IgG and IgA)
^{13}C or ^{14}C urea breath tests
Stool antigen
Histology of gastric biopsy with Giemsa stain or Warthin-Starry silver stain
Culture of gastric biopsy
Rapid urease test

Gastric and duodenal inflammation results from infection by the organism, but the exact mechanism is undetermined. *Helicobacter pylori* produces several enzymes which may allow penetration into the gastric mucosa. It also produces urease which converts urea (present in the gastric epithelium) to ammonia and bicarbonate. This raises the pH around the organism and allows back diffusion of H^+ ions into the mucosa resulting in epithelial damage. *Helicobacter pylori* is found almost exclusively in gastric mucosa, including areas of gastric metaplasia in the duodenum or esophagus.

The extent to which *H. pylori* causes disease (Table 17) is still under investigation. Colonization does not uniformly result in development of peptic disease; however, infected adults and children have a much higher incidence of duodenal ulcers and gastritis. It also appears that colonization may more frequently result in upper gastrointestinal pathology in children than in adults.

Approximately, 90% to 100% of adults with duodenal ulcers and 60–90% with gastric ulcers are found to have *H. pylori*. Children with peptic disease are less likely than adults to have *H. pylori* isolated. In reported studies, about 50% of children with gastritis and 60% with duodenitis were found to be colonized. Symptoms of peptic disease associated with *H. pylori* do not differ from that without the organism.

Diagnosis can be made by several methods, including serologic testing (Table 18). In an untreated patient, high titers of antibody to *H. pylori* are likely to represent current infection. Titers usually decline after treatment but may be slow to fall and difficult to interpret. A positive ^{14}C test urea breath test is present only with infection; however, these tests are not readily available and the ^{14}C test causes low radiation exposure. Other methods are invasive and require endoscopy. However, many patients with gastrointestinal symptoms and suspected infection will undergo endoscopy during evaluation of their symptoms. Histologic stains of the gastric mucosa, usually the antrum, or biopsy culture are sensitive and specific. The rapid ^{14}C urea breath test is less expensive and has excellent ability to detect the organism.

Treatment protocols are still a matter of discussion and research. Most often, patients are treated with a combination of a proton pump inhibitor and two antibiotics for 14 days (Table 19).

HEPATITIS

The clinical presentation of jaundice, following a prodrome of anorexia, nausea, vomiting, and right upper quadrant pain, suggests a diagnosis of acute hepatitis and dictates a serologic evaluation for etiology (Table 20). Hepatitis is often asymptomatic in children, particularly hepatitis C in all ages and hepatitis A in infants under 18 months of age.

Hepatitis A virus (HAV) is the most common cause of hepatitis in children in the United States. Transmission through the fecal-oral route often occurs in daycare centers, school, institutional settings, and among household members. The incubation period is 30 days and the virus is excreted for 1 week before clinical symptoms occur. Patients often remain anicteric but other symptoms last approximately 2 weeks. The presence of anti-HAV IgM confirms the diagnosis. Treatment is supportive, although acute fulminant hepatitis can occur. Patients with hepatitis A may be contagious for as long as 1 week after the onset of jaundice. Chronic liver disease does not occur. Universal immunization with hepatitis A vaccine is now recommended

TABLE 19   Treatment of Helicobacter Infection

Clarithromycin 15 mg/kg/day PO div. b.i.d. (max. 1 g) + *either* amoxicillin 40 mg/kg/day PO div. q 8 hr (max. 1.5 g/day) or metronidazole 20 mg/kg/day PO div. q 8 hr (max. 1.5 g/day) + proton pump inhibitor (lansoprazole, omeprazole, esomeprazole, rabeprazole, or pantoprazole).

Alternatives:
Metronidazole (as above) + tetracycline 40 mg/kg/day PO div. q 6 hr (max. 2 g/day) + bismuth subsalicylate 2 tablets PO q 6 hr (1 tablet or liquid for smaller children) + either a protein pump inhibitor or an H$_2$ blocker (cimetidine, famotidine, nizatidine, or ranitidine) for 3 weeks.

TABLE 20   Differential Etiology of Hepatitis

Hepatitis, A, B, C, D, E
Epstein-Barr virus
Cytomegalovirus
Leptospirosis
Noninfectious
    Drug induced (INH, erythromycin)
    Obstructive jaundice

with the initial dose given at 12 months of age followed by a second dose 6 to 12 months later. Older children and adults should receive the 2 dose vaccine as soon as possible (see Chapter 4).

Hepatitis B virus (HBV) infection is less common in the United States but endemic in many parts of the world, particularly Southeast Asia. Prior to the routine use of vaccine, approximately 300,000 new cases of hepatitis B occurred each year in the United States. Transmission occurs by percutaneous exposure to contaminated blood, through sexual transmission, and vertically from mother to child. The incubation period is 60 to 180 days. Serologic testing detects various parts of the virus which include: HBsAg (inner core antigen), HBeAg (a non-structural core antigen which indicates replication), and DNA polymerase (a DNA repair enzyme that indicates replication). Antibodies to Hbc and Hbs are found at a later stage of infection, and the patient has eliminated the virus when antibodies to Hbs appear. Infection with HBV can also be confirmed by polymerase chain reaction (PCR) detection of hepatitis B DNA. Individuals with hepatitis B are infective while they are seropositive for HBsAg or have antibodies to Hbc but lack antibody to HB. Chronic hepatitis B occurs in <5% of adult infections, but in 50% of children with infection acquired during the first year of life, and in 80% to 90% of perinatal infections. Chronic liver disease consists of chronic antigenemia, chronic persistent hepatitis, chronic active hepatitis, cirrhosis, and hepatocellular carcinoma. Interferon α-2b and peginterferon α-2a are approved for treatment of adults with chronic HBV infection, but have not been adequately studied in children. Recommendations for HB vaccine in high-risk groups and for childhood immunization are reviewed in Chapter 4.

Hepatitis C virus (HCV) infection is an increasing concern in the United States but the incidence has been significantly reduced following the routine screening of blood donors. The use of intravenous drugs of abuse now account for the majority of new cases with a smaller number resulting from sexual and perinatal transmission.

The incubation period is 6 to 12 weeks. A pattern of fluctuating liver transaminases is common. An enzyme linked immunosorbent assay (ELISA) test is used for screening to identify antibody to the virus while confirmation of ongoing infection is determined with a RIBA (recombinant immunoblot assay) or PCR. Our understanding of the clinical course of HCV is incomplete, but it appears that chronic infection is very common and progression to cirrhosis or hepatocellular carcinoma may be high. Treatment with a combination of interferon α-2b and oral ribavirin is available for chronic active hepatitis but results are variable. Because this therapy is largely investigational in children, patients should be managed by experienced pediatric gastroenterologists.

Hepatitis D virus (delta, HDV) is a defective virus that only coinfects with HBV. It is endemic in the Middle east and Mediterranean areas and seen epidemically in other parts of the world. HDV infection is more commonly associated with fulminant or chronic hepatitis B. Serologic markers include anti-HDV IgM and IgG, HDAg, and HDV RNA.

Hepatitis E virus (HEV) is transmitted by the fecal–oral route via contaminated water or food. It is more common in North Africa, Asia, India, and Russia. The incubation period is approximately 6 weeks and clinical symptoms are usually mild except in pregnant women where mortality may be as high as 20%. Diagnosis can be made by testing for IgM and IgG anti-HEV or by identification of viral RNA in serum or stool with a PCR assay.

The serologic markers available to detect many forms of hepatitis are given in Table 21. Etiologic diagnosis is made by serologic evaluation and should be accomplished rapidly so that decisions for prophylactic administration of hepatitis A or B vaccine or hyperimmune human immunoglobulin (for HBV) to family members can be made (see Chapter 4). If a delay in laboratory testing is anticipated, family members should receive hepatitis A vaccine because this is inexpensive and must be given early to protect against HAV.

Therapy for patients with acute hepatitis is supportive and can be managed at home. Indications for hospital admission include intractable vomiting, an elevated prothrombin time, and altered neurologic status. While contagious, patients should be advised as to stool and/or blood precautions and sexual transmission of disease.

PSEUDOMEMBRANOUS COLITIS

Pseudomembranous colitis (PMC) is an inflammatory condition of the colon associated with antibiotic use. The etiology has been determined to be *Clostridium difficile* toxin.

Virtually all antibiotics have been associated with PMC. In children, more cases have been reported following administration of ampicillin or amoxicillin, but this probably reflects the widespread use of these antibiotics and their broad-spectrum coverage. The route (parenteral, enteral, and topical antibiotic use), dose, and length of treatment for the antibiotic are not related to the development of PMC.

The diarrhea associated with PMC is usually of rapid onset and patients may experience 10 to 20 stools per day, although children tend to have less severe diarrhea. At least half of patients have blood and/or fecal leukocytes in the stool. Abdominal pain and tenderness can occur and may mimic an acute abdomen. Fever, anorexia, nausea, and vomiting are also part of the symptom complex (Table 22).

The onset of disease is usually within 4 to 10 days of initiation of antibiotics. Onset has occurred within 4 h of starting an antibiotic, and as late as 10 weeks after stopping the antibiotic. At least one-third of these patients have onset of disease after the antibiotic has been stopped. The exact incidence of PMC is unknown, but it appears to be less common in children than in adults.

Diagnosis is usually established by testing the stool for the presence of *C. difficile* toxin or by endoscopic examination of the colon. The distribution of PMC is predominately in the descending and sigmoid colon and rectum, and is easily viewed by colonoscopy or flexible

TABLE 21 Serologic Diagnosis of Acute Hepatitis

Hepatitis A virus	Anti-HAV IgM
Hepatitis B virus	HBs Ag, anti-HBcIgM
Hepatitis C virus	Anti-HCV (ELISA)
Epstein-Barr virus	Heterophil test; anti-VCA, anti-EA, anti-EBNA for younger children
Cytomegalovirus (CMV)	Anti-CMV IgM

Abbreviations: EA, early antigen; EBNA, Epstein-Barr nuclear antigen; VCA, viral capsis antigen.

TABLE 22 Clinical and Laboratory Findings in Pseudomembranous Colitis

Symptoms
  Watery stools
  Hematochezia
  Fever
  Tenesmus
  Nausea and vomiting
  Anorexia
  Abdominal pain and tenderness
  Dehydration
  Toxic megacolon
  Perforation of the bowel
Laboratory findings
  Guaiac-positive stools
  Fecal leukocytes
  Elevated white blood cells with elevation of
      polymorphonuclear leukocytes

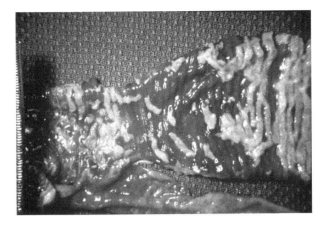

FIGURE 3 (*See color insert.*) Pseudomembranous colitis with resulting peritonitis, shock and death in an infant on cephalothin. Autopsy specimen of the colon.

sigmoidoscopy. Pseudomembranous colitis has a characteristic profile of raised, well-circumscribed lesions (Fig. 3). Toxin is present in 97% to 100% of patients with endoscopic evidence for PMC. *Clostridium difficile* produces two toxins: toxin A, an enterotoxin that causes colitis and toxin B, which is less enterotoxic. Newer ELISA techniques detect both toxin A or B, and a cell culture cytotoxicity assay is preferred for toxin B detection. Because toxin is present in about 25% of infants <1 year of age, interpretation of results is difficult in this age group. Stool cultures are of little diagnostic use because asymptomatic colonization with this organism is common, particularly in neonates and infants.

General supportive care with fluids are important aspects of treatment (Table 23). Antiperistaltic medications should not be used as they may prolong colonization with *C. difficile*. If the patient is hospitalized, simple isolation or enteric precautions should be observed. If possible, the offending antibiotic should be discontinued and in one-third to one-half of cases this is the only intervention necessary. Oral metronidazole and vancomycin are effective in the elimination of *C. difficile* for patients who do not respond to simple discontinuation of the offending antibiotic. However, drugs used in the therapy of PMC are efficacious even when used concurrently with the offending antibiotic. Drugs may be given intravenously in the presence of an ileus or in patients who are critically ill. Oral vancomycin is minimally absorbed and very effective for treatment of PMC but is expensive, and induces antibiotic resistance, particularly among *Enterococci*. For mild to moderate forms of PMC metronidazole is usually adequate. Cholestyramine has also been used to bind the toxin in mild cases of the disease.

The relapse rate is 12% to 20% and usually begins 4 to 20 days after the initial treatment. Clinically, the patients experience the same signs and symptoms as during their initial bout of PMC. *Clostridium difficile* and its toxin can again be isolated, even though during the period between initial treatment and relapse they may not have been detectable. Patients who have

TABLE 23   Treatment of Pseudomembranous Colitis

Fluids, supportive care
Avoidance of antiperistaltic medications
Discontinue offending antibiotic
Simple isolation
If diarrhea persists after stopping antibiotics or disease is severe:
Metronidazole 30 mg/kg/day (max. 2 g) PO div. q 6 hr for 10 days
Vancomycin 40 mg/kg/day (max. 2 g) PO div. q 8 hr for 10 days should only
be considered for patients who have not improved with metronidazole

diverticulitis or who are granulocytopenic are more likely to relapse. The ability of the organism to undergo sporulation is probably the most important factor in relapse as the spore form is less sensitive to antibiotics and therefore may not be eradicated with treatment. Reinfection from the environment is also a possibility as *C. difficile* can readily be cultured in the room of patients hospitalized for PMC. It also can be found in their home environment and on the hands of hospital personnel. *Clostridium difficile* inoculated into a carpet can be recovered for up to 5 months and is resistant to many routine methods of cleaning.

Treatment for relapse involves a second course of antibiotics at the original dosage but continues for a longer duration, generally 2 to 3 weeks. Use of foods or preparations containing *Lactobacillus* can help suppress the growth of *C. difficile*. Also, vancomycin can be used at one-half of the original dose or on an alternate day schedule. This allows regrowth or normal bowel flora while suppressing the growth of *C. difficile*, which is extremely sensitive to vancomycin. In Europe, *Saccharomyces boulardii*, a non-pathogenic yeast which may be taken in capsule form, has been used to help prevent the growth of *C. difficile*.

ROTAVIRUS

Rotavirus is most common in infants, accounting for up to one-half of all cases of viral gastroenteritis. Rotavirus strains are divided into 7 antigentic groups A–G, with group A being responsible for the majority of human infections. There are also subgroups and serotypes within this grouping system. Rotavirus is an RNA virus with two outer layers which contain antigens detectable by immunologic techniques. These glycoprotein antigens allow classification of the rotavirus into subgroup types. Polyacrylamide gel electrophoresis patterns can also separate rotavirus strains and are used in epidemiological studies.

Rotavirus is spread by the fecal–oral route. Children can have asymptomatic shedding of the virus which enhances its spread. A respiratory route of infection has been postulated.

Rotavirus may be a clinically significant infection in young infants while older children are less severely affected. As infants are more likely to have both vomiting and diarrhea, dehydration is common. Patients may also become intolerant of their formula secondary to disaccharidase deficiency or protein intolerance. Up to 13% of hospitalized patients with rotavirus infection have another infectious agent identified (e.g., *Salmonella* or *Shigella*) Tables 24 and 25 provide clinical aspects of rotavirus infection.

Diagnosis of a rotavirus infection is usually made by detection of the virus (antigen) in the stool. Several commercial kits, using ELISA or latex agglutination methodologies, are available and are the most clinically applicable. Other techniques include electron microscopy, immunoelectron microscopy, and antibody titers performed by several methods.

TABLE 24   Clinical Aspects of Rotavirus Gastroenteritis

Incubation	48–72 hrs
Seasonality	Winter
Peak age of illness	6–24 months
Transmission	Fecal-oral, possibly respiratory
Duration of illness	5–8 days
Diagnostic tests	ELISA, latex agglutination

TABLE 25   Clinical Signs and Symptoms of Rotavirus Infection

Signs and symptoms
  Foul smelling stools
  Vomiting
  Diarrhea
  Fever
  Dehydration (usually isotonic)
  Pharyngeal redness
  Rhinitis
  Otitis media
  Irritability
Complications
  Intussusception
  Necrotizing enterocolitis
  Sudden infant death syndrome

Treatment is symptomatic and usually based upon correction or maintenance of body fluid balance. A live, oral, pentavalent vaccine that contains 5 live re-assortment rotaviruses is now available and recommended for routine administration to infants (see Chapter 4).

SALMONELLOSIS

Salmonella sp. are pathogens which commonly cause bacterial gastroenteritis in children. Although there are over 2000 serotypes, 10 of these account for approximately two-thirds of total isolates. Clinically, *Salmonella* sp. are divided into those strains that cause enteric fever, such as *S. typhi*, *S. paratyphi A*, *S. paratyphi B*, and *S. cholerae-suis*, and those more commonly associated with other forms of disease (Table 26).

Gastroenteritis is the most common form and accounts for most *Salmonella* infections in the United States. In other countries, enteric fever (typhoid) is more common as *S. typhi* is the predominant species. Bacteremia tends to occur in the young and the old, with approximately 40% of cases arising in children under 5 years of age. Neonates account for the highest proportion of this group, despite breast feeding providing protection against salmonellosis. Localized infections (Table 27) are frequently due to *S. cholerae-suis*.

A chronic carrier state can also occur. This predominantly occurs following enteric fever in adults with gallbladder disease. One study demonstrated that a chronic carrier state (defined as excretion for over 1 year) was seen in 2.6% of patients who were infected with nontyphi *Salmonella*. Most chronic carriers were under 5 years of age (Table 28).

Salmonella may be introduced into food by a food handler or processor. It is resistant to mild refrigeration, and thus, undercooked food is a potential source of contamination and transmission of the disease.

Symptoms can begin quite abruptly (Tables 28 and 29). The distal small bowel and colon are the predominant sites of involvement. Salmonellae invade the lamina propria, induce an inflammatory reaction and release of prostaglandins; this stimulates cyclic AMP, which in itself causes secretory diarrhea. An endotoxin of *Salmonella* can be isolated but may not be associated with the pathogenesis of disease. The damage to cells is not as extensive as with *Shigella*, and thus, the resulting colitis and enteritis are not as destructive. The organism is limited to the superficial layers of the gut mucosa; therefore, normal mechanisms of elimination allow clearance of *Salmonella* in a rapid manner.

Salmonella gastroenteritis is, in general, a self-limited disease. However, there are several conditions that may influence its ability to cause sepsis or other complications (Table 30).

Because neonates and infants under 3 months of age are more prone to sepsis and meningitis than other age groups, a 14-day course of antibiotics is recommended for this group. Patients with sickle cell anemia have a higher incidence of osteomyelitis due to *Salmonella*. The ability of *Salmonella* to cause extra-intestinal and focal infections is partly dependent upon the state of the host, the species of *Salmonella* involved, and the inoculum dose. Studies of febrile children in emergency departments have documented *Salmonella* in as many as 10% of blood cultures. There is no clear evidence that the clinical course for patients

TABLE 26   Clinical Forms of Salmonellosis

Gastroenteritis
Enteric fever
Bacteremia/occult bacteremia
Localized infection
Chronic carrier

TABLE 27   Focal Infections of Salmonellosis

Meningitis	Abdominal abscess
Brain abscess and empyema	Cholecytitis
Prosthetic valve encodarditis	Salpingitis
Endocarditis	Urinary tract infection
Pericarditis	Arthritis
Mycotic aneurysm	Osteomyelitis
Myocardial abscess	Reiter's syndrome
Septic thrombophlebitis	Pharyngeal abscess
Necrotizing enterocolitis	Pneumonia and empyema
Appendicitis	Endophthalmitis

TABLE 28   Characteristics of Salmonella Gastroenteritis

Incubation	8–72 hrs
Seasonality	Warm weather
Transmission	Via food, animals, marijuana, fomites, flies, insects, person-to-person
Sites of involvement	Distal small bowel, colon
Duration of symptoms	2–7 days

TABLE 29   Symptoms and Laboratory Findings in *Salmonella* Gastroenteritis

Symptoms
  Diarrhea
  Fever >102°F
  Abdominal pain
  Abdominal distension
  Vomiting
  Constitutional symptoms
  Tenesmus
  Hematochezia
Laboratory findings
  Elevated white blood cell count
  Guaiac-positive stools
  Polymorphonuclear leukocytes in stool smears (85%)
  Positive stool culture

with *Salmonella* gastroenteritis and positive blood cultures is different from those with negative blood cultures, but most experts still recommend antibiotics for blood culture positive cases.

Although gastroenteritis and localized infections are by far the most common forms of salmonellosis, enteric fever still occurs in the United States (Table 31). The term 'typhoid fever' has been mostly abandoned since organisms other than *S. typhi* can cause identical symptoms.

Salmonella typhi is somewhat unique in that there is no natural host in nature other than humans. The main route of transmission is via food or water contaminated by human fecal material. There are some instances of possible transmission by insect vectors; however, this has not been firmly established.

There are four phases of typhoid fever. The first is a flu-like illness, during which the patient may also have symptoms of gastroenteritis. The second phase reflects multisystem invasion by the organism. Patients show encephalopathic changes, bronchitis, and evidence of reticuloendothelial system involvement with hepatosplenomegaly and lymphadenopathy. Relative bradycardia usually occurs during this period, which begins approximately 2 to 3 weeks after ingestion of the organism. High fever may be seen and without treatment can persist for 2 to 3 weeks. Due to gastrointestinal involvement, perforation or hemorrhage is a risk. If the disease does not abate, a third phase is entered, during which metastatic phenomena such as myocarditis occur. The fourth phase is the carrier state which occurs in approximately 3% of patients. The presence of gallbladder disease markedly enhances the chances of becoming a chronic carrier. Chronic carriage is more common in adult women, but this may be related to the fact that gallbladder disease is more common in this group.

Diagnosis of enteric fever is made on clinical grounds, serologic measurement (*Salmonella* O and H antibodies), and cultures. During the initial phases of enteric fever, stool cultures may be positive; however, there is an increasing yield from the stool culture

TABLE 30   Factors Associated with Severe Salmonellosis

Age below 3 mos
Decreased gastric acidity
Stress (cold, malnutrition)
Antibiotics
Depressed immune function
Hemolysis

TABLE 31   Enteric Fever in Salmonellosis

Organism	*Salmonella typhi* and paratyphoid strains
Transmission	Via human reservoirs, contaminated food or water, insect vectors
Seasonality	All
Incubation	3–56 days (mean 10 days)
Symptoms	Fever, headache, chills, diarrhea, vomiting, abdominal pain, cough
Signs	Rose spots, hepatosplenomegaly, neurologic signs, relative bradycardia

TABLE 32 Indications for Treatment of *Salmonella* Gastroenteritis

Infants under 3 mos of age
Toxic or severe disease
Bacteremia
Immunodeficiency (acquired, primary, or secondary)
Malignancy
Patients on immunosuppressive medications

TABLE 33 Treatment of Salmonellosis

Clinical form	Treatment
Gastroenteritis (if indicated)	Ampicillin 100 mg/kg/day PO or IV div. q.i.d. 7 (max. 6 g) for 5–7 days
	Amoxicillin 40 mg/kg/day PO div. t.i.d. for 5–7 days
	Trimethoprim/sulfamethoxazole 10 mg/kg/day TMP/50 mg/kg/day SMX PO div. b.i.d. (max. 320 mg TMP/1600 mg SMX) for 5–7 days
Enteric fever Bacteremia or HIV	Ceftriaxone 50–75 mg/kg/day × 14 days
	Cefotaxime 200 mg/kg/day IV div. b.i.d. (max. 12 g) for 14 days
	Trimethoprim/sulfamethoxazole 20 mg/kg/day TMP/100 mg/kg/day SMX PO or IV div. b.i.d. (max. 320 TMP/1600 mg SMX) for 14 days
	Ciprofloxacin 20–30 mg/kg/day PO div. b.i.d. (max. 1.5 g)
Localized or focal infection	As directed by infectious process and location.

between 3 and 4 weeks of disease. Initially, blood cultures are positive in 80% to 90% of patients. Other sites that can be cultured are bone marrow and rose spot biopsies. Antibody titers for febrile agglutinins become positive after the first week of illness.

Salmonella gastroenteritis is not usually treated as antibiotics are ineffective in improving the course and may prolong excretion of the organism. However, there are specific instances when treatment is indicated (Table 32). These include patients who are highly prone to invasive disease or already have established severe disease.

Ampicillin, amoxicillin, chloramphenicol, and trimethoprim/sulfamethoxazole are all effective for susceptible organisms (Table 33). Amoxicillin or trimethoprim/sulfamethoxazole are the drugs of choice but selection is dependent upon local sensitivities. Third generation cephalosporins and ciprofloxacin, for patients over 18 years of age, are also effective against most strains of *Salmonella*. Patients with AIDS or altered immunity are best treated with ampicillin or a third generation cephalosporin. Eradication of the chronic carrier state is often unsuccessful even after 4 to 6 weeks of therapy.

Detection of *Salmonella* in stool cultures following therapy does not necessitate a second course of treatment unless the patient remains symptomatic. The local public health department should be notified of all cases of *Salmonella* infection.

SHIGELLOSIS

Shigella is a nonmotile gram-negative rod. It has 32 serotypes divided into four groups: group A, *Shigella dysenteriae*; group B, *S. flexneri*; group C, *S. boydii*; and group D, *S. sonnei*. In the United States and many developed nations *S. sonnei* is responsible for the majority of gastrointestinal infections. Virulence is related to genetically determined properties that allow the organism to invade gastrointestinal cells, multiply within a cell, escape from host defenses, and spread from cell to cell. Plasmids code for proteins on the organism's outer membrane, permitting these activities by the bacteria.

Toxins also contribute to pathogenicity. The toxin of *S. dysenteriae* (the most intensely studied) is an exotoxin and produces transudation of fluid in ileal loops of experimental animals. It is also a cytotoxin, inducing cell death by suppression of cell protein synthesis. Damage to intestinal villus cells inhibits sodium and water absorption and leads to accumulation of fluid in the intestinal lumen.

Transmission of *Shigella* occurs via the fecal-oral route. Humans are the major reservoir for this bacteria and, unlike other enteric pathogens, only a very small number of organisms

(200) are needed to produce disease. Contaminated food and water are the primary sources associated with epidemics of shigellosis; however, houseflies may also transmit disease. *Shigella* can be cultured from toilet seats for up to 17 days postinoculation. There may be asymptomatic carriers that contribute to spread of the disease.

The incubation period of *Shigella* is 1 to 3 days and the duration of illness, if uncomplicated, is 3 to 7 days. There is an increased incidence during winter months in the United States, but in other countries, more cases are reported during hot, dry weather. The majority of patients are under 10 years of age with a peak incidence at 2 years (Table 34).

In children, the diarrhea is watery and voluminous with blood usually noted 24 to 48 hours after initial symptoms (Table 35). Stool volume may then decrease with a frequent stooling pattern. Respiratory symptoms and fever are prominent features. Endoscopic examination of the colon reveals intense inflammation with crypt abscesses most prominent in the rectum and decreasing proximally. In severe dysentery, a pseudomembrane can be seen.

There are several culture media able to support the growth of *Shigella*. Stool specimens should be plated as soon as possible to achieve optimum results. The stool smear typically shows a large amount of white blood cells with predominant polymorphonuclear leukocytes and bands. Leukocytosis is also seen with the band count greater than the neutrophil count in 32% to 85% of patients. A high absolute band count may also be seen with *Campylobacter* and *Salmonella* infection.

There are many complications of shigellosis (Table 36) primarily associated with *S. dysenteriae*. Dehydration can be seen with any of the *Shigella* species. Protein loss in stools can contribute to the development of clinically significant malnutrition in the child with a marginal premorbid nutritional state. Hemolytic uremic syndrome with progression to renal failure can develop, usually after 1 week of clinical disease when the patient may have shown improvement.

The incidence of bacteremia is quite low but clinical sepsis with shigellosis ranges from 0.6% to 7%. The majority of children affected are under 5 years of age and there is 35% to 50% morality with bacteremia. Children with bacteremia more frequently present with dehydration, are afebrile, and malnourished. Blood cultures are most often positive during the first 2 days of disease. Another complication is seizures, which are associated with all species of *Shigella*. Seizure incidence varies from 10% to 45% in children up to 7 years of age. The mechanism for the seizure is most likely fever related and not a neurotoxin as previously thought.

There is presently a high incidence of ampicillin resistance among isolates of *Shigella*. Drug selection therefore, depends on local sensitivities to ampicillin and trimethoprim/ sulfamethoxazole (Table 38); however, some isolates have become resistant to both of these

TABLE 34 *Shigella* Gastroenteritis

Incubation	1–3 days
Seasonality	Varies depending upon worldwide location
Age of illness	Before 10 years of age (peak at 2 years)
Transmission	Person-to-person, food, water, housefly
Site of involvement	Colon (primarily distal segment)
Duration of illness	3–7 days

TABLE 35 Clinical Signs and Symptoms of *Shigella* Infection

Symptoms
    Watery stools (10–25 times per day)
    Blood and mucus in stools
    Abdominal cramps and tenesmus
    Fever
    Malaise
    Anorexia
Laboratory findings
    Blood and WBCs in stool smear
    Guaiac-positive stools
    Leukocytosis with increased absolute band count
    Positive stool culture
    Protein loss in stools

TABLE 36 Complications of Shigellosis

Dehydration	Hemolytic-uremic
Hyponatremia	syndrome
Bacteremia-sepsis	Urinary tract infeciton
Toxic megacolon	Pneumonia
Intestinal	Eye involvement
perforation	Seizures
Rectal prolapse	Reiter's syndrome

TABLE 37 Treatment of Shigellosis

Strain	Treatment
Susceptible strains	Trimethoprim/sulfamethoxazole 10 mg/ kg/day TMP/50 mg/kg/day SMX PO or IV div. b.i.d. (max. 320 mg TMP/ 1600 mg SMX)
	Ampicillin (not amoxicillin) 80–100 mg/ kg/day PO or IV div. q.i.d. (max. 2 g)
Resistant strains	Ceftriaxone 50–75 mg/kg/day div. q.i.d.
	Ciprofloxacin 20–30 mg/kg/day (max. 1.5 g) PO div. b.i.d.

medications. Nalidixic acid is often used in developing nations, and third generation cephalosporins are frequently effective for treatment of multiply-resistant strains. Additionally, quinolones are excellent options for adults, but their potential toxicity to epiphysial cartilage in children must be considered (Table 37).

Fever should defervesce within 12 to 20 hours with therapy and improvement of diarrhea should be seen in 1 to 3 days. *Shigella* is eliminated within the first 2 days of therapy but, if therapy is not instituted, it can be cultured from stools for up to 1 month. This finding may influence the decision to treat children with mild enteritis. Antidiarrheal drugs should be discouraged as they prolong fever, diarrhea, and excretion of the organism. Mortality in uncomplicated gastroenteritis is less than 1%. Chronic carriage of *Shigella* in stools is very unusual unless the patient was initially malnourished.

VIRAL GASTROENTERITIS

Viral gastroenteritis is one of the most common illnesses in childhood with numerous etiologic agents identified in sporadic and epidemic cases (Table 38). Rotavirus (see individual section) and enteric adenovirus are most identified as the cause of infection (Table 38).

Entereic adenovirus gastroenteritis usually occurs in children under 2 years of age and at any time of the year. The incubation period is up to 7 days and transmission is through the fecal–oral route. Respiratory symptoms and vomiting are common, and diarrhea can last up to 2 weeks. Viral detection kits using techniques similar to rotavirus detection are available. Treatment is symptomatic and supportive.

Nora virus usually affect school-age children and adults throughout the year. Incubation is 18 to 48 hours and symptoms usually last only 1 to 2 days. Vomiting is the most common symptom in children, often with comcomitant diarrhea, nausea, and abdominal pain. Treatment is supportive.

TABLE 38 Viral Etiology of Gastroenteritis

Rotavirus
Enteric adenovirus
Nora virus
Coronavirus
Astrovirus
Calicivirus

TABLE 39   Characteristics of *Yersinia* Infection

Incubation	1–11 days
Seasonality	Cool weather
Peak age of illness	Any
Transmission	Food, milk, oysters, raw chitterlings, water, wild and domestic animals, person-to-person, blood transfusion
Duration of illness	5–14 days (longer for systemic disease)

TABLE 40   Clinical Signs and Symptoms of *Yersinia* Infection

Fever
Diarrhea
Blood in stools
Vomiting
Severe abdominal pain
    Including signs and symptoms of appendicitis
Increased absolute band count on complete blood count (infants under 6 mo of age)
Guaiac-positive stools
White blood cells on stool smear

YERSINIA

Yersinia enterocolitica is a small gram-negative facultative anaerobic coccobacillus responsible for large numbers of gastroenteritis cases in Europe and Canada, but less commonly in the United States. There are numerous serotypes with types 0:3 and 0:9 being most common in human infections in Europe. Serotype 0:3 is most common in Canada and 0:8 in the United States, although many cases of serotype 0:3 have now been reported in the United States.

The pathogenicity of this organism is genetically determined by the presence of plasmid-encoded proteins on its outer membrane. These proteins permit resistance of *Yersinia* to several host-defense mechanisms including opsonization and neutrophil phagocytosis. Iron is a growth requirement for several bacteria and it appears to play an important role in the development of infections with *Yersinia*. Treatment of experimental animals with iron, or deferoxamine (which allows iron to be more readily utilized by the bacteria), significantly increases the virulence of *Y. enterocolitica*.

The mode of transmission in sporadic cases is unclear. In epidemic cases, person-to-person transmission (within families or hospital personnel) and food-borne transmission have been identified (Table 39).

Clinically, there are several forms of disease which include enterocolitis, pseudoappendicitis, autoimmune-like disease, sepsis, and metastatic disease. Younger children have a milder form of disease with diarrhea being the predominant symptom (Table 40); however, several cases of sepsis and metastatic disease have been reported in infants.

A profile of pseudoappendicitis is usually seen in older children and young adults and is due to acute mesenteric adenitis. Older adolescents and young adults may also have symptoms of an acute enteritis resembling Crohn disease with localization of disease to the terminal ileum.

Several groups of patients are at higher risk of developing systemic infection with *Y. enterocolitica* (Table 41). A group somewhat uniquely affected by this organism are patients with iron overload, such as in thalassemia or hemochromatosis.

TABLE 41   Risk Factors for Development of Systemic Disease in *Yersinia* Infection

Infants under 3 mos of age
Disease associated with iron overload
    Hemoglobinopathies
    Hemosiderosis
    Hemochromatosis
    Accidental iron overdose
Immunodeficeincy
Malignancy

Yersinia is readily isolated from uncontaminated sources such as joint fluid or blood. It is difficult to isolate on routine stool cultures because it appears as a very small colony which is easily overgrown. Selective media have been developed to facilitate identification of the organism. Serologic techniques for diagnosis are available, including RIA and ELISA, but have their limitations.

Acute gastroenteritis is usually a self-limited disease that does not require therapy except in immunosuppressed patients. Patients with chronic gastrointestinal symptoms have responded to antibiotics, but controlled studies have not been performed. Metastatic infections, such as osteomyelitis or hepatic abscesses, should be treated with antibiotics and the duration of treatment dictated by the site of involvement. Antibiotic therapy has not been proven beneficial in mesenteric adenitis; however, septicemia is an absolute indication for therapy.

Yersinia is generally sensitive to trimethoprim/sulfamethoxazole, aminoglycosides, third generation cephalosporins, fluoroquinolones, and tetracycline. Most strains are resistant to the penicillin group and first generation cephalosporins due to the production of β-lactamase. Other useful drugs include aminoglycosides, chloramphenicol, quinolones, and third generation cephalosporins. Focal or gastrointestinal infections in susceptible hosts may be treated with a single drug, such as trimethoprim/sulfamethoxazole or tetracycline. Septicemia is generally treated with aminoglycosides, doxycycline, chloramphenicol, or trimethoprim/ sulfamethoxazole. Combination therapy, such as doxycycline plus an aminoglycoside, may be needed. The necessary duration of therapy in septicemia has not been established; several weeks of therapy may be needed (see Chapter 20 for dosages of antibiotics).

10 | Bone and Joint Infections

INTRODUCTION

Infectious agents are introduced into bone by: (a) hematogenous infection from bacteremia, (b) local spread from contiguous foci such as cellulitis or infected varicella lesions, and (c) direct inoculation following trauma, invasive procedures, or surgery. The incidence of osteomyelitis is greater in males (2.5 times more often than females) and approximately 40% of cases occur in patients less than 20 years of age.

HEMATOGENOUS OSTEOMYELITIS

The pathogenesis of hematogenous osteomyelitis begins in the metaphysis of tubular long bones adjacent to the epiphyseal growth plate. Thrombosis of the low-velocity sinusoidal vessels due to trauma or embolization is considered the focus for bacterial seeding in this process. This avascular environment allows invading organisms to proliferate while avoiding the influx of phagocytes, the presence of serum antibody and complement, the interaction with tissue macrophages, and other host defense mechanisms. The proliferation of organisms, release of organism enzymes and by-products, and the fixed volume environment contribute to progressive bone necrosis. The signs, symptoms, and pathologic progression vary by age (Table 1).

Tubular long bones are primarily involved, especially of the lower extremities; the common sites of bone involvement in children demonstrate this predilection (Table 2).

TABLE 1 Hematogenous Osteomyelitis: Signs and Symptoms

Newborn		Older infant and young child (2 wks–4 yrs)	Older child and adolescent (4–16 yrs)
Systemic symptoms[a]	Clinical sepsis, irritable, especially to touch; pseudo-paralysis	Pain, limp, refusal to use affected limb	Focal symptoms, less restriction of movement; local pain; mild limp; fever, malaise
Signs	Red, swollen, discolored local site; massive swelling	Marked focality; point tenderness; well localized pain	Focal signs; point tenderness very localized
Pathology	Thin cortex; dissects into surrounding tissue	Cortex thicker; periosteum dense	Metaphyseal cortex thick; periosteum fibrous and dense
Progression	Nidus (purulent) rapidly progresses[b]; subperiosteal purulence spreads; secondary septic arthritis	Subperiosteal abscess and edema; metaphyseal involvement	Cortical rupture rare
Roentgenograph	Useful early—periosteal and bony changes	Later findings confirmatory; early changes—deep soft tissue swelling	Bony changes apparent only after 7–10 days of involvement

[a] May be subclinical; constitutional symptoms (fever, malaise, anorexia, and irritability) are no different among the different age groups; also no correlation with severity of constitutional symptoms and ultimate severity of subsequent osteomyelitis.
[b] Residual effects may be anticipated in up to 25% of newborns.

TABLE 2   Site of Bone Involvement

Site	Frequency (%)
Femur	36
Tibia	33
Humerus	10
Fibula	7
Radius	3
Calcaneus	3
Ilium	2

The bacterial etiology of hematogenous osteomyelitis demonstrates an age-specific pattern (Table 3). Other epidemiologic factors, predisposing chronic diseases and exposure history may suggest unusual pathogens (Table 4).

The differential diagnosis of hematogenous osteomyelitis includes: pyomyositis, cellulitis, toxic synovitis, septic arthritis, thrombophlebitis, or in a sickle cell disease patient, a bone infarction. The diagnosis of osteomyelitis is confirmed with isolation of organisms from bone, subperiosteal exudate, or contiguous joint fluid. Needle aspiration through normal skin over involved bone at a subperiosteal site or at the metaphyseal area combined with a potentially involved joint aspiration should be performed by an orthopedic surgeon. Aspirates of involved focal areas yield positive cultures in only 50% to 60% of cases that have not been pretreated with antibiotics. However, because early institution of antimicrobial therapy is so common, even fewer of suspected cases are culture positive.

Blood cultures have been reported to be positive in as many as 50% of cases so should be obtained routinely prior to initiation of antimicrobial therapy.

Diagnosis

The most sensitive radiographic procedure for establishing a diagnosis of osteomyelitis, localizing disease, and determining the need for surgical intervention is magnetic resonance imaging (MRI). However, many experts still prefer a technetium bone scan since it is less expensive and will identify multifocal disease. Routine plain X-rays should initially be obtained (Fig. 1) since they are readily available and may identify other etiologies of bone pain. The diagnosis of osteomyelitis on routine roentgenographs can be subtle to obvious (Table 5) depending on the duration of disease and are adequate for differentiating patients with trauma, including physical abuse. X-rays are also fairly sensitive for identifying leukemic infiltrates which represent one important cause of bone pain.

Diagnosis of bone infection is enhanced with the use of MRIs which can be completed in minutes or technetium scanning which requires 2 hours to complete. One of these studies should be obtained for any patient who has obvious evidence of focal bone pathology, fever of

TABLE 3   Bacterial Etiology in Hematogenous Osteomyelitis

Neonates	Infants and children
Organisms	
Staphylococcus aureus 40%	*S. aureus* 80%
Group B streptococci 30%	Group A streptococci 7%
Coliforms 10%	*Salmonella* sp. 6%
Others 20%	Others 7%
Neisseria gonorrhoeae	Coliforms
Pseudomonas aeruginosa Candida sp.	*Streptococcus pneumoniae*
	Candida sp.
	Anaerobes

TABLE 4 Specific Etiologies of Osteomyelitis

Clinical circumstances	Probable etiology
Human bite	Anaerobes
Dog or cat bite	*Pasteurella multocida*
Puncture wound of foot	*P. aeruginosa*
Sickle cell disease	*Salmonella* sp.
Rheumatoid arthritis	*S. aureus* (from joint)
	P. multocida
Diabetes mellitus	Fungi
Newborns	Group B streptococci
	E. coli
	Salmonella sp.
Uncommon etiologies	
Facial and cervical area; in the jaw; sinus drainage; lytic bone changes with "egg shell" areas of new bone	*Actinomyces* sp.
Vertebral body or long bone abscesses; systemic signs and symptoms	*Brucella*
Regional distribution; systemic findings; vertebral body, skull, long bone involvement	*Salmonella* *Coccidioides*
Skin lesion; pulmonar involvement; skull and vertebral bodies most common, but long bone involvement is reported	*Blastomyces*
Very distinct, slowly progressive bony lesions can occur	*Cryptococcus*
Exposure to cats, FUO, liver granulomas, chronic adenitits	*Bartonella henselae* (cat scratch disease)

undetermined etiology with bone tenderness on physical exam and an elevated C reactive protein or sedimentation rate, or suggestive findings on routine roentgenographs. Both imaging procedures can also aid in directing aspirate procedures for diagnosis and culture.

In situations where osteomyelitis is suspected on physical examination but the technetium bone scan is equivocal or non-diagnostic, secondary radionuclide imaging including MRI may be performed. In selected cases, including pelvic, vertebral or small bone (hands/feet) osteomyelitis, the use of MRI or computerized tomography (CT) is useful in establishing a diagnosis or directing surgical intervention. A technetium or indium labeled WBC scan using tagged autologous leukocytes requires 24 hours of imaging for completion and has only limited usefulness. Gallium scanning requires 24 to 48 hours, may be difficult to read (midline scans) due to uptake in the bowel, and has been replaced by MRI, CT, and WBC scans.

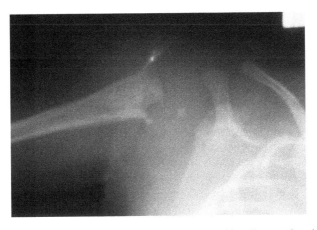

FIGURE 1 Group B streptococcal osteomyelitis. Destructive bone changes of the proximal humerus in this 29-day-old infant whose symptoms began 14 days earlier with fever and refusal to move the left arm (pseudoparalysis).

TABLE 5 Roentgenographic Diagnosis of Hematogenous Osteomyelitis

Day	Changes
0–3	Local, deep soft-tissue swelling; near metaphysical region or with localized findings
3–7	Deep soft-tissue swelling; obscured translucent fat lines (spread of edema fluid)
10–21	Variable–bone specific; bone destruction, periosteal new bone formation

NONHEMATOGENOUS OSTEOMYELITIS

Bone involvement arises through spread from a contiguous focus of infection or direct inoculation. The following are the more common types of non-hematogenous osteomyelitis.

Pseudomonas Osteochondritis

The predilection of *Pseudomonas* to involve cartilaginous tissue and the relative amount of cartilage in children's tarsal-metatarsal region are the reasons for this infection being classified as an "osteochondritis." The classic history is a nail puncture through a tennis shoe. This entity is seen as early as 2 days postinjury but frequently requires up to 21 days to manifest clinically. The proper initial management of this trauma is vigorous irrigation and cleansing of the puncture wound in conjunction with tetanus prophylaxis. Upon diagnosis of *Pseudomonas* osteochondritis from wound, drainage culture or surgical curettage culture, intravenous antibiotics should be initiated and guided by antibiotic sensitivity testing. The crucial factor in successful therapy is complete evacuation of all necrotic, infected bone and cartilage. If this is accomplished, only 7 to 10 days of parenteral antibiotics are necessary (depending on soft tissue healing and appearance) for completion of therapy. *Pseudomonas* osteochondritis of the vertebrae or pelvis should lead one to suspect intravenous drug abuse as an etiology.

Patellar Osteochondritis

Patellar Osteochondritis is seen in children 5 to 15 years of age when the patella has significant vascular integrity. Direct inoculation via a puncture would yields symptoms within 1 week to 10 days. Constitutional symptoms are uncommon. *Staphylococcus aureus* is the most common etiology. Roentgenographs may take 2 to 3 weeks to show bone sclerosis or destruction.

Contiguous Osteochondritis

Infection is uncommon in children compared to adults. It is associated with nosocomial-infected burns or penetrating wounds. The clinical course characteristically includes two to four weeks of local pain, skin erosion, ulceration, or sinus drainage. Multiple organisms are common and draining sinus cultures correlate well with bone aspirate or biopsy cultures. *S. aureus*, streptococci, anaerobes and nosocomial Gram-negative enterics are the etiologic organisms; peripheral leukocyte count or erythrocyte sedimentation rates are usually normal. It is important to be aware of predisposing conditions (Table 6).

PELVIC OSTEOMYELITIS

The frequency of bone involvement (highest to lowest) is: ilium, ischium, pubis, and sacroiliac areas. The tendency for multi-focal involvement is high in the pelvis compared to other sites. The symptoms may be poorly localized with vague onset; hip and buttock pain with a limp are

TABLE 6   Predisposing Conditions for Contiguous Osteochondritis

Closed fractures	Osteomyelitis 1 to several weeks postfracture; after postfracture pain subsides, the pain recurs with progression, local erythema, warmth, and fluctuation; fever common; osteomyelitis applies to this circumstance
Open fractures	Thorough debridement and wound cleansing paramount; lower infection rates have been reported in patients receiving prophylactic first-generation cephalosporin for open fractures; the consequence of infection can be significant; staphylococci, streptococci, anaerobes and *Clostridia* sp. or gram-negative enterics depending on the environment related to the trauma should be considered; tetanus prophylaxis vital (see Chapter 4)
Hemodialysis	Increased risk due to multiple procedures with intravascular cannulae; ribs, thoracic spine, and bones adjacent to indwelling catheters; *S. aureus* and *S. epidermidis* commonly found

frequently the only findings. Tenderness to palpation in the buttocks, the sciatic notch, or positive sacroiliac joint findings suggest this diagnosis. The differential diagnosis includes mesenteric lymphadenitis, urinary tract infection, and acute appendicitis. Patients with inflammatory bowel disease have an increased risk for the development of pelvic osteomyelitis.

VERTEBRAL OSTEOMYELITIS

The vertebral venous system is valveless with a low velocity bidirectional flow, likely the predisposing factors for vertebral body osteomyelitis. It is common for two adjacent vertebrae to be involved while sparing the intervertebral disc. Spread to the internal venous system (epidural abscess) or the external venous system (paraspinous abscess) are complications of this infection.

The symptoms of vertebral osteomyelitis include constant back pain (usually dull), low-grade fever, and pain on exertion; the signs may include paraspinous muscle spasm, tenderness to palpation or percussion of the spinal dorsal processes, and limitation of motion. The symptoms can frequently be present for 3 to 4 months without overt toxicity or signs of sepsis. Roentgenographs show rarefaction in one vertebral edge as early as several days and progress to marked destruction, usually anteriorly, followed by changes in the adjacent vertebrae and new bone formation.

Staphylococci are the infecting organisms in 80% to 90% of cases with gram-negative enterics (associated with UTI), *Pseudomonas* sp. (IV drug abusers), and a small percentage of miscellaneous organisms (see Table 3). Parenteral antibiotic therapy for presumed staphylococcal involvement should be initiated with the consideration for a needle aspirate or bone biopsy for culture and sensitivity testing. Antibiotic therapy should be continued for a minimum of 6 weeks but no data are available for the optimal duration; the clinical course should be considered for decisions of therapy beyond this limit. Treatment should also include surgical drainage (especially if cord compression is present) and immobilization (bed rest versus casting).

DISCITIS

Non-infectious disc necrosis versus bacteremic seeding of the disc space during the loss of blood supply are difficult to separate clinically. Intervertebral disc infection demonstrates some important characteristics: male sex predominance, peak incidence under 5 years of age, occurrence nearly always in the lumbar area (L4–L5 then L3–L4 most common), peripheral leukocytosis in only one-third of patients, and consistently elevated erythrocyte sedimentation rate (ESR). The symptoms include backache, progressive limp, irritability and refusal to sit (non-ambulatory infants), hip pain, and low-grade fever. These are present 1 to 18 months (median 10 to 12 weeks) prior to diagnosis. Signs include back stiffness, tenderness to spine palpation, and limitation of movement. *S. aureus* is the most frequent organism; needle aspirate and bone biopsy have been reported as culture positive in up to 50% of cases. Less

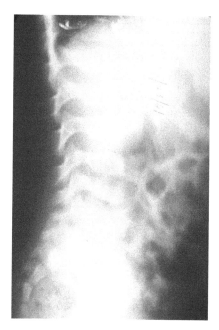

FIGURE 2 Discitis. Narrowing of the L3/L4 disc space, with irregularity of the adjacent vertebral body endplates. This 2-year-old developed severe back pain with spinal rigidity over 3 weeks. He was afebrile and comfortable except when moved. There was marked spasm of the paraspinal muscles and a positive Gowers' sign.

common isolates include pneumococcus and gram-negative organisms. Roentgenographs (Fig. 2, lateral view of lumbar spine) may show disc space narrowing by 2 to 4 weeks after onset of symptoms. This is followed by destruction of adjacent vertebral edges; vertebral body compression is rare.

The benefit of antimicrobial therapy remains controversial. Oral antibiotics may be given following a short course (3 to 5 days) of parenteral therapy depending on the organism and the clinical situation. Prolonged periods (4 to 6 months) of oral antibiotics may be prudent for patients with extensive disc damage. The prognosis varies, but, in general, young children reconstitute and heal the disc space whereas older children are more likely to have spontaneous spinal fusion.

TREATMENT OF OSTEOMYELITIS

The treatment of hematogenous osteomyelitis should be guided initially by Gram stain and subsequently by susceptibilties of organisms recovered from bone or joint aspirates. Empiric therapy on an age- and disease-related basis administered parenterally should be initiated once a diagnosis is confirmed and cultures have been obtained (Table 7). Initial empiric antibiotics should be selected to cover *Staphylococcus aureus*, including methicillin-sensitive (MSSA) and methicillin-resistant (MRSA) strains (clindamycin, vancomycin, or linezolid), and in children with sickle cell disease, to provide treatment for *Salmonella* (ceftriaxone or cefotaxime).

Parenteral therapy should be continued until a clinical response is documented, usually 3 to 5 days. Total parenteral antibiotic therapy in acute bacterial hematogenous osteomyelitis is indicated if: physiologic and constitutional changes are not ideal for oral antibiotic absorption; there is dissemination and abscess formation (especially for *S. aureus*); or compliance cannot be assured. Otherwise, oral absorption is adequate for the continuation of therapy (Table 8). The duration of antibiotic therapy (parenteral and oral) should generally be 3 weeks with the

TABLE 7   Simplified Management of Osteomyelitis

Phase	Management
Initial Day 0–3 inpatient	Obtain CBC and CRP Begin IV antibiotics (e.g., clindamycin)Repeat CBC and CRP when afebrile and clinical response observed CRP <3 mg/dL or returning to normal
Continued therapy Day 4–21 outpatient	PO antibiotics, e.g., linezolid (or cephalexin if susceptible) at 2–3 times the usual dose
Completion Day 21 (ESR <30 mm/ hr)	Obtain erythrocyte sedimentation rate (ESR); if <30 mm/hr stop antibiotics

Delayed response
Day 21–42 (ESR
>30 mm/hr)
	ESR >30 mm/hr
	Obtain MRI
	  Surgical debridement if bone inflammation and destruction identified
	Continue PO antibiotics
	Repeat ESR at 42 days
	  <30 mm/hr: stop antibiotics
	  >30 mm/hr: repeat MRI consider continued surgical and/or medical
	    management × 6 wk

exception of vertebral osteomyelitis and may have to be extended longer depending on the sites of infection and clinical response. The use of home intravenous antibiotics for selected cases can substitute for part of the initial therapy or for the entire course if oral continuation therapy is felt to be suboptimal for age, site or severity (*Pseudomonas* osteochondritis following puncture would of the foot and surgical debridement is an exception). Surgical drainage or debridement of subperiosteal abscesses or soft tissue abscesses should be considered. Immobilization of an affected extremity is necessary for pain relief and to enhance healing.

Duration of Treatment

Most cases of hematogenous osteomyeltis are culture negative after 21 days of therapy (Table 7). Exceptions are vertebral osteomyeltitis which should be treated for 6 weeks and puncture wound osteochondritis caused by *Pseudomonas* which only requires 7 to 10 days of antimicrobial therapy following adequate surgical debridement.

SEPTIC ARTHRITIS

With the production of joint fluid by the synovial membrane, the kinetics of capillary diffusion of fluid into the joint space and the effective blood flow of the joint space, the relatively high frequency of joint infections is not surprising. Bacteria can enter the joint space by direct inoculation (kneeling on a needle, trauma), contiguous extension (osteomyelitis), or via a hematogenous route. In children the lower extremities account for over 80% of cases (Table 9).

The diagnosis of septic arthritis is made earlier than in osteomyelitis due to the onset of constitutional symptoms within the first few days of the infection. Patients almost always have fever, focal findings in the joint (swelling, tenderness, heat, limitation of motion), and placement of the joint in a neutral, non-stressed position. In infants the hip may have an absence of focal findings with the exception of positioning. Infants are observed with the involved leg abducted, slightly flexed, and externally rotated. Resistance to movement or pain should be evaluated for a possible septic hip. There is often an associated dislocation in this setting. An obvious portal of entry in septic arthritis is uncommon.

The diagnosis of suspect joint infection by roentgenograms depends on finding evidence of capsular swelling. In the case of hip involvement, roentgenograms can be valuable; placement of the child in the frog-leg position for an anteroposterior radiograph shows

TABLE 8   Antimicrobial Therapy for Osteomyelitis and Septic Arthritis

Infection	Antimicrobial agents
Osteomyelitis and septic arthritis	
Empiric therapy	
Neonate (0–28 days)	Vancomycin + cefotaxime or ceftriaxone
Infants and children	Clindamycin, vancomycin or linezolid
Puncture wound to foot	Gentamicin[a] tobramycin or amikacin + ceftazidime, ticarcillin, or meropenem + clindamycin, vancomycin, or linezolid[b]
Specific therapy[c]	
S. aureus—MSSA	Cefazolin, clindamycin, oxacillin, nafcillin
S. aureus—MRSA	Clindamycin, vancomycin, or linezolid
Group B streptococci	Penicillin
Group A streptococci	Penicillin
S. pneumoniae	Penicillin sensitive—penicillin
	Penicillin resistant—ceftriaxone, cefotaxime
	Penicillin/cephalosporin resistant—clindamycin, vancomycin, or linezolid
Enterobacteriaceae	Meropenem, cefepime
	alternative: aminoglycoside or third generation cephalosporins depending on sensitivities
N. gonorrhoeae	Ceftriaxone
P. aeruginosa	Aminoglycoside + cefepime, ceftazidime or ticarcillin;
Salmonella sp.	Third generation cephalosporins
C. albicans	Amphotericin B ± 5-flucytosine or liposomal AmpB or fluconazole
Anaerobes	Penicillin, clindamycin, or metronidazole
Continuation oral therapy[d]	Clindamycin or linezolid
S. aureus	Cephalexin if susceptible
Streptococci (group A)	Penicillin or amoxicillin
S. pneumoniae	Penicillin or amoxicillin; third generation cephalosporins; clindamycin
Enterobacteriaceae	Ampicillin or trimethoprim/sulfamethoxazole
N. gonorrhoea	Cefixime
P. aeruginosa	Ciprofloxacin or other quinolones
Salmonella sp.	Amoxicillin, TMP/SMX, or third generation cephalosporins
C. albicans	Fluconazole
Anaerobes	Penicillin, metronidazole, or clindamycin
Culture negative	Coverage for S. aureus (see above)

[a]Aminoglycoside choice guided by *Pseudomonas* sensitivities in your hospital.
[b]Concomitant wound infection, Gram stain positive.
[c]Inpatient or home intravenous therapy.
[d]Oral continuation (modified by sensitivity testing).
Abbreviations: MRSA, methicillin resistant *Staphylococcus aureus*; MSSA, methicillin sensitive *Staphylococcus aureus*; TMP/SMX, trimethoprim/sulfamethoxazole.

displacement of fat lines. Obliteration or lateral displacement of the gluteal fat lines or a raised position for Shenton's line with widening of the arc are consistent with hip joint effusion under pressure. The presence of a significant joint effusion by hip ultrasound is adequate to dictate a joint aspiration. Radionuclide imaging or MRI (see "Osteomyelitis" in this chapter) may be a useful adjunct in a complex or uncharacteristic case for early diagnosis. The use of hip ultrasound followed by a technetium bone scan (or CT/MRI) in selected cases is a reasonable progression of tests based on usefulness, cost and radiation exposure.

The confirmatory procedure for diagnosis is a joint aspiration with Gram stain, culture, and cytology–chemistry evaluation. Joint aspiration of knees (most common joint involved) should be a procedure for all primary care physicians; aspiration of hips or shoulders should be limited to an experienced orthopedist (under fluoroscopic control for hip aspirations). Joint fluid should be processed for Gram stain and aerobic and anaerobic cultures. The fluid should

TABLE 9 Joint Involvement in Septic Arthritis

Joint[a]	Percentage
Knee	38
Hip	32
Ankle	11
Elbow	8
Shoulder	5
Wrist	4
Small joints	2

[a] 2–5% of cases have multiple joint involvement.

be analyzed for glucose concentration (compared to a concomitant blood glucose), leukocyte count and differential, ability to spontaneously clot, and mucin clot test. Joint fluid should be obtained in a heparinized syringe to assure leukocyte analysis. To perform the mucin clot test, glacial acetic acid is added to the joint fluid while stirring; normal fluid reacts with a white precipitate (rope) that clings to the stirring rod with a clear supernatant (Table 10).

Etiologic diagnosis of septic arthritis can be aided by blood cultures; some series have reported up to 20% to 30% of sterile joint fluids with concomitant positive blood cultures. Additional laboratory studies include a hemogram to screen for anemia (hemoglobinopathy), ESR (usually elevated in septic arthritis), serum or urine for bacterial antigen detection (only in partially treated cases with suspect group B streptococci, *H. influenzae*, pneumococcus, or meningococcus), and accessory cultures: wound, infected skin lesions (secondarily infected varicella lesions over the involved joint), cellulitis, or urethral–cervical–rectal cultures in sexually active adolescents (gonorrhea). CSF analysis should be included when meningitis is clinically suspected and in newborns.

The differential diagnosis of septic arthritis includes joint fluid inflammation due to a variety of etiologies (Table 11).

The causative bacteria in most cases of septic arthritis are Gram-positive aerobic organisms particularly since the introduction of *H. influenzae* vaccine. *S. aureus* remains the most frequent single pathogen. The causative organisms differ for neonates, infants, and older children (Tables 12 and 13).

TREATMENT OF SEPTIC ARTHRITIS

The empiric choice of antimicrobial therapy in septic arthritis should be guided by the age of the patient, site of involvement, underlying disease and the Gram stain of joint fluid but should consider: *S. aureus* in all cases; declining incidence of *H. influenzae* in fully immunized children; group B streptococci, and to a lesser extent Gram-negative organisms and *Candida* sp. in neonates, and *N. gonorrhoeae* in newborns and sexually active adolescents (Table 8). The other etiologies and age-related incidence include *Mycoplasma* (>10 years), *Ureaplasma* (>5 years), Lyme arthritis (Borrelia-type organism; >6 months), hepatitis B (>1 year), rubella (>10 years), mumps (<12 years), varicella (<5 years), HSV, CMV, and parvovirus (all ages).

TABLE 10 Joint Fluid Analysis

	Septic arthritis	JRA	Reactive arthritis
Spontaneous clotting	Large clot	Large clot	Small clot
Mucin clot	Curdled milk	Small friable masses	Tight rope; clear supernatent
Glucose concentration (% of blood glucose)	30	75	75–90
Leukocytes total	50,000–200,000	5000–20,000	15,000–30,000
Leukocytes % PMNs	90	60	50

TABLE 11 Differential Diagnosis of Septic Arthritis

Infectious	Viral, mycobacterial, fungal or mycoplasma, bacterial endocarditis, deep cellulitis, Lyme disease, congenital syphilis
Hypersensitivity	Serum sickness (drug, postinfectious), anaphylactoid purpura
Oncologic	Leukemia, neuroblastoma, pigmented villonodular synovitis, primary bone tumor
Metabolic	Gout, hyperparathyroidism
Immunologic	Agammaglobulinemia, Behçet's syndrome, hepatitis
Neurogenic	Diabetes mellitus, peripheral nerve or spinal cord injury, leprosy
Bleeding	Trauma (to include physical abuse), skeletal trauma due to birth, hemophilia
Orthopedic	Toxic synovitis, aseptic necrosis, osteochondritis, bursitis
Miscellaneous	Kawasaki disease, collagen vascular disease, polyarthritis nodosa, sarcoidosis, inflammatory bowel disease, familial Mediterranean fever, Tietze's syndrome, reactive arthritis

Antibiotic therapy should be directed in cases with negative Gram stains and negative bacterial antigen assays for the most likely organisms for age (see Table 8). Nearly all antibiotics that have been studied penetrate readily into joint fluid, averaging 30% to 40% of peak serum concentration. The penicillins, cephalosporins (first, second, and third generation), macrolides, aminoglycosides, and chloramphenicol attain effective concentrations in joint fluid. Intraarticular antibiotics add no benefit. Larger joints may require open drainage. The duration of antibiotic therapy should be 3 weeks minimum with the first 3 to 5 days administered parenterally followed by oral continuation therapy as long as the following criteria are met: no GI disorder to underlying disease that would diminish oral absorption, clinical response to parenteral antibiotics and surgical management has been established; the organism is sensitive to a class of antibiotic in oral form and compliance can be guaranteed. Some experts administer a trial dosage of oral antibiotics during inpatient management.

To evaluate the effectiveness of antibiotic therapy in more difficult cases, serial joint aspirations can be performed. Although cultures may be positive for up to 5 to 7 days in non-surgically drained joint fluid, a decrease in leukocyte density should be seen by 1 to 2 weeks of therapy. In studies using serial joint aspirations, by days 1 through 10 of antibiotic therapy those patients who subsequently recover had less than 5000 cells/mm^3 compared to those with recrudescent infection who had more than 60,000 cells/mm^3. The best predictor of outcome and complications is the duration of signs and symptoms prior to diagnosis and effective therapy.

Septic arthritis in neonates and infants and most cases of hip or shoulder involvement, should be drained as soon as the diagnosis is established. Any joint should be considered for

TABLE 12 Etiology of Septic Arthritis

	Newborns and infants		Older children
	Community acquired (%)	Nosocomial (%)	Combined series (%)
Staphylococcus aureus	25	62	77
Staphylococcus epidermidis		4	
Group B streptococci	50	4	
Group A streptococcus	3	1	7
Pneumococcus	5	1	6
Enterobacteriaceae	5	9	7 (predominantly immunocompromised patients)
Candida sp.		17	
N. gonorrhoeae	10		
Miscellaneous	2	2	3

TABLE 13 Special Considerations

Neonatal septic arthritis	Subtle presentation
	Unusual organisms
	Use of umbilical catheters
	Difficulty in evaluating hips, shoulders
	Potential catastrophic outcome
Adolescents, monoarticular	Sexual contact history increases possibility of gonococcal etiology
	Disseminated gonorrhea (perihepatitis, endocarditis, meningitis, sepsis)
Reactive arthritis	Predisposition in HLA-B27 positive patients
	Occurs following *Shigella* sp., *Salmonella* sp., *Yersinia*, and *Campylobacter* enteric infections
	May mimic rheumatic fever, collagen vascular disease, or serum sickness
Reiter's syndrome	Urethritis, conjunctivitis, with or without rash and arthritis (ankles, knees) associated with chlamydia infection
Lyme disease	Early diagnosis and treatment with penicillin or amoxicillin can prevent arthritis
Kawasaki disease	Arthritis, most common non-cardiac complication
	Occurs in 20–30% of cases
	Large joints most common, multiple joints
	Respond to salicylates

open drainage when loculation, high fibrin content, or tissue debris prevents adequate drainage by needle aspiration.

LYME DISEASE

There are 3 stages of Lyme disease based on timing and severity: (1) early localized; (2) early disseminated, and (3) late disease. Arthralgia may be seen with both forms of early disease while recurrent arthritis is the most common manifestation of late disease. The arthritis is most commonly pauciarticular involving the knees and other large joints. In children, treatment of early disease usually prevents late onset arthritis as well as other manifestation of late disease.

Diagnosis is best made clinically during the early stages of disease by observing the unique rash, erythema migrans (Fig. 3). For late disease, a 2-step approach for serologic diagnosis is recommended in guidelines published by the Infectious Disease Society of

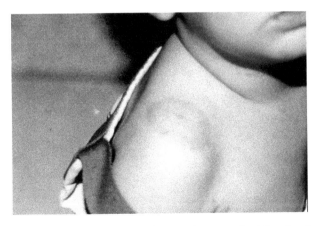

FIGURE 3 (*See color insert.*) Erythema migrans rash at the site of a tick bite in an 18-month-old with acute Lyme disease. This lesion with central clearing measured 6×7 cm in diameter.

TABLE 14   Treatment of Lyme Disease

Disease stage	Antibiotic
Early localized disease	Doxycycline, 4 mg/kg/day (max. 200 mg/day) div. b.i.d. PO 14 days
<8 yrs of age who have received 5 previous courses (30 days) of tetracyclines	Amoxicillin, 50 mg/kg/day (max. 1.5 g) div. t.i.d. PO × 14 days or Cefuroxime, 30 mg/kg/day (max. 1 g) div. b.i.d. × PO 14 days
Early disseminated and late disease	
Multiple erythema migrans lesions and isolated facial palsy	Same as above × 21 days
Arthritis	Same as above × 28 days
Persistent or recurrent arthritis, meningitis and carditis	Ceftriaxone 75 mg/kg/day (max. 2 g) div. q.d. IV or IM × 14 days or Penicillin 300,000 U/kg/day (max. 20 million) div. q 4 hr IV × 14 days

America (1). A screening test, enzyme immunoassay or immunofluorescent antibody, should first be done. If positive, results should be confirmed with a Western immunoblot assay. No further testing is recommended if the screening assay is negative. A positive Western blot is defined as detection of IgG antibody to 5 or more of the following antigens (bands): 18, 23/24, 28, 30, 39, 41, 45, 60, 66, and 93 kDa polypeptides. An IgM immunoblot assay is positive if antibody (bands) is detected for 2 of 3 antigens (23/24, 39, and 41 kDa polypeptides).

Doxycycline is the drug of choice for children except perhaps those younger than 8 years who have previously received 5 courses of tetracyclines (Table 14).

REFERENCE

1.   Wormser GP, Nadelman RB, Dattwyler RJ, et al. Practice guidelines for the treatment of Lyme disease. Clin Infect Dis 2000; 31(Suppl. 1): S1–14.

11 | Urinary Tract Infections

Over the previous decade, considerable progress has been made in the management of urinary tract infections (UTI), resulting from a better understanding of host factors and bacterial virulence. Additionally, radiographic imaging of the urinary tract has advanced, simplifying evaluation of the child with documented infection. On the other hand, most surgical procedures for correction of anatomic defects that predispose to UTI, particularly reimplantation of ureters, have not been shown to offer benefit.

Covert (asymptomatic) bacteriuria should be distinguished from symptomatic UTI, as it is a benign entity mostly in girls requiring no treatment nor follow-up. In infants and young children, symptomatic UTIs are commonly encountered, with an aggregate risk of 3.0% to 7.8% for girls and 1.1% to 1.7% for boys. The shorter urethra and greater potential for perineal colonization accounts for this higher incidence in girls. The predominant mechanism of UTI for both sexes is ascent of bowel organisms but, during the neonatal period, hematogenous seeding of the kidney from bacteremia may also play a role.

Pyelonephritis may lead to irreversible renal scarring and end-stage renal disease. Successful diagnosis involves a high index of suspicion and awareness of optimal techniques to diagnose UTI. It is possible to prevent renal damage with prompt diagnosis and treatment.

The American Academy of Pediatrics, Subcommittee on Urinary Tract Infection, has published guidelines for the diagnosis, treatment, and evaluation of the initial UTI in febrile infants and children ages 2 months to 2 years. The 11 recommendations contained in this document are summarized in Table 1 and represent an appropriate starting point for discussing management of UTI in children.

CRITERIA FOR DIAGNOSIS

Clinical Criteria

Cystitis classically presents with urgency, frequency, dysuria, secondary enuresis, and foul-smelling urine. Spiking fever, flank or abdominal pain, and irritability suggest pyelonephritis. The clinical manifestations of chronic pyelonephritis are most commonly recurrent abdominal pain, unexplained febrile episodes, and failure to thrive.

A urine culture must be obtained in infants in whom fever, lethargy, or unexplained irritability are the only presenting signs and symptoms. It is important to recognize that many children with urethral or perineal irritation may present with voiding symptoms (Table 2) in the absence of UTI.

Laboratory Testing

A positive dipstick or microscopic urinalysis result is suggestive of UTI (Table 3), but confirmation must be obtained by culture with a quantitative colony count. Identification of the organism is essential, especially with recurrent UTI.

Pyuria is poorly correlated with UTI. Approximately 40% of children with UTI have a white blood cell count <10 per high-power field in centrifuged sediment. Conversely, children with pyuria frequently do not have bacteriuria (Table 4). Therefore, culture of urine collected by bladder catheterization remains the "gold standard" for diagnosis.

Specimen collection greatly influences the accuracy of UTI diagnosis. When a specimen is carefully collected by clean-catch midstream technique (in the older child), catheterization,

TABLE 1   AAP, Subcommittee on UTI: Recommendations on the Diagnosis, Treatment, and Evaluation of the Initial UTI in Febrile Infants and Young Children[a], 1999

1. The presence of UTI should be considered in children with unexplained fever
2. In children with unexplained fever, the degree of toxicity, dehydration, and ability to retain oral intake must be carefully assessed
3. If a child with unexplained fever warrants immediate antimicrobial therapy, a urine specimen should be obtained by SPA or catheterization; the diagnosis of UTI cannot be established by a culture of a bagged urine
4. If a child with unexplained fever does not require immediate antimicrobial therapy, there are 2 options:
   I: Obtain and culture a urine specimen collected by SPA or catheterization
   II: Obtain a urine specimen by the most convenient means and perform a urinalysis. If the urinalysis is positive, culture a urine specimen collected by SPA or catheterization: if urinalysis is negative, it is reasonable to follow closely, recognizing that a negative urinalysis does not rule out a UTI
5. Diagnosis of UTI requires a urine culture.
6. If the child with suspected UTI is assessed as toxic, dehydrated, or unable to retain oral intake, initial antimicrobial therapy should be administered IV, and hospitalization should be considered
7. In the child who may not appear ill but who has a culture confirming a UTI, antimicrobial therapy should be initiated, IV or po
8. Children with UTI, who have not defervesced within 2 days of antimicrobial therapy, should be reevaluated and recultured
9. Children, including those whose initial treatment was administered IV, should complete a 7- to 14-day course of po antibiotics
10. After a 7- to 14-day course of antibiotics and sterilization of the urine, children should receive antibiotics until imaging studies are completed
11. Children with UTI who do not defervesce within 2 days of antimicrobial therapy should undergo ultrasonography and cystography promptly. Children who have the expected response to antimicrobials should have a sonogram and cystography performed at the earliest convenient time

[a]Refers to infants and young children 2 months to 2 years of age.

or suprapubic aspiration, substantial bacteriuria on urinalysis usually correlates with a high colony count of a single organism (Table 5). Multiple organisms or a low colony count suggest a contaminated specimen rather than a true UTI.

Urine specimens collected by bag technique carry a high risk (50%) of contamination, especially in female infants and uncircumcised males with nonretractable foreskins. A positive urinalysis on such a specimen must be confirmed by catheterization or suprapubic aspiration, but a negative specimen collected by bag technique is helpful in excluding UTI. Girls should be instructed to carefully cleanse the perineum and to straddle the toilet facing backward in

TABLE 2   Causes of Urinary Tract Symptoms in the Absence of Bacteriuria

Urethritis
Meatal irritation
Vulvovaginitis
Balanitis
Topical irritants
   Bubble bath or soap
   Laundry detergents
   Lotions
   Dyes/scents in clothing or toilet tissue
Medications
Vaginal foreign body
Pinworms
Emotional stress
Trauma (including masturbation and sexual abuse)
Daytime frequency syndrome
Candida
Trichomonas

TABLE 3 Screening Tests for Urinary Tract Infections

Routine urinalysis
  White blood cell count ≥10 per high-power field
  Urine (10 mL) centrifuged for 5 min at 3000 rpm
    and viewed at 45× magnification
  Leukocyte esterase
    Correlates with pyuria
    Positive predictive value of 50%
Nitrite
  Bacteria slowly reduce nitrate to nitrite
  Overnight or concentrated urine optimal
  Negative result with high fluid intake or frequency
  Negative result with *Pseudomonas* UTI
Bacteria
  Presence in unspun urine correlates with
    10^5 bacteria/ml
White blood cell casts
  Indicative of pyelonephritis
Serum C-reactive protein
  Elevated with pyelonephritis

TABLE 4 Causes of Pyuria Without Bacteriuria

Febrile systemic illness
Concentrated urine (dehydration)
Irritation from catheter or instrument
Inflammation of neighboring structures (e.g., acute
  appendicitis)
Calculi
Acute glomerulonephritis
Interstitial nephritis
Nonbacterial infection (e.g., *Candida, Mycobacterium
  tuberculosis, Ureaplasma*)
Previous reconstructive surgery using an intestinal
  patch

order to abduct the labia and reduce voiding of urine into the vagina. A midstream specimen can then be obtained. In uncircumcised boys, the foreskin should be retracted sufficiently to allow cleansing of the meatal region. Urine culture should be plated within 30 minutes or refrigerated if the culture will be delayed. Storage of urine at room temperature promotes bacterial multiplication, resulting in higher colony counts. On a temporary basis, urine specimens may be stored in a refrigerator or in a basin of ice water to reduce bacterial multiplication.

RISK FACTORS FOR URINARY TRACT INFECTION

Failure of host defenses resulting in UTI may arise from defects at the cellular, organ, or functional level. Increased bacterial adherence to the urothelium of children with recurrent UTI has been attributed to a mucin layer deficiency. The nonsecretor phenotype for blood group antigens is an additional, hereditary risk factor. The nonsecretor status is associated with reduced excretion of water-soluble glycoproteins and alteration of the terminal oligosaccharide configuration on the exterior of epithelial cells. This deficiency facilitates bacterial adherence and results in an increased incidence of recurrent UTI. Other host defenses such as urinary inhibitory glycoproteins have been identified.

    Organ-specific risk factors include poor vulvar hygiene in females or the presence of a foreskin in males (Table 6), both of which predispose to bacterial colonization of the perimeatal region and subsequently the urethra. Numerous studies have documented the increased risk

TABLE 5 Criteria for Culture Diagnosis of Urinary Tract Infections (Single Organism)

Specimen collection	Intermediate result (colonies/mL urine)	Positive result (colonies/mL urine)
Suprapubic aspiration	Any growth	>100
Catheterized urine	10,000–50,000	>50,000
Clean-voided (male)	≥10,000 (foreskin retracted or absent, glans penis well cleansed)	>100,000
Clean-voided (female)	>50,000	>100,000
Bagged urine	>100,000	Indeterminate

TABLE 6   Factors Predisposing to Urinary Tract Infection

Urothelial deficiency
Increased bacterial adherence due to nonsecretor phenotype
Organ-specific deficiencies
Anomalies with hydronephrosis or obstruction
Nephrolithiasis
Vesicoureteral reflux
Indwelling catheter or foreign body
Nonretractable foreskin
Fecal incontinence
Poor perineal hygiene
Functional factors
Bladder dysfunction with detrusor hypertonicity
Constipation

(5- to 20-fold) of UTI in the uncircumcised male. In one study, 95% of male infants with UTI were uncircumcised, and the majority of these were under 3 months of age. Of all the structural abnormalities, vesicoureteral reflux (VUR) are the most frequent and significant predisposing abnormality for recurrent UTI and renal scarring.

Obstruction of the ureter may occur at the upper end (ureteropelvic junction [UPJ]) or the lower end (ureterovesical junction [UVJ]). Significant dilatation of the upper urinary tract will result in stasis, which predisposes to infection. Duplication of ureters is commonly associated with reflux into the ureter, which drains the lower segment of the kidney. Obstruction of the ureter draining the upper kidney segment (ectopic ureter/ureterocele) also occurs. With an ectopic ureter, which drains outside the bladder, the abnormal renal segment may become infected. In such cases, urine collected directly from the bladder by catheterization or suprapubic aspiration, may show reduced colony counts, delaying the diagnosis of UTI. In males, obstruction is most commonly caused by posterior urethral valves, which highly predispose these children to UTI; the initial indication of this anatomic anomaly is most commonly infection.

Functional factors, which protect against UTI include regular, complete bladder emptying and low-pressure bladder filling. Bacterial multiplication may be increased by voluntary postponement of voiding due to children's normal lack of interest in routine bodily functions. When bladder capacity is increased, or the child interrupts urination, bladder emptying may be incomplete and residual urine predisposes to UTI. Two main categories of lower urinary tract dysfunction may result in UTI with or without incontinence: bladder instability with increased intravesical pressure and incomplete sphincter relaxation during voiding. Neurogenic bladder due to spinal cord injury, spina bifida, or cerebral palsy can result in either or both of these types of lower urinary tract dysfunction.

After toilet training, the pattern of an "unstable bladder" may persist due to a maturational delay and may be associated with involuntary bladder contractions. Other children demonstrate inappropriate voiding habits with voluntary contraction of the sphincter during micturition and higher residual urine. Both of these functional abnormalities occur in association with VUR. Unless these dynamic problems are identified and treated, UTI is likely to recur.

Severe constipation or fecal retention with soiling are associated with bladder dysfunction. Improvement in bowel habits is necessary to prevent recurrence of UTI.

LOCALIZATION OF URINARY TRACT INFECTION

The location of UTI may influence the type of therapy selected (intravenous vs. oral) but does not alter the need for radiologic investigation. Clinical criteria to separate pyelonephritis from cystitis are imprecise but differentiation is rarely essential. High fever, flank pain, leukocytosis and white blood cell casts in the urine all suggest pyelonephritis and an elevated C-reactive protein even more strongly supports upper tract infection. The most sensitive test to identify pyelonephritis is a radionuclide scans, using dimercaptosuccinic acid (DMSA). Ureteral catheterization or percutaneous aspiration of the renal pelvis is rarely necessary except when an organism cannot be identified or when infection in a specific renal moiety may influence subsequent management; for example, the need for surgery with a congenital anomaly.

BACTERIAL ETIOLOGY

Escherichia coli is the primary uropathogen, both in neonates and older children. Other organisms of the *Enterobacteriaceae* group, such as *Proteus, Klebsiella, Enterobacter, Pseudomonas, Acinetobacter,* and *Serratia,* also cause infection (Table 7). These less common organisms may be seen in cases of recent antibiotic exposure. Enterococcus is seen in 5% to 15% of UTI in adults and sexually active adolescent females but is rare in young children.

A positive urine specimen will have a high colony count of a single bacterium. Specimens showing intermediate growth may be confirmed by repeat culture of a sample obtained by catheterization or suprapubic aspiration prior to starting antibiotic therapy.

Falsely low colony counts in the presence of true UTI are encountered with high fluid intake (dilute urine), severe urinary frequency, concomitant intake of antibiotics, or sequestered UTI (e.g., obstructed, infected segment, or abscess).

TREATMENT

The goals of treatment of UTI are to provide relief of symptoms as well as to prevent future episodes and renal damage. Untreated, symptomatic patients with a history of fever for 3 days or more are at risk of developing renal scarring. More intensive therapy with parenteral antibiotics should be considered in cases of vomiting with inability to retain oral medications, suspected sepsis, dehydration, poor parental compliance with oral treatment, or a urologic anomaly with poor response to oral therapy. Gram stain of urine assists in the selection of an antibiotic having a predominant gram-negative/gram-positive spectrum. In children with compromised renal function, nephrotoxic antibiotics should be used with caution and serum creatinine and peak and trough concentrations of antibiotics monitored.

In the outpatient setting, UTI is usually treated with amoxicillin, sulfonamide antibiotics, or a cephalosporin (Table 8). Emerging resistance of *E. coli* to ampicillin (amoxicillin) may render this drug less effective. In infants under 2 months of age, sulfonamide antibiotics or nitrofurantoin should be avoided as they have the potential to displace bilirubin from albumin. Antibiotics that are excreted in high concentrations in urine but do not achieve therapeutic concentrations in the bloodstream, such as nalidixic acid or nitrofurantoin, are less effective in acute pyelonephritis. Antibiotic sensitivity is most commonly determined by the

TABLE 7 Etiology of Urinary Tract Infection

Organism	Incidence (%)
Escherichia coli	80
Klebsiella sp.	10
Proteus	3
Pseudomonas	1
Enterococcus	1
Staphylococcus spp.	1

TABLE 8 Oral Antibiotics for the Treatment of Lower Urinary Tract Infections

Antibiotic Dosage
Amoxicillin 20–40 mg/kg/day div. q 8 h
Trimethoprim/sulfamethoxazole 6–12 mg TMP/
  30–60 mg SMX/kg/day div. q 12 h
Sulfisoxazole 120–150 mg/kg/day div. q 6 h
Cephalosporins
  Cefdinir (Omnicef®) 14 mg/kg/day div. q 24 h
  Cefixime (Suprax®) 8 mg/kg/day div. q 12 h
  Cefpodoxime (Vantin®) 10 mg/kg/day div. q 12 h
  Cefprozil (Cefzil®) 30 mg/kg/day div. q 12 h
  Loracarbef (Lorabid®) 15–30 mg/kg/day div. q 12 h
  Ciprofloxacin (Cipro®) 20–30 mg/kg/day div. q 12 h

TABLE 9   Parenteral Antibiotics for the Treatment of Pyelonephritis

Antibiotic	Dosage[a]
Ampicillin	100 mg/kg/day div. q 6 h
Ticarcillin	300 mg/kg/day div. q 6 h
Ceftriaxone	75 mg/kg/day div. q 24 h
Cefotaxime	150 mg/kg/day div. q 6 h
Ceftazidime	150 mg/kg/day div. q 6 h
Cefazolin	50 mg/kg/day div. q 8 h
Gentamicin	7.5 mg/kg/day div. q 8 h
Tobramycin	5 mg/kg/day div. q 8 h
Ciprofloxacin	20 mg/kg/day div. q 12 h
Meropenem	60 mg/kg/day div. q 8 h

[a] See Chapter 20 for dosages in neonates.

disk method, using the usual serum rather than urine antibiotic concentration breakpoints. Since antibiotics are excreted in urine in extremely high concentrations, even a pathogen resistant to an antibiotic based on blood concentration criteria may be rapidly eradicated. Still antibiotic susceptibility testing is required to select the most appropriate agent.

With initiation of appropriate antibiotic therapy, a clinical response is usually seen within 24 to 48 hours. The optimal duration of treatment in uncomplicated cystitis is controversial. Single dose or short course antibiotic therapy may be associated with a higher risk of recurrence and thus a course of 7 days, in uncomplicated UTI, is appropriate. With pyelonephritis, effective treatment should be instituted as soon as possible. With delay in treatment of greater than 3 days, the risk of renal scarring is increased. For acute pyelonephritis, therapy should be continued for 7 to 14 days (Table 9).

Any toxic-appearing child or infant with suspected pyelonephritis should be hospitalized for intravenous antibiotic treatment. Oral antibiotics may be substituted for intravenous therapy when the patient has been afebrile for 24 to 48 hours.

RECURRENT URINARY TRACT INFECTION

Recurrence is observed in 30% to 50% of children with UTI, with approximately 90% of recurrences seen within 3 months of the initial episode. Eighty percent of recurrences are new infections by different fecal-colonic bacterial species that have become resistant to recently administered antibiotics. The recurrence rate is not altered by extending the duration of initial treatment. A daily prophylactic dose is recommended until imaging studies are obtained.

The anatomic status of the upper urinary tract or the presence or absence of VUR can have an important bearing on the long-term treatment chosen in recurrent UTI (Table 10).

Children having more than 2 UTI episodes in a 12-month period with normal X-rays may need chronic prophylactic antibiotic therapy for 3 to 6 months to allow repair of intrinsic bladder defense mechanisms. Girls with frequent UTI tend to have asymptomatic recurrences. Resistance to antibiotics commonly develops due to R1 factors in fecal-colonic bacteria in patients on long-term suppressive therapy. Children with recurrent UTI and anatomic defects or reflux may need prophylactic antibiotics as long as the defect exists (Table 11).

During antimicrobial prophylaxis for recurrent UTI, girls and less commonly boys may experience breakthrough infections. There is a high incidence of voiding dysfunction or constipation in these children. The number of breakthrough infections can be reduced by placing these children on a regimen of frequent, timed voiding and double antimicrobial prophylaxis consisting of nitrofurantoin 2 mg/kg each morning and trimethoprim/sulfamethoxazole 2/10 mg/kg at bedtime.

Other methods for reducing reinfection of the lower urinary tract in girls include: intense therapy of any constipation, avoiding bubble bath and detergents in bath water, wiping

TABLE 10 Long-Term Management of Recurrent Urinary Tract Infection

Clinical findings/management	Prophylaxis
With vesicoureteral reflux	
Surgical correction	Prophylaxis until resolution of reflux
No surgical correction	Prophylaxis until 10 years of age, and risk of renal scarring is reduced, or until reflux resolves
Without vesicoureteral reflux	
Investigate other genitourinary abnormalities: obstructive uropathy, neurogenic bladder, bladder dysfunction, ureter duplication, calculi	
Investigation findings positive	Prophylaxis for at least 1 year or until surgical correction
Investigation findings negative(with three or more episodes of urinary tract infection over past 12 months)	Prophylaxis for 6 months and assess any dysfunction of the lower urinary tract

perineal area from front to back after voiding or defecation, ingesting 1 to 2 L of water per day, emptying the bladder every 3 to 4 h during the day, and wearing cotton rather than nylon underwear.

PERSISTENT URINARY TRACT INFECTION

Failure to eradicate an organism from the urine suggests an anatomic or physiologic defect (Table 12). Such patients require continuous antibiotics until the underlying abnormality resolves or is corrected surgically.

INDICATIONS FOR RADIOGRAPHIC EVALUATION

Guidelines for radiographic evaluation of the upper and lower urinary tract following UTI differ among authoritative sources; however, a reasonable approach is to evaluate the urinary tract after the first culture-proven infection in all boys and younger girls (Table 13). The only exception is for cystitis in older females, especially if sexually active. Renal scarring and damage are most common before 5 years of age in children with recurrent infection associated with anatomic or functional abnormalities. In girls with VUR, the incidence of renal scarring is increased 3- to 4-fold if a second UTI has occurred prior to recognition and management of reflux.

Cystography, either radiographic or radionuclide, is the only way to detect reflux with certainty. A standard contrast voiding cystourethrogram (VCUG) is preferred for the initial

TABLE 11 Antibiotic Prophylaxis for Recurrent Urinary Tract Infections

Antibiotic	Dosage
Trimethoprim/sulfamethoxazole	2 mg TMP/10 mg SMX/kg/day as a single bedtime dose or 5 mg TMP/25 mg SMX/kg twice/wk
Nitrofurantoin	1–2 mg/kg/day div. q 24 h
Sulfisoxazole	10–20 mg/kg/day div. q 12 h
Nalidixic acid	30 mg/kg/day div. q 12 h
Methenamine mandelate	
Amoxicillin	75 mg/kg/day div. q 12 h
Cephalexin	10 mg/kg/day div. q 12 h

TABLE 12   Factors Causing Persistent Urinary Tract Infections

Anatomic defects (obstruction or vesicoureteral reflux)
Foreign bodies (catheters, stones)
Dysfunction of the lower urinary tract
Constipation

TABLE 13   Recommendations for Radiographic Evaluation

Upper urinary tract
Renal ultrasound
Lower urinary tract
Radiographic contrast voiding cystourethrogram in males
Contrast voiding cystourethrogram or radionuclide cystogram in females
Special studies
Intravenous pyelography (IVP)
Anatomical detail
Dimercaptosuccinic acid (DMSA) scan
Early diagnosis of pyelonephritis
Vesicoureteral reflux
Scar detection
Assessment of renal function
Computerized tomography
Suspected abscesses
Flourourodynamic Study (FUDS)
Assess associated lower urinary tract dysfunction

study, especially in males because it best defines the anatomy of the bladder and urethra and detects posterior urethral valves. Renal ultrasound will demonstrate hydronephrosis of one pole or the entire collecting system and will show ureteral dilatation with a high degree of accuracy. If both of these tests are negative, a structural defect is unlikely.

If the child has symptoms of incontinence with or without constipation, a flourouro-dynamic study (FUDS) may be done in place of the VCUG. FUDS will elucidate any detrusor or sphincter dysfunction as well as demonstrate reflux and urethral anatomy (Fig. 1).

Appropriate timing of radiographic studies is variable. A child hospitalized with pyelonephritis should undergo renal ultrasound as early as possible, since results might influence management. A voiding cystogram can be obtained at any convenient time during treatment. Antimicrobial therapy should be continued in therapeutic or prophylactic doses as the radiographic assessment is being performed and evaluated. Any degree of VUR is sufficient to warrant treatment and long-term observation (Table 10). Obtaining the cystogram in closer proximity to the episode of UTI may reveal marginal VUR, since some children only demonstrate reflux while infected.

Renal scintigraphy to confirm pyelonephritis by demonstration of a photopenic area is not necessary unless it would alter the management of the patient.

VESICOURETERAL REFLUX

The path of the ureter through the bladder wall and submucosa follows an oblique course. This configuration creates a flap-valve mechanism which normally prevents the reascent of urine into the upper urinary tract. When the UVJ is deformed due to a congenital defect or high bladder pressure, a bladder contraction will cause urine to ascend into the ureter and pelvis. VUR therefore allows bacteria access to the kidney.

The different configurations of the renal papillae include both simple and compound types. Compound papillae have more circular openings to the collecting ducts, which allow easier access of bacteria into the renal parenchyma.

VUR is graded according to the degree of filling of the ureter, renal pelvis, and calyces and the presence of dilatation—a scale of I to V has become standard (Fig. 2). The majority of children will show low-grade reflux (I or II) and 85% of these cases resolve spontaneously over

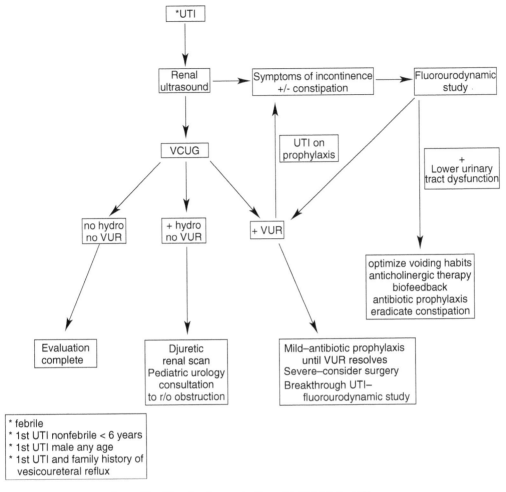

FIGURE 1 Algorithm for the evaluation of initial febrile UTI.
Abbreviations: UTI, urinary tract infection; VCUG, voiding cystourethrogram; VUR, vesicoureteral reflux.

a period of several years. Those children with higher grade reflux show lower rates of resolution. All children with VUR should initially be maintained on prophylactic antibiotic therapy until the reflux resolves, in order to reduce the risk of renal scarring. In children older than 5 years who have not demonstrated breakthrough UTI, a period of observation without

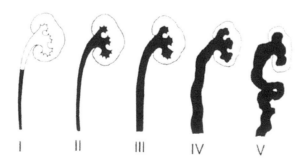

FIGURE 2 The grading of vesicouretheral reflux as defined by The International Study classification; blacked-out areas show extent of reflux.

antibiotics may be considered, provided that compliance is optimal. Cystograms with X-ray contrast material or radionuclide agents should be obtained every 1 to 2 years to monitor the resolution of reflux. Renal growth, as well as any degree of renal scarring, should be assessed on an annual basis with renal ultrasound or radionuclide scanning. Children with recurrent UTI, poor renal growth, progressive renal scarring, or persistent high-grade reflux (IV or V) may be candidates for ureteral reimplantation. The inheritance of VUR has not been defined, but VUR is a familial disorder. One-third of asymptomatic siblings will also have this disorder and should be evaluated for VUR.

LOWER URINARY TRACT DYSFUNCTION

Bladder dysfunction, as already outlined, may be due to maturational factors, or neurogenic disorders, or the dysfunctional elimination syndrome. Children with recurrent UTI should be questioned carefully about voiding habits, daytime incontinence, posturing to defer voiding, or constipation. Unstable bladder contractions should be suspected in children with symptoms of detrusor instability, urgency incontinence, squatting or posturing to defer voiding. Anticholinergic therapy (oxybutinin, propantheline, or imipramine) may be required for long-term control of UTI in addition to prophylactic antibiotic therapy. Causes of fecal soiling or constipation should also be addressed.

Dysfunctional elimination syndrome is a relatively new term established to describe the interplay between functional constipation and bladder dysfunction, and should be considered in children with recurrent UTI. Any child being evaluated for recurrent UTI should be questioned specifically about bowel habits. No standard definition of constipation exists, but symptoms indicative of constipation include a greater than 72 h interval between bowel movements, encopresis, small hard stools, fecal retention as determined by rectal exam after defecation, or the appearance of stool throughout the colon on X-ray. Constipation has been implicated as a major cause of failure of medical treatment of UTI. In addition, constipation has been found to cause uninhibited bladder contractions that result in incontinence or enuresis.

Constipation should be aggressively treated with dietary fiber supplementation. The grams of fiber needed daily can be calculated by the simple formula of age $+ 5 =$ grams of fiber daily, which is approximately 0.5 g/kg/day. Laxatives, enemas, and reconditioning of normal bowel habits by timed toilet sitting are also used to treat constipation. Progressively, as constipation resolves, medications may be titrated down and eventually discontinued. Physicians should be aware that anticholinergic therapy, which may be used for bladder instability can predispose to constipation. Several studies have found that successful treatment of constipation can cure recurrent UTI in patients without anatomic abnormalities.

CLEAN INTERMITTENT CATHETERIZATION

In children with neurogenic bladder dysfunction requiring clean intermittent catheterization, asymptomatic bacteriuria may persist. In such cases, repeated treatment of positive urine cultures in the absence of symptoms may result in selection of progressively more resistant organisms. Treatment should thus be reserved for symptomatic UTI, such as fever, new onset of wetting between catheterizations, or otherwise unexplained abdominal pain.

URINARY TRACT OBSTRUCTION

Hydronephrosis may be detected on initial ultrasonography following a UTI. If VCUG fails to demonstrate VUR, a diuretic renal scan should be obtained to assess the degree of obstruction at the UPJ or UVJ. When hydronephrosis is detected prenatally, asymptomatic infants with certain categories of milder urinary tract obstruction and good renal function may be observed for spontaneous improvement. Close urologic surveillance with frequent imaging studies of the upper urinary tract and prophylactic antibiotics is recommended. Accurate documentation of any episodes of UTI is essential to determine whether corrective surgery

TABLE 14   Treatment of Candiduria

Removal or change of catheter
Fluconazole 3–6 mg/kg/day p.o. × 2–5 days
or
Bladder irrigation with amphotericin B 5–15 mg/100 mL D$_5$W
Treatment failures: Intravenous antifungal agents
    Fluconazole 12 mg/kg/day div. q 12 h
    Amphotericin B 0.3 mg/kg/day ix. div. q.d. for 2–5 days

may be required. In patients with severe urinary tract obstruction, sufficient antibiotic concentrations may not be achieved in the urine due to poor renal function. In such cases, failure to respond to antibiotics suggests the need for retrograde or percutaneous drainage of the infected system.

CANDIDURIA

Immunosuppression, prematurity, debilitation, prolonged antibiotic therapy, and catheterization are risk factors for candiduria. Infection may present with tissue invasion or obstruction of the urinary tract secondary to fungus balls. Urine culture containing 10,000 colonies/mL of *Candida* defines significant infection, and visualization of hyphae on urinalysis suggests tissue invasion. Investigation of candiduria consists of ultrasound of the kidneys and bladder to detect any fungus balls. *Candida* spreads to the kidneys hematogenously as well as ascending infection from the bladder.

Asymptomatic candiduria occurs as a consequence of isolated colonization of the urinary tract. Any predisposing factors should be removed and the urine should be alkalinized to a pH of 7.5 because *Candida* grows best in an acidic urine.

If candiduria is confined to the bladder, both oral fluconazole and irrigation with amphotericin B (100–300 mL solution, 5–15 mg/100 mL D$_5$W) have been shown to sterilize the bladder. Removal of an indwelling catheter is required to eradicate *Candida* and intermittent catheterization is an option in patients needing continued bladder drainage. Bladder irrigation should not be performed in the presence of VUR with high bladder pressures, as systemic absorption of amphotericin B may result. Systemic therapy for *Candida* may be required if multiple sites of infection are documented (Table 14). In cases of systemic candidiasis, the renal parenchyma is involved in 88% of cases.

PERINEPHRIC AND RENAL ABSCESSES

A renal abscess may be caused by ascending infection of mainly gram-negative organisms or hematogenous seeding by gram-positive infections during episodes of bacteremia. Patients present with spiking temperatures, flank pain, abdominal distention, or other abdominal symptoms. Renal abscess is often a difficult diagnosis to make, but it should be considered in cases of prolonged fever refractory to antimicrobial therapy. CT is the diagnostic test of choice in cases of renal abscess because it delineates the extent of the abscess. Confirmation of a renal abscess warrants continued intravenous antibiotic therapy until full resolution of the abscess is documented by repeat radiographic studies. If there is no concomitant infection in the renal collecting system and the pathogen has not been determined, percutaneous aspiration of the abscess may be performed to obtain a specimen for culture. Failure to respond to continued intravenous antibiotics dictates the need for drainage of the abscess. A cortical abscess may rupture into the perinephric space, and remain confined within the fascia surrounding the kidney. The evaluation and treatment of a perinephric abscess is similar to that of a renal abscess. Multiloculated perinephric abscesses usually require surgical drainage.

12 | Skin and Soft-Tissue Infections

ABSCESSES

Skin and soft tissue abscesses occurring in the normal child are often managed simply with incision and drainage, debridement and irrigation. There is no clear evidence that antibiotics offer any benefit in the treatment of abscesses that can be drained. When medical therapy is considered necessary such as with nonfluctuant subcutaneous abscesses or cellulitis, systemic antimicrobial therapy should be given. Persistent or severe infections should alert the physician to the possibility of other underlying conditions. Occasionally, streptococcal and staphylococcal skin abscesses result in toxic shock syndrome (see Chapter 2) and skin infections caused by exotoxin producing *Staphylococcus aureus* evolve to staphylococcal scalded skin syndrome with its characteristic Nikolsky sign (Fig. 1).

ACNE

The pathogenesis of adolescent acne involves a combination of sebaceous follicle obstruction, increased sebum production and overgrowth of the common skin bacterium, *Proprionibacterium acnes*.

Therapy is directed at skin cleansing, drying, removal of comedones, and reduction in bacterial colonization (Table 1).

ADENOPATHY

Lymph node enlargement in children may reflect either a localized or a generalized systemic process. Adenitis (see Chapter 3) should be differentiated from adenopathy since etiologies and management varies considerably. Multiple bacteria have been recognized as etiologic agents of adenitis and therapy should be aimed at these organisms (see Table 4 of Chapter 3). Diagnosis may require needle aspiration, fine needle, or excisional biopsy.

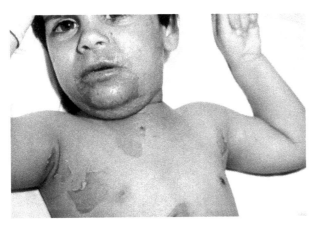

FIGURE 1 Nikolsky sign in a child with staphylococcal scalded skin syndrome. The upper layer of the dermis is wrinkled and has peeled back with light stroking, "like wet tissue paper."

TABLE 1   Treatment of Acne

Initial
Topical benzoyl peroxide 5% bid plus
Topical antibiotic b.i.d. (morning and afternoon)
Clindamycin 1% gel or erythromycin 3%
If no response seen or acne vulgaris
Add tretinoin q.d. (at night before bed) 0.025%
cream or 0.01% gel
Stop topical antibiotics
Begin p.o. antibiotics
Doxycycline 100 mg b.i.d. or
Minocycline 50 mg b.i.d.

TABLE 2   Causes of Persistent or Generalized Adenopathy

Infectious
Tuberculosis (scrofula)
Infectious mononucleosis
Cat scratch disease
CMV
Toxoplasmosis
Other viruses
Tularemia
Kawasaki disease
Syphilis
Hepatitis
Brucellosis
Noninfectious
Leukemia
Lymphoma
Neuroblastoma
Other malignancies
Sarcoidosis

When adenopathy is persistent, there are other important diagnostic considerations, both infectious and noninfectious. Most important is ruling out diagnoses where early intervention is of major clinical benefit (Table 2).

With persistent adenopathy, the primary concern centers around the possibility that an oncogenic process may be the etiology. If the patient is younger than 8 years, leukemia is the most likely malignancy and this can be screened with a complete blood count (CBC), lactic dehydrogenase, and uric acid (see Chapter 3). If the child is older than 8 years, lymphoma is a possibility and can only be ruled out with a fine needle or excisional biopsy. Prior to this procedure, other aspects of the differential diagnosis may be evaluated during a 30-day observation period as outlined in Table 3.

TABLE 3   Approach to Persistent Adenopathy

Initial evaluation
History (pertinent exposure)
Physical examination (measure lymph nodes; if fluctuant see Table 4 of
Chapter 4)
CBC
Bartonella henselae serology (if exposure to kittens)
Mono spot test (if CBC supportive)
TB skin test
Throat culture
Chest X-ray
Serum to hold (acute serum)
Initial management (above laboratory results negative)
Penicillin or other p.o. antibiotic × 14 days
Remeasure node in 14 days
14 days
Node smaller: no further evaluation
Node unchanged, larger or additional nodes
Serum (convalescent, paired with acute)
EBV
CMV
toxoplasma
30 days (all tests negative)
Fine-needle biopsy
If not definitive
Excisional biopsy

TABLE 4   Etiologic Agents of Blepharitis

Staphylococcus aureus
Moraxella lacunata
Pediculus pubis
Pediculus capitis
Demodex follicularum

TABLE 5   Most Common Sites of Decubitus Ulcers

Sacrum
Heel
Ischium
Lateral malleolus

BLEPHARITIS

Recurrent inflammation of the eyelid margins frequently occurs in persons with poor personal hygiene or hypersensitivity. Complaints include redness, irritation, and burning. Diagnosis may require culture and scrapings from the inflamed eyelid margins. Gram stains demonstrate polymorphonuclear leukocytes and bacteria (Table 4).

Treatment consists of daily debridement with warm, moist compresses, and generalized improved personal hygiene. Topical antibiotic ophthalmic drops (sulfacetamide, bacitracin, chloramphenicol, or gentamicin) may be used 3 to 4 times per day. Local corticosteroids are employed for allergic blepharitis. Systemic antibiotics are only necessary in resistant cases.

For pediculus infestation, remove the parasites and ova with forceps and apply 3% ammoniated mercury ointment or 1% physostigmine ointment 4 times per day for 7 days. Another alternative is smothering the lice with petrolatum, applied 2 or 3 times daily for 7 to 10 days. Other areas of infestation must also be treated.

DECUBITUS ULCERS

Decubitus ulcers occur when soft tissues have suffered prolonged pressure, friction, and shearing force. Pressure over body sites first results in erythema. Once skin and soft tissue breakdown progresses, bacterial colonization and subsequently deeper invasion occur. Bacterial etiology can be determined by standard culture techniques, which usually reveals multiple pathogens. Occasionally biopsy is required to obtain meaningful culture material (Tables 5 through 7).

EXANTHEMATOUS DISEASES

The exanthematous diseases may be difficult to diagnose. Features to consider include: immunization history, exposure, prodromal period, nature and distribution of rash, diagnostic and pathognomonic signs, and laboratory confirmation (Table 8). A unique centrifugal vesicular eruption is Gianotti–Crosti syndrome (Fig. 2), previously associated with hepatitis B infection in 25% of cases, but now more commonly seen with enteroviruses, hepatitis C, Epstein-Barr virus (EBV), and AIDS.

HORDEOLUM AND CHALAZION

A hordeolum is an infection of the glands of Zeis. Most frequently it results from a staphylococcal infection of the ciliary follicle and associated sebaceous glands.

TABLE 6   Etiologic Agents Recovered from Decubitus Ulcers

S. aureus
S. epidermidis
Pseudomonas
Gram-negative enterics
Anaerobic organisms

TABLE 7   Treatment of Decubitus Ulcers

Relieve pressure, friction, and shearing force
Removal of devitalized tissue, whirlpool for large or deep areas
Keep surrounding areas of skin clean and dry
Topical and systemic antibiotics should be selected on the basis of culture and sensitivity patterns and used only for more severe cases
Ciprofloxacin plus clindamycin when multiple pathogens recovered

TABLE 8   Classification of Rashes

Maculopapular	Sunburn
Miliaria	Papulovesicular
Measles	VZV
Rubella	Coxsackie virus infections
Scarlet fever	Rickettsialpox
Enteroviral	Disseminated herpes simplex
Infectious mononucleosis	Impetigo
Erythema infectiosum	Insect bites
Exanthem subitum	Gianotti-Crosti (hepatitis B in 5%)
Toxoplasmosis	Petechial
Kawasaki disease	Rocky mountain spotted fever
Scalded-skin (*Staphylococcus*)	Meningococcemia
Meningococcemia	Ehrlichiosis
Rocky Mountain spotted fever	Infectious mononucleosis
Other tick fevers	*Haemophilus influenzae* sepsis
Typhus	Papular urticaria
Toxic erythemas	Drug eruptions
Drug eruption	Molluscum contagiosum

A chalazion is a granulomatous process caused by retention of Meibomian gland secretions. Although it usually resolves spontaneously, excision is occasionally required (Table 9).

IMPETIGO

Impetigo is a superficial infection of the skin caused primarily by *Staphylococcus aureus*. Group A streptococcus is also recovered in 20% to 30% of cases. The localized skin infection may follow

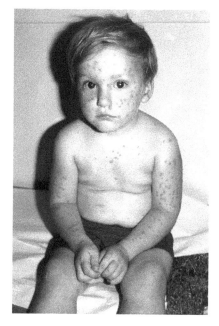

FIGURE 2   (*See color insert.*) Gianotti-Crosti syndrome, also known as papular acrodermatitis of childhood, is characterized by the rapid development of symmetrical flat-topped (lichenoid) skin-colored or erythematous papules in a centrifugal distribution.

TABLE 9   Treatment of Hordeolum and Chalazion

Hordeolum	Warm compresses
	Topical antistaphylococcal ointment
	Resistant cases may require incision and drainage and systemic antibiotics
Chalazion	Similar to hordeolum but may require excision

minor trauma. Disease first appears as discrete papulovesicular lesions surrounded by erythema, which become purulent and form an amber-colored crust (Fig. 3). These lesions are only mildly contagious but care must be taken to prevent spread to other individuals (Table 10).

LACERATIONS AND PUNCTURE WOUNDS

Trauma to the skin and soft tissues, particularly lacerations or puncture wounds, have the potential of developing secondary bacterial infection. Often the most likely bacterial etiology depends on the nature of the wound and location (i.e., *Staphylococcus* and *Streptococcus* with lacerations and *Pseudomonas* with puncture wounds to the feet). Initial antibiotic therapy depends on assessment as to the most likely organisms while definitive therapy is guided by culture results (Table 11).

MOLLUSCUM CONTAGIOSUM

Molluscum contagiosum is a disease of the skin caused by a pox virus. It appears that the virus is spread by direct contact and sexual abuse is one consideration in the infected child. Diagnosis is established by biopsy, stained smears of the expressed molluscum body, or viral cultures. Mild cases usually resolve without medical intervention (Table 12).

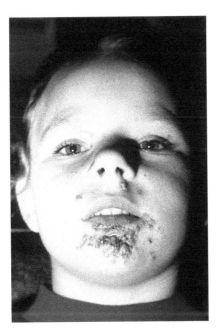

FIGURE 3   Impetigo. Pustular, honey-crusted or bullous skin lesions due almost exclusively to *Staphylococcus aureus* and less frequently (20%) to Group A streptococci.

TABLE 10   Treatment of Impetigo

Careful cleansing with soap and water
Cephalexin 25–50 mg/kg/day div. q 8 h; clindamycin 10–30 mg/kg/day
   div. q 8 h; or erythromycin 35–50 mg/kg/day div. q 6 h × 10 days
or
Mupirocin ointment q.i.d. × 10 days

TABLE 11   Treatment of Lacerations and Puncture Wounds

Irrigation
Careful debridement and removal of foreign material
Suturing as indicated for cosmetic repair and to
   prevent fluid collection
Antibiotics should be used only if infection has
   occurred
Initiate tetanus prophylaxis as indicated

TABLE 12   Treatment of Molluscum Contagiosum

Often no treatment is necessary
Shaving to unroof and apply imiquimod 5% cream
   or cantharidin collodion 0.7%
Extraction or curettage
Liquid nitrogen freezing

MYOSITIS AND PYOMYOSITIS

Myositis is inflammation of large muscles usually associated with a viral infection (Table 13). Muscle pain is the initial symptom, followed by local swelling. Diagnosis is made by identifying the underlying infectious agent but may require needle aspiration, blood cultures, or muscle biopsy (Table 14).

PEDICULOSIS CAPITIS (HEAD LICE)

The prevalence of head lice has increased over the past decade, attributable primarily to the increased resistance of *Pediculis humanus capitis* to many over-the-counter medications. The presence of head lice does not suggest poor hygiene but simply exposure to another infested individual. Infestation is much less common in African Americans because of the characteristics of their hair. "No-nit" school and day-care policies are inappropriate and nits need not be

TABLE 13   Etiology of Myositis

Myositis
  Viruses
    Influenza B
    Coxsackie B
  Other enteroviruses
    Herpes simplex
  Bacteria
    Leptospirosis
    Meningococcus
  Parasites
    Cysticercosis
    Toxoplasmosis
    Trichinosis
Pyomyositis
  S. aureus
  Group A β-hemolytic streptococci
  Coliforms
  Anaerobes

TABLE 14   Treatment of Pyomyositis

Therapy is determined by etiologic agent
   (usually systemic vancomycin
   penicillinase-resistant penicillin: nafcillin
   (or oxacillin) or cephalosporin)
Incision and drainage
Analgesics as needed

TABLE 15   Treatment of Pediculosis Capitis

Over-the-counter
  1% permethrin—apply to scalp for 10 min
  Repeat in 7–10 days
  Pyrethrin plus piperonyl butoxide—apply to dry hair
  Repeat in 7–10 days
Prescription
  5% permethrin cream—apply to scalp and leave
    overnight covered with shower cap
  Repeat in 7–10 days
  Trimethoprim-sulfamethoxazole p.o. × 10
    days—combine with topical therapies
  Ivermectin—200 mcg/kg single dose
  Malathion 0.5% (>6 yr of age)—apply to hair
    overnight
  Lindane 1% shampoo—apply for 4 min
  Crotamiton 10% lotion—apply to scalp for 24 h
Combing nits—only if casts are less than 5 mm
    from the scalp
  Prepare hair with regular mayonnaise
    (not fat free), mineral or olive oil;
    use a close-toothed nit comb

TABLE 16   Treatment of Scabies

Bed linens and clothes need laundering at the start of
  treatment. All infected family members should be
  simultaneously treated
Shower and shampoo prior to treatment
Apply 5% permethrin (Elimite®) cream to the entire
  body
Spare the face but include the scalp, temple and
  forehead; rub in gently
Leave on for 8–14 hours and then remove by
  washing (shower or bath)
Repeat treatment only if reinfection occurs
Severe (Norwegian scabies) or refractory cases:
  single oral dose of ivermectin (200 μg/kg)

removed unless they are less than 5 mm from the scalp since a protein matrix further from the scalp is almost always an empty benign hair cast. All household members should be examined and those infested need treatment as well as anyone who sleeps in the same bed as an infested individual (Table 15).

SCABIES

Sarcoptes scabiei, the itch mite, causes a pruritic rash classically involving the sides and webs of the fingers, flexor surface of the wrist, elbow, anterior axillary folds, female breasts, abdomen, penis, and buttocks. In infants and young children atypical sites, such as the scalp, neck, palms, and soles, may be involved.

Identification of the mite in skin scrapings is accompanied by placing a drop of mineral oil on a suspected lesion and scraping the lesion with a scalpel blade. The best area is the webs of fingers. The scrapings are examined under the light microscope (Table 16).

WARTS (VERRUCAE)

Warts or verrucae are a common viral disease of the skin caused by a papillomavirus. Transmission is thought to be by direct contact. Spontaneous resolution often occurs.

Shaving overlying skin to unroof the columns of viral particles followed by the topical application of 5% imiquimod cream, podophyllin, 40% salicylic acid, or 90% trichloroacetic acid 3 times weekly or periodic electrodesiccation or liquid nitrogen freezing are usually curative. Covering with duct tape has also been shown to be effective. Such treatments need to be repeated until lesions have resolved, which takes 4 to 16 weeks.

13 | Central Nervous System Infections

BRAIN ABSCESS AND CEREBRITIS

The diagnosis and management of intracranial bacterial suppurative disease has evolved remarkably with the advent of CT, MRI, and modern antibiotics. However, brain abscesses, subdural empyema, and other suppurative intracranial disorders remain life-threatening and are frequently associated with significantly disabling neurologic deficits.

Brain abscesses begin as focal bacterial encephalitis or cerebritis, characterized by neutrophilic infiltration and edema. Over several days fibroblastic proliferation and increased vascularity surround an increasingly necrotic core of liquified brain tissue forming the "encapsulated" abscess. The source of infection of the abscesses varies with 30% secondary to contiguous spread (sinusitis, mastoiditis, etc.), 25% being hematogenous, and 25% related to trauma. Approximately 20% have no apparent predisposing factor. Typically, brain abscesses arising from contiguous spread develop adjacent to the initiating site. Abscesses arising from hematogenous spread frequently, occur in areas of middle cerebral artery distribution (namely at the cortical grey-white junction or within the basal ganglia). Factors, which may contribute to brain abscess formation, are given in Table 1.

Brain abscesses present initially with poorly localizable and vague neurologic complaints. Dull headache and low-grade fever associated with predisposing factors are sufficient to clinically raise the suspicion of an intracranial suppurative process. Typical signs and symptoms of brain abscess (Table 2) are variable and systemic signs of sepsis may be absent.

The present availability of CT and MRI has dramatically changed the timescale in which brain abscesses are diagnosed and treated. Initial confirmation of suspected cases as well as longitudinal follow-up can be achieved with serial enhanced CT or MRI scans. Ring enhancement does not necessarily correlate with surgical encapsulation. In the early stages of cerebritis (days 1–3), focal areas of cortical edema may appear on CT without evidence of contrast enhancement. As the lesion evolves into late cerebritis (days 4–9) and early encapsulated phases (days 10–13), contrast diffuses into the center of the lesion. After 2 weeks, CT imaging reveals an enhancing ring and a nonenhancing necrotic center (Fig. 1). In all phases, periabscess edema may produce a significant mass effect. CT and MRI also allow accurate localization of abscesses for neurosurgical interventions, including open or needle drainage with stereotactic instrument guidance.

Lumbar Puncture

Lumbar puncture may be significantly hazardous in patients with brain abscesses or other focal mass lesions. Increased intracranial pressure with focal masses may produce tangential forces, which can herniate brain tissue across fixed structures, such as the tentorium cerebelli or other dural surfaces, when lumbar puncture is performed and spinal fluid removed. In most cases of unruptured brain abscesses, cerebrospinal fluid (CSF) examination does not contribute significantly to the diagnosis. Frequently, few or no inflammatory cells are present and often cultures of CSF do not reveal responsible microorganisms. The opening pressure at the time of lumbar puncture may be significantly elevated indicating a potential for subsequent brain herniation.

TABLE 1 Predisposing Factors for Brain Abscess

Via contiguous spread:
  Sinusitis
    Frontal
    Ethmoidal
    Maxillary
  Mastoiditis and otitis media
  Trauma
    Cribriform plate fractures
    Middle cranial fossa/basilar skull fractures
      (across mastoid air cells, middle ear, etc.)
    Penetrating head injuries
  Postoperative (neurosurgical)
  Meningitis
  Infections of the face or scalp
  Dental infections
  Congenital anomalies of the skull (e.g., encephaloceles)
Via hematogenous spread:
  Cyanotic heart disease
    Right-to-left shunts
    Valvular disease
    Septal defects
  Lung disease
    Bronchiectasis
    Lung abscess or empyema
    Rarely, cystic fibrosis
    Drug abuse (i.v.)
    Other distant focus of infection
Immunosuppression:
  Steroids
  Antimetabolite therapy
  Congenital immunodeficiency disorders
  Acquired immunodeficiency syndrome
Neonates (particularly with *Citrobacter* meningitis)
Sickle cell disease
Congenital CNS malformations
  Dysraphic sites (myelomeningoceles, neurenteric cysts, etc.)
  Sinus tracts associated with dermoids, etc.

Radiographs of the Skull

Radiographs of the skull contribute very little to the diagnosis of brain abscess. Occasionally, exudate may be detected in the frontal, ethmoid, or sphenoid sinuses. Evidence of mastoiditis may be present. The pineal gland is seldom calcified in children and thus, mass shifts across the dura are difficult to detect.

Echoencephalography and Electroencephalography

Echoencephalography and electroencephalography have very little or no current usefulness in the diagnosis and management of brain abscesses. Although electroencephalography (EEG) may aid in the identification of abscesses, changes are generally nonspecific. Localization is better achieved with CT or MRI.

Other studies to be considered for detecting potential predisposing factors or sources of infection in patients with brain abscesses should include echocardiography, which may indicate valvular defects or vegetations. Although a complete blood count (CBC) is routinely performed, it contributes little to the clinical differentiation of brain abscesses. Blood cultures,

TABLE 2   Signs and Symptoms of Brain Abscess

Headache (80%)
　Poorly localizable
　　Dull
　　Worsened by valsalva maneuver or position change
Fever (80%)
　　Prolonged course
　　Absent in 20% of cases
Expanding mass and increased intracranial pressure
　　Vomiting
　　Somnolence, confusion
　　Papilledema (late, and present <50% of cases)
　　Focal signs; aphasia, hemiparesis, ataxia, lower cranial nerve findings,
　　　focal seizures with or without secondary generalization
　　Presentations may be either insidious or "stroke-like"

both for aerobic and anaerobic bacterial and fungal agents such as *Candida* sp. should be obtained, particularly when valvular heart disease and right-to-left shunts are present. Bacteria responsible for brain abscesses are listed in Table 3.

　　Treatment. Early diagnosis and medical management of brain abscess and other intracranial suppurative lesions are now possible with CT and MRI. For this reason, the criteria for surgical intervention have changed. The size and stage of brain abscess encapsulation, amount of edema and mass effect on CT, and the general medical state of the patient often dictate modifications in the standard treatment approach (Tables 4 and 5).

FUNGAL INFECTIONS

Fungal infections of the central nervous system (CNS) may account for both acute and subacute deteriorations in neurologic function, particularly in children with factors predisposing them to opportunistic infections (Table 6). Even with a high index of clinical suspicion, the diagnosis of fungal infection is frequently delayed. Details of treatment are included in Chapter 18, Tables 1-15.

　　Insidious changes in neurologic function, such as unexplained lethargy, psychosis, or irritability, may be the earliest symptoms of fungal infection. More alarming features, including focal or generalized seizures, meningismus, single or multiple cranial neuropathies,

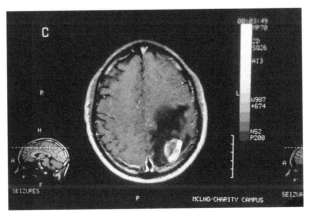

FIGURE 1 Brain abscess with an enhancing surrounding ring and necrotic center.

TABLE 3   Bacterial Organisms Causing Brain Abscess

Common causes	Causes of barrier disruption
Anaerobes[a]	Indwelling ventricular reservoir
Staphylococcus aureus[a]	External ventriculostomy
Streptococcus pyogenes[a]	Cranial surgery
Streptococcus viridans[a]	Hyperalimentation
Streptococcus pneumoniae[a]	Loss of cutaneous integrity
Citrobacter sp. (neonates)	
Mycobacterium tuberculosis	
Less common causes	
Enterobacter sp.[a]	
Klebsiella sp.[a]	
Escherichia coli	
Proteus sp.	
Staphylococcus epidermis[a]	
Haemophilus sp.	
Nocardia sp.	
Listeria monocytogenes	
Aspergillosis fumigatus[a]	
Candida albicans[a]	
Crytpococcus spp.	

[a] Indicates those organisms more often seen in patients with barrier disruption.

hemiparesis, and papilledema, occur as fungal diseases progress in the brain. It is crucial that patients be diagnosed early (Table 7), partly because of preexisting and debilitating disorders and, in part, due to the prolonged therapy with relatively toxic agents that is required following diagnosis. Emphasis must be placed on a high clinical index of suspicion.

The typical pathological patterns of fungal CNS infections accounting for the evolution of signs and symptoms in these disorders are quite variable and usually subtle (Table 8).

Specific fungal organisms associated with CNS infections are numerous (Table 9). Only in unusual circumstances (e.g., mucormycosis), in which orbital and sinus complications are prominent, are characteristic features noted.

Treatment of fungal infections of the CNS is crucially dependent on early recognition and alleviation of predisposing factors. The most widely used intravenous antifungal agent remains amphotericin B. It must be diluted with a 5% dextrose solution to a concentration no greater than 1 mg/10 mL and given as a 4 to 6 h infusion. Amphotericin B is highly nephrotoxic and has limited CNS penetration when used systemically. For that reason,

TABLE 4   Management of Brain Abscesses

Immediately begin broad spectrum antibiotics
   Vancomycin
   Metronidazole and
   Ceftriaxone (Ceftazidime if brain abscess is associated with chronic sinusitis, chronic mastoiditis, or chronic
      middle ear infection)
Neurosurgical intervention within 24 hours
   Needle aspiration if abscess 1 cm or larger
   Drainage or excision when possible for abscesses >4 cm
Repeat enhanced CT or MRI as indicated to determine need for additional surgery
Continue antibiotics, guided by culture results, for a minimum of 6 wk
Repeat enhanced CT or MRI after 6 wk of antibiotics
   Good resolution, no evidence of continued inflammation—stop antibiotics
   Inflammation present—continue antibiotics for 6 more weeks
   Repeat enhanced CT or MRI

TABLE 5 Dosages of Antibiotics for Brain Abscesses

Vancomycin 60 mg/kg/day IV div. q 6 hrs
Metronidazole 30 mg/kg/day IV div. q 8 hrs
Ceftriaxone 80 mg/kg/day IV div. q 24 hrs
Cefotaxime 300 mg/kg/day IV div. q 6 hrs
Ceftazidime 300 mg/kg/day IV div. q 8 hrs
Meropenem 120 mg/kg/day IV div. q 8 hrs
Penicillin 400,000 U/kg/day IV div. q 6 hrs
Ampicillin 400 mg/kg/day IV div q 6 hrs

TABLE 6 Factors Predisposing Children to Fungal CNS Infections

Primary immunodeficiency
Secondary immunodeficiency
Corticosteroid therapy
Antimetabolite therapy (e.g., azothioprine)
Cytotoxic therapy (e.g., cyclophosphamide)
AIDS
Chronic disease
Diabetes mellitus
Leukemia or lymphoma
Chronic renal disease
Cystic fibrosis
Organ transplantation
Intravenous therapy or drug abuse
Hematogenous spread from other foci
Valvular heart disease
Primary pulmonary fungal disease
Primary cutaneous fungal disease
Contiguous spread
Orbital, sinus, or cutaneous spread (e.g., mucormycosis)

intraventricularly administered amphotericin B is often used, particularly in coccidioidal infections. Added CNS toxicity occurs with intraventricular administration.

When administered orally, flucytosine has excellent penetration into the CNS. Generally it is used in combination with amphotericin B in patients with moderate to severe fungal CNS infections, and in neonates. Recent studies in adult patients with AIDS and cryptococcal meningitis have supported the use of amphotericin B in conjunction with flucytosine for better CSF sterilization than with amphotericin B alone.

TABLE 7 Diagnostic Approach to Fungal CNS Infections

Fungal cultures
CSF
Blood
Sputum
Tissue aspirates
CSF analysis
Cell count
Glucose
Protein
Culture (a large volume of CSF is required)
Serum and CSF cryptococcal antigen titers
Special stains (e.g., India ink)
Immunoglobulin electrophoresis or oligoclonal banding
Serum serologic assays
Tissue biopsy for histology and culture
Meninges
Brain
Skin
Lung

Abbreviation: CSE, cerebrospinal fluid.

TABLE 8 Tissue Reactions to Fungal CNS Infections

Meningitis: acute, subacute, or chronic
Meningoencephalitis
Abscess: solitary, multiple, or microabscesses
Granulomas
Arterial thrombosis

TABLE 9   Fungal Organisms Associated with CNS Infection

Aspergillus fumigatus	Aspergillosis
Blastomyces dermatitidis	Blastomycosis, North American
Candida albicans	Candidiasis
Coccidioides immitis	Coccidioidomycosis
Cryptococcus neoformans	Cryptococcosis (torulosis)
Histoplasma capsulatum	Histoplasmosis
Pseudallescheria boydii	Maduromycosis
Rhizopus sp.	Mucormycosis
Sporothrix schenckii	Sporotrichosis

Fluconazole and itraconazole have selected indications in sensitive fungal invasive infections such as blastomycosis, coccidioidomycosis, histoplasmosis, cryptococcosis, and candidiasis. One may be the drug of choice in certain fungal infections poorly responsive to amphotericin B, including *Pseudallescheria* sp. In CNS infections, intrathecal administration may be required because antifungal agents have poor CNS penetration.

Symptomatic care of children with CNS fungal infections includes clinical and laboratory evaluation for the syndrome of inappropriate secretion of antidiuretic hormone (SIADH),

TABLE 10   Currently Recommended Antifungal Therapy for CNS Infections

Aspergillus
 Voriconazole 6–8 mg/kg i.v. q 12 hrs on day one, then 7 mg/kg i.v. q 12 hrs
 plus
 Caspofungin 70 mg/m^2 on day one, then 50 mg/m^2/day q 24 hrs
 or
 Amphotericin B 0.25–0.5 mg/kg/ initially, increase as tolerated to 1.0–1.5 mg/kg/day; infuse as a single dose over 2 hrs
Blastomyces
 Amphotericin B 0.25–0.5 mg/kg initially, increase as tolerated to 0.5–1.5 mg/kg; infuse as a single dose over 2 hrs
Candida
 Amphotericin B 0.25–0.5 mg/kg initially, increase as tolerated to 0.5–1.5 mg/kg; infuse as a single dose over 2 hrs
 plus
 Flucytosine 100–150 mg/kg/day p.o. div. q 6 hrs maximum 150 mg/kg q 24 hrs—adjust for serum levels of 40–60 mcg/mL
 Duration: 30 days minimum, guided by enhanced CT or MRI
Coccidioides
 Fluconazole 12 mg/kg/day i.v. div. q 24 hrs × 30 days
Cryptococcus
 Amphotericin B 0.5–0.8 mg/kg/day i.v. div. q 24 hrs
 plus
 Flucytosine 100 mg/kg/day p.o. div. q 6 hrs
 Duration: 6 weeks
 Followed by: Fluconazole 100 mg/kg/day p.o. div. q 24 hrs
 Duration: 10 weeks
Histoplasma
 Amphotericin B 0.25–0.5 mg/kg initially, increase as tolerated to 0.5–1.5 mg/kg; infuse as a single dose over 2 hrs for 2–3 weeks
 Followed by: Fluconazole 12 mg/kg/day p.o. div. q 24 hrs × 6 months
Mucor
 Surgical debridement
 Amphotericin B 1.5 mg/kg/day i.v. div. q 24 hrs until completing a total dose of 50 mg/kg
 Topical amphotericin B
 Hyperbaric oxygen
Pseudallescheria
 Voriconazole 6–8 mg/kg i.v. q 12 hrs on day one, then 7 mg/kg i.v. q 12 hrs

insidiously developing hydrocephalus, and thrombotic infarctions. Seizures frequently occur and require therapy adapted to impaired renal and hepatic function (Table 10).

VENTRICULITIS (SHUNT INFECTION)

Shunt obstruction and infection are the most frequent and serious complications following placement of ventriculoperitoneal shunts. As many as 20% to 40% of shunts ultimately become infected. In particular, shunts placed in neonates and young infants appear highly susceptible. There may also be an increased incidence of ventriculitis in children with hydrocephalus associated with myelomeningoceles (Arnold-Chiari malformation). The presence of intracranial infections or bacteremia is absolute contraindications to initial shunt placement, and frequently neurosurgeons consider any infection, including otitis media, a relative contraindication. In particular, prolonged operative time for shunt placement appears to correlate best with risk of infection.

Immediately following shunt placement—and for the first 1 to 2 months postoperatively—the risk of infection is highest. Skin contamination is the likely source of colonization of the shunt. For this reason, by far the most common infective agent is *Staphylococcus epidermidis* or less commonly, *Staphylococcus aureus*, diphtheroids, and fungal organisms in particular *Candida* sp. Occasionally, gram-negative bacilli including *Escherichia coli*, *Pseudomonas*, *Klebsiella*, and *Proteus* sp. may cause infection (Table 11).

Usually, clinical recognition of shunt infection is not difficult and occasionally, the operative incision may appear frankly purulent, erythematous, and indurated. Fever, hypotension, or other clinical signs of sepsis may be present in these cases. Alternatively, shunt infection may occasionally present with abdominal distention and signs of bacterial peritonitis. On the other hand, infection with *S. epidermidis* may be more insidious, with local infection over the shunt incision site being the only sign.

In either case, shunt infections frequently present with signs and symptoms of shunt malfunction (decompensated hydrocephalus) with or without fever or other signs of infection. Findings of shunt malfunction/infection include lethargy or irritability, papilledema, cranial nerve palsies (especially 6th nerve palsies), impaired upgaze, and cortical spinal tract dysfunction. Preexisting seizure disorders may worsen with the presence of shunt infection or obstruction.

The examination of CSF by shunt bulb aspiration is the most sensitive and safest procedure for documenting the etiology of shunt infection. Surgically preparing the site of the

TABLE 11   Bacterial Organisms Associated with Shunt Infections

Staphylococcus epidermidis
Staphylococcus aureus
Diphtheroids
Escherichia coli
Pseudomonas sp.
Klebsiella sp.
Proteus sp.
Haemophilus influenzae

TABLE 12   Intraventricular Antibiotics for Shunt Infection

Antibiotic	Daily dose (mg)[a]
Amikacin	5–50
Ampicillin	10–25
Carbenicillin	25–40
Cephalothin	25–50
Chloramphenicol	25–50
Colistin	10
Gentamicin	1–8
Kanamycin	4–10
Methicillin	25–100
Polymyxin B	5
Quinupristin/dalfopristin	2–5
Teicoplanin	5–40
Tobramycin	5–20
Vancomycin	5–20

[a] Higher dosages for large ventricles (hydrocephalus).

shunt bulb, and using a 26-gauge needle, permits aspiration of sufficient CSF for Gram stain, bacterial and fungal cultures, chemical analysis, and cell count. Alternatively, a lumbar puncture may be performed in those instances where decompensated hydrocephalus is not clinically suspected. However, in the presence of complaints of an individual's typical decompensated hydrocephalus symptoms and physical findings of increased intracranial pressure on examination, lumbar puncture is usually contraindicated secondary to concerns of inducing brainstem herniation. Interval increased ventricle size on nonenhanced CT scans of the brain may aid in the diagnosis of decompensated hydrocephalus. However, the absence of increased ventricle size does not rule out shunt malfunction or infection as up to 1/3 of surgically proven shunt malfunctions do not show interval changes on CT scan. Blood cultures should always be obtained as other abnormal laboratory findings may include prominent leukocytosis.

A difficult problem is the presence of positive cultures of shunt hardware removed electively at the time of surgery in the absence of evidence of CSF infection. At times, these shunt colonizations are considered asymptomatic and no antibiotic therapy may be warranted.

The approach to the treatment of ventriculitis depends somewhat on the causative organism. Traditionally, high-dose i.v. antibiotics for 14 days combined with immediate shunt removal have been the treatment of choice. In about 15% of cases of *S. epidermidis* ventriculoperitoneal (VP) shunt infections, high-dose i.v. antibiotics or combined intra-ventricular and i.v. antibiotics without shunt removal are sufficient.

Initial medical management of shunt infection includes vancomycin i.v. (40 mg/kg per day div. q 6 hours) pending the return of cultures. Particularly in cases of staphylococcal infection, an adherent and sticky layer of mucus may be embedded on the shunt tubing, preventing total sterilization of the ventricle and shunt system by i.v. antibiotics alone. Where, after the first 48 h of treatment, clinical or bacteriologic improvement is not achieved, it is recommended that i.v. antibiotics be combined with shunt removal. Antibiotic therapy, at this point, should be tailored to the specific culture results and bacteriologic sensitivities.

Prophylactic therapy for shunt infections should be routinely used, particularly in those patients most susceptible to infection (e.g., neonates, those with Arnold-Chiari malformation, or debilitated patients). The most popular regimen is vancomycin, one pre-op and one or more post-op doses of 10 mg/kg. Other suggested prophylactic regimens include antistaphylococcal agents such as oxacillin or nafcillin in doses of 30 to 50 mg/kg given 2 hours preoperatively and then repeated postoperatively. Vancomycin i.v. preoperatively, and rifampin i.v. pre- and postoperatively have also been used (Tables 12 and 13). No widespread consensus exists regarding recommendations for prophylactic antibiotic therapy. There is widespread agreement, however, that thorough skin preparation, reduced operative time, and other aspects of meticulous surgical care minimize the chance of wound and shunt infection.

VIRAL DISEASE OF THE CNS

Viral and postviral neurologic diseases are frequent in pediatric practice. Although the majority of these disorders are benign and self-limited, notable exceptions occur, including herpes encephalitis, some equine encephalitides, postinfectious encephalomyelitis, Guillain-Barré syndrome, and Reye syndrome.

TABLE 13   Intravenous Antibiotics for Shunt Infection[a]

Staphylococcus epidermidis or *Staphylococcus aureus*
  Nafcillin or oxacillin 200–400 mg/kg/day div. q 6 h
  Vancomycin 60 mg/kg/day div. q 6 h (for nafcillin-resistant organisms)
Gram-negative coliforms
  Ceftriaxone 100 mg/kg/day div. q 24 h
  Cefotaxime 200 mg/kg/day div. q 6 h

[a] Removal of the shunt may be necessary if prompt response to antimicrobial therapy is not obtained.

Several viruses that cause meningoencephalitis (Table 14) appear clinically similar. Seasonal occurrence and associated systemic signs and symptoms may suggest a specific viral cause. Endemic causes of encephalitis include Japanese B equine virus (the most common cause of encephalitis outside of the United States) and the arboviruses. Sporadic encephalitis is usually caused by the enterovirus group. Equine encephalitis, a mosquito-borne viral disease, typically occurs in the warm months whereas herpes encephalitis is sporadic. The presence of gastrointestinal signs and symptoms may suggest an enteroviral agent whereas upper or lower respiratory tract infections may suggest adenovirus as a potential etiology. CNS infectious and postinfectious disorders may occur with common childhood disorders, such as varicella.

The clinical signs and symptoms of viral meningoencephalitis are dependent on the age of the child, severity of illness, and to a lesser extent, the specific viral agent. In general, mental-status changes ranging from coma to delirium, focal or generalized seizures, meningismus, and fever, are typical presenting features. Diagnosis is usually confirmed by examination of CSF and exclusion of other bacterial, protozoan, or fungal organisms. Exceptions to this rule are chemical meningoencephalitis and Mollaret meningitis, the latter being a disorder of recurrent aseptic meningitis associated with herpes simplex virus (HSV) and perhaps other herpes group viruses. Routine studies of CSF include measurement of the opening pressure, cell count and differential, protein and glucose determination (with comparison to the serum glucose level), and viral, bacterial, and fungal cultures when appropriate. Polymerase chain reaction (PCR) diagnostic testing has been developed to detect a variety of pathogens including HSV-1, HSV-2, varicella zoster virus, JC virus, cytomegalovirus (CMV), enterovirus, tuberculosis, and Lyme disease. PCR analysis of the CSF for HSV-1 and HSV-2 has a diagnostic sensitivity and specificity of well over 90%.

In general, treatment of viral meningoencephalitis involves supportive management, whether the patient is hospitalized or followed at home. Complications in treatment are summarized in Table 15. Analgesics, in selected cases, and fluid and electrolyte therapy are usually sufficient. More fulminant causes of viral meningoencephalitis, in particular herpes encephalitis, may rapidly progress and leave the child with severe morbidity or death.

TABLE 14   Viruses Associated with Meningoencephalitis

Arboviruses
   St. Louis encephalitis
   Western equine encephalitis
   Eastern equine encephalitis
   California encephalitis
   Japanese B equine encephalitis
   Venezuelan equine encephalitis
Enteroviruses
   Polio types 1, 2, and 3
   Coxsackie groups A and B
   Enteric cytopathogenic human orphan (ECHO) virus
Herpes viruses
   Herpes virus types 1 and 2
   Varicella-zoster
   Cytomegalovirus (CMV)
   Epstein-Barr
Miscellaneous viruses
   Mumps
   Measles
   Adenovirus
   Influenza A and B
   Lymphocytic choriomeningitis virus

TABLE 15 Possible Complications of Viral Meningoencephalitis

Acute disseminated encephalomyelitis (ADEM)
Acute development of the syndrome of inappropriate secretion of antidiuretic
   hormone (SIADH)
Vomiting and dehydration
Seizure disorder
Behavior disturbances: hyperactivity, delirium, attention deficits

Herpes Encephalitis

Encephalitis caused by HSV-1 or HSV-2 presents with the acute onset of fever and altered consciousness, often associated with seizures and focal neurologic findings. Untreated the course is fulminant, rapidly progressing to coma and death. Erythrocytes in the CSF are seen in approximately 25% of patients so this finding is suggestive of HSV. The best imaging study is T2-weighted MRI, most sensitive for picking up areas of focal edema in patients with encephalitis. MRI reveals edematous changes much sooner and with better delineation than does CT, which may remain normal for several days into the clinical course. CT eventually reveals focal edema and possible hemorrhage in unilateral or bilateral temporal and orbitofrontal regions of the brain. EEG often reveals focal epileptiform activity and/or background slowing over the temporal lobes, ipsilaterally or bilaterally. The finding, when present, is not specific to HSV as other viruses and bacteria can affect the brain in a focal fashion.

CSF should be obtained for culture and PCR. While cultures become negative as early as 24 h of antiviral therapy, PCR may still be useful for up to 10 days of acyclovir. The use of PCR has replaced brain biopsy (Fig. 2) or serologic studies to confirm HSV encephalitis. Gram stain of the CSF should be carefully examined. Although the presence of gross or microscopic blood in CSF strongly suggests herpes, equine encephalitis also produces this change.

The treatment for herpes encephalitis is acyclovir (30 mg/kg/day i.v. div. q 8 h) for 21 days.

Postviral Disorders

Postviral disorders of the CNS often occur in children recovering from seemingly mild, common viral illnesses. The presence of signs and symptoms of optic neuritis, focal seizure activity, myelitis, ataxia, and other motor disturbances such as hemiparesis, monoparesis, or

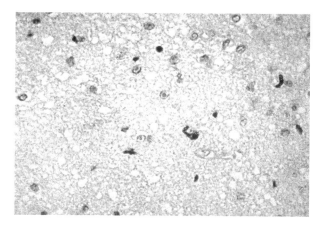

FIGURE 2 (*See color insert.*) Brain biopsy in a 6-year-old showing scattered areas of cells containing cytoplasmic viral inclusions characteristic of herpes simplex encephalitis.

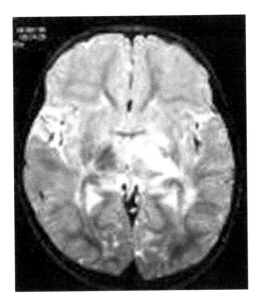

FIGURE 3 Acute disseminated encephalomyelitis (ADEM). Cranial MRI with abnormal increased high-density signals on T2-weighted images, involving white matter within the medial aspect of the temporal lobes, brain stem, basal ganglia, thalamus, and medial cerebellar hemispheres.

paraparesis suggests this neurologic disorder. The chronologic progression of postviral encephalitis may be insidious or fulminant. In addition to the studies used for the evaluation of acute meningoencephalitis, cerebrospinal immunoglobulin electrophoresis, and oligoclonal banding are useful. CT scans, EEG, and the assessment of visual, auditory, and spinal pathways by evoked potentials permit adequate localization and documentation of multiple lesions in the neuraxis.

Acute Disseminated Encephalomyelitis (ADEM)

ADEM is an inflammatory demyelinating disease of the CNS associated with an antecedent viral infection and thought to be immune-mediated. The initial presentation is that of aseptic meningoencephalitis with a CSF pleocytosis and elevated protein. Diagnosis is made by MRI, which characteristically demonstrates multiple areas of increased signal intensity in the white matter on T2-weighted imaging (Fig. 3). Clinical illness lasts 2 to 4 weeks. Although controlled clinical trials are not available, reports have suggested benefit with intravenous immunoglobulin (IVIG) (400 mg/kg/day for 5 days, total 2 g/kg), methylprednisolone, 15 to 30 mg/kg/day, and plasmapharesis.

14 | Surgical Infections

Infection, either endogenous or nosocomial, is a significant factor in the management of surgical care in children. Proper selection of preoperative management, intraoperative judgment and technique, and postoperative care of actual or potential infections can reduce the risk of complications.

A constant flux of new antibiotics may entice the physician into believing that their use alone provides a panacea for all surgical infections. Instead, use of percutaneous or open drainage in consort with antimicrobials should be preferred. Antibiotic choice demands a comprehensive knowledge of the signs and symptoms of common surgical infectious processes and their likely etiologies.

GENERAL PRINCIPLES

The development and progression of surgical infections require a colonizing organism, an appropriate nutritional milieu for that organism, and lack of an appropriate host defense. The number of pathogens and their virulence affects the infectious potential of an inoculum although chronologic and species interactions will affect the gravity of a surgical infection, particularly in cases of aerobic–anaerobic synergism (e.g., *Escherichia coli* and *Bacteroides fragilis*). In addition, nutritional status, length of preoperative stay, perioperative cleansing and skin preparation, duration of the procedure, the immunologic status of the child, and the use of cautery will significantly affect the incidence of infection.

Endogenous infections originate from altered skin or mucosal barriers. Bacterial translocation from the gut occurs following phagocytic ingestion of bacteria in the gut, lymphatic transport of these viable bacteria to extraintestinal tissue, and generation of sepsis from that locus. Although, historically, gut rest following accidental or operative trauma has been strongly advocated, clearly mucosal damage and subsequent microbial translocation can be prevented by early enteral diet. There is increased risk for translocation following prolonged shock, prolonged fast, protein malnutrition, and total parenteral nutrition thus mandating an enhanced awareness of patient nutrition. Glutamine-supplemented diets decrease bacterial translocation and infection. While short-chain fatty acids from fermentable fiber decrease colonic mucosal atrophy and Ω-6 polyunsaturated fatty acids promote survival of sepsis in animal models.

Preoperative hospital stay must be minimized. Preoperative shaving is deleterious and should be abandoned as a practice. Treating remote infections before operation reduces surgical infection risk. Personnel should wash their hands before and after taking care of a surgical wound. The surgeon should not directly touch a fresh wound or drainage without the use of sterile gloves. Any wound drainage should be cultured and examined with Gram's stain. Rigid aseptic technique and rapid but careful completion of the operation provides the greatest protection against postoperative infection. Despite these precautions, high rates of infection may occur without antimicrobial use. Seventy-5% of antibiotic orders on a surgical service, both appropriately and inappropriately, are for prophylaxis as an effort to improve outcome.

ANTIMICROBIAL PROPHYLAXIS

Parenteral antimicrobial prophylaxis is recommended for operations associated with a high risk of infection or not frequently associated with infection but with severe or life-threatening consequences should they occur. Currently, the most common use of antibiotics in hospitals is surgical prophylaxis, which have been shown to be safe and effective against organisms likely to contaminate the operative wound. Antimicrobial prophylaxis is initiated before the procedure, ideally within 60 min prior to the surgical incision, and promptly discontinued after operation. Oral prophylactic antibiotics should not be used to supplement parenteral prophylaxis. Oral antibiotics are used as prophylaxis for colorectal surgery to decrease the bacterial colony count in the gut flora for the purpose of minimizing potential exposure in the operating field. Their use, however, should be limited to the 24 h period before operation.

Several guidelines for antimicrobial prophylaxis in surgery have been published and there is considerable agreement for antimicrobial selection and timing. Recommendations from these groups have been summarized and consolidated in Tables 1 and 2. The goal of antimicrobial prophylaxis is to achieve serum and tissue drug levels that exceed, for the duration of the operation, the mean inhibitory concentrations (MICs) for pathogens most likely to cause postoperative infections.

Other Specific Procedures

Abundant randomized clinical trials have well demonstrated the benefit of antimicrobial prophylaxis for specific surgical procedures. This includes clean, clean contaminated, contaminated, or infected surgical procedures. Major shortcomings are risk of drug toxicity, emergence of resistant organism, and superinfections. Most surgical procedures require specific regimens directed at pathogens previously shown to cause postoperative infection (Table 3).

Dosing, appropriate intervals, and maintaining appropriate blood levels are essential for maximum efficacy. Implementation of these recommendations must balance potential benefit against the risk of complications, including allergy, toxicity, and creation of drug-resistant bacteria. Prophylactic antimicrobials are to be used only if the risk of infection outweighs the risk of complications. Risk of surgery can be quantitated by classification of operative procedures (Table 4).

TABLE 1 Surgical Infection Prevention Guidelines

General dosing:	
Antibiotic timing	Infusion of the first antimicrobial dose should begin within 60 mins before the surgical incision
Duration of prophylaxis	Prophylactic antimicrobials should be discontinued within 24 hrs after the end of surgery
Antimicrobial dosing	An additional antimicrobial dose should be provided intraoperatively if the operation is still continuing 2 half-lives after the initial dose
Antibiotic selection, by procedure:	
Abdominal or vaginal hysterectomy	Cefotetan therapy is preferred; cefazolin or cefoxitin are alternatives. Metronidazole monotherapy is also used. If the patient has a β-lactam allergy, use clindamycin combined with gentamicin or ciprofloxacin or aztreonam; metronidazole with gentamicin or ciprofloxacin; or clindamycin monotherapy
Hip or knee arthroplasty	Use cefazolin or cefuroxime. If the patient has a β-lactam allergy, use vancomycin or clindamycin
Cardiothoracic and vascular surgery	Use cefazolin or cefuroxime. If the patient has a β-lactam allergy, use vancomycin or clindamycin
Colon surgery	For oral antimicrobial prophylaxis, use neomycin plus erythromycin base or neomycin plus metronidazole. For parenteral antimicrobial prophylaxis, use cefotetan, cefoxitin, or cefazolin plus metronidazole. If the patient has a β-lactam allergy, use clindamycin combined with gentamicin, ciprofloxacin, or aztreonam, or use metronidazole combined with gentamicin or ciprofloxacin

Source: From Ref. 1.

TABLE 2   Initial Dose and Time to Redosing for Antimicrobial Drugs Commonly Utilized for Surgical Prophylaxis

Antimicrobial	Renal half-life (h) Patients with normal renal function	Recommended infusion duration	Weight-based dose recommendation	Recommended redosing interval (h)
Aztreonam	1.5–2	3–5 min, 20–60 min	30 mg/kg	3–5
Ciprofloxacin	3.5–5	60 min	10 mg/kg	4–10
Cefazolin	1.2–2.5	3–5 min, 15–60 min	20–30 mg/kg; max. 1 g	2–5
Cefuroxime	1–2	3–5 min,15–60 min	50 mg/kg	3–4
Cefoxitin	0.5–1.1	3–5 min, 15–60 min	20–40 mg/kg	2–3
Cefotetan	2.8–4.6	3–5 min, 20–60 min	20–40 mg/kg	3–6
Clindamycin	2–5.1	10–60 min (do not exceed 30 mg/min)	If <10 kg, 37.5 mg; if >10 kg, 3–6 mg/kg	3–6
Erythromycin base	0.8–3	NA	9–13 mg/kg	NA
Gentamicin	2–3	30–60 min	2.5 mg/kg	3–6
Neomycin	2–3 (3% absorbed under normal gastrointestinal conditions)	NA	20 mg/kg	NA

A classification-specific wound infection rate should be surveyed for all operations. Clean procedures do not require prophylaxis unless the risk of infection during surgery is life-threatening. Prophylactic antibiotics are used in procedure classification clean/contaminated or greater.

Antibiotics given to patients whose wounds are classified as dirty and infected are strictly therapeutic not prophylactic. Although guidelines are unclear, discontinuation of therapeutic antibiotics after the patient is clinically improved and afebrile for a minimum of 48 h is an acceptable use of these agents. Conversely, the child who remains ill and febrile is seldom likely to be helped by unguided changes in antibiotics and there is no rationale for conversion to oral therapy to allow discharge.

WOUND INFECTION

Children have a lower incidence of wound infection than adults; however, a substantial number still occur. Surgical wounds are considered to be noninfected if there is no discharge during healing and infected if there is discharge of pus. Inflamed wounds or culture-positive serous fluid may signify infection. Criteria for infection generally exclude stitch abscess. Clean wound infection rates should be less than 1.5%. This rate may exceed 40% in contaminated or dirty cases. The lower incidence of wound infection in children is probably due to the fact that their delicate tissues require gentle handling, operations are brief, and postoperative stay is brief reducing nosocomial infections. Wound infection rates are highest for abdominal operations and lowest for those on the extremities.

Sutures themselves are foreign bodies; however, absorbable monofilament sutures without interstices provide the least nidus for bacteria. Although leaving the skin open in contaminated cases is advocated by adult surgeons, the technique need not be used in most pediatric wound infections. For example, most pediatric surgeons today primarily close all wounds in patients with perforated appendicitis.

Wound infection may occur as early as the first postoperative day up until many weeks after operation (Table 5). Group A streptococcus infection presents with rapidly advancing erythema and serous drainage. It is often unnecessary to immediately open the wound but high-dose intravenous penicillin or cefazolin should be given and if there is not the expected

TABLE 3   Recommended Antimicrobial Prophylaxis for Certain Surgical Procedures

Surgical procedure	Prophylactic antibiotic
Tonsillectomy and adenoidectomy	No available data
Tympanostomy	Gentamicin eardrops
Cleft palate repair	p.o. TMP/SMX, sulfisoxazole, or ampicillin
Major head and neck surgery	Cefazolin, ampicillin, or gentamicin plus clindamycin
Eye surgery	Gentamicin or tobramycin ophthalmic drops or cefazolin subconjunctival injection
Cardiovascular prosthetic implant	Vancomycin for methicillin-resistant staphylococcus
Cardiothoracic and vascular surgery	Vancomycin
Inguinal hernia repair	No available data
Appendectomy	IV cefoxitin, cefazolin, or metronidazole
Colon surgery	Cefoxitin, gentamicin for ampicillin-resistant enteric gram-negative bacteria
Gastroduodenal surgery	IV cefazolin
Biliary tract surgery	IV cefoxitin; gentamicin for ampicillin-resistant enteric gram-negative bacteria
Elective splenectomy	Pneumococcal vaccines (both Prevnar® and Pneumovax®) before the procedure
Penetrating abdominal trauma	Cefoxitin
Urinary tract obstruction	p.o. TMP/SMX, ampicillin, or nitrofurantoin
Ruptured viscus	Aztreonam or mezlocillin or ampicillin/sulbactam plus metronidazole; aztreonam or gentamicin plus mitronidazole if penicillin-resistant organisms identified
Abortion	
First trimester	IV/IM penicillin G or p.o. doxycycline
Second trimester	Cefazolin, IV/IM penicillin G, or p.o. metronidazole
Orthopedic surgery	Cefazolin or vancomycin
Cerebrospinal fluid shunting	Vancomycin Vancomycinv
Gastrostomy	Cefazolin, vancomycin, or clindamycin
Burns	IV or p.o. penicillin plus 0.5% silver nitrate or 10% afenide acetate cream
Skin surgery	Cefazolin; penicillin; vancomycin if methicillin-resistant *S. aureus* identified

immediate improvement, the wound must be opened. *Clostridia* related cellulitis presents with pain, foul-smelling exudate, and skin crepitus from subcutaneous emphysema and can rapidly progress to widespread necrotizing fasciitis. In addition to rapid institution of penicillin and clindamycin, a surgeon must open the wound and prepare for possible wide incision and debridement. Staphylococcal infection occurs 3 to 7 days after operation with gradual onset of fever, tenderness, induration, swelling, and erythema. Palpation may elicit drainage but if not, the wound should be gently separated, all sutures removed, the wound irrigated with saline, and packed with saline damp to dry dressings. Use of iodoform-impregnated gauze for packing primary or secondary-infected wounds used by many surgeons can cause wound-edge cytotoxicity and is thus far without definable benefit.

Infections caused by enteric bacteria occur from one to many weeks after operation. Erythema is limited, suppuration less prominent, and drainage watery-brown and foul smelling. Besides local signs, there is often systemic toxicity and an intraabdominal source should be aggressively sought for where applicable.

HIV, HEPATITIS B, AND SURGERY

Hepatitis B virus and HIV remain threats to the operating surgeon's career and health. When health care workers follow recommended infection control procedures, the risks of acquiring disease from patients or transmitting these viruses to patients are quite small. Strict adherence to universal precautions, including the appropriate use of handwashing, protective barriers,

TABLE 4 Classification of Operative Procedures

Clean
  Nontraumatic
  Noninflammatory
  No break in technique
  Respiratory, genitourinary, gastrointestinal tract not entered
Clean/contaminated
  Minor break in technique
  Oropharynx entered
  Respiratory or gastrointestinal tract entered without significant spillage,
    i.e., appendectomy, colorectal surgery with prior oral antibiotic therapy
    for gut flora prophylaxis
  Biliary tract entered (without infected bile) i.e. cholecystectomy for
    cholelthiasis or treated cholecystitis
  Vagina entered
  Genitourinary tract entered (without infected urine)
Contaminated
  Major break in technique
  Fresh traumatic wound
  Gross gastrointestinal spillage
  Biliary tract entered (infected bile) i.e., cholangitis
  Genitourinary tract entered (infected urine)
Dirty
  Bacterial inflammation encountered
  Transection of clean tissue for access to purulence
  Traumatic wound from "dirty" source
  Traumatic wound with retained devitalized tissue, foreign body and/or
    fecal contamination
  Perforated viscus

and care in the use and disposal of needles and other sharp instruments, is essential. The recent mandatory use of needleless systems in many hospitals has reduced the incidence of sharp instrument-related exposures. Open dermatitis should restrict the surgeon from patient care and handling of equipment and devices used in performing basic procedures until the condition resolves. Surgeons infected with HIV or HBV (HB$_s$Ag-positive) should not perform exposure-prone procedures without advice from an expert review panel.

BURNS

Infection in children with burns results from multiple systemic and local factors. Endogenous organisms grow easily in the burn eschar and invasion of viable tissue with subsequent systemic infection can follow. Fever is very common in the first 3 days following the burn and, therefore, only persistent hyperpyrexia (>39.5°C) is considered abnormal. Observation of such children for changes in clinical behavior (e.g., increasing fever, poor appetite, or decreased sensorium) will optimize early recognition of infection. Sepsis presents with hypothermia or hyperthermia, trachypnea, mental changes, oliguria, ileus, and hypotension. Crystalloid infusion, ventilatory support, and inotropes (along with antibiotic therapy against cultured organisms) are the cornerstones of sepsis management. Children with recurrent bacteremia should be examined for otitis media, urinary tract infections, tracheobronchitis, pneumonia, and cellulitis and treated accordingly.

    Timely closure of the burn wound by excision and grafting with interim protection by topical antimicrobials are the essentials of burn wound treatment and will prevent most infections. The initial step is twice daily application of manfenide, which has increased eschar penetration. Tangential excision and perioperative vancomycin will minimize colonization by staphylococci. Gram-negative infections should be additionally treated with appropriate

TABLE 5   Characteristics of Wound Infections

Organism	Onset (Days)	Signs	Therapy
Streptococcus	<1–2	Rapid spread of erythema and cellulitis	Penicillin G
Clostridia	<1–2	Erythema, brown foul-smelling drainage, skin crepitus	Pencillin G, clindamycin
Staphylococcus	47	Crepitus, erythema, tenderness, cellulitis, purulent drainagev	Open, debride, and pack wound; PO clindamycin or linezolid; IV vancomycin, clindamycin, or linezolid if cellulitis severe
Enteric gram- negative	7–14	Induration, seropurulent drainage, systemic toxicity	Open, debride, and pack wound Broad-spectrum antibiotics if cellulitis or toxicity severe

culture-guided antibiotics. Pseudomonas infection is best managed by subeschar injection of broad-spectrum β-lactam penicillin before operation (i.e., piperacillin sodium 200–300 mg/kg in 50 mL of saline).

Approximately two-thirds of burn wound infections are now of fungal origin (*Candida* sp. 25%, *Aspergillus* 15%, *Mucor* 8%, and other fungi 19%). Histologic biopsy examination is the most reliable means for diagnosis of fungal infections. Excision of involved tissue usually eliminates *Candida* and *Aspergillus*. Phycomycetes, however, cross-tissue planes, have vascular invasion, and produce expanding necrosis. Systemic acidosis favors dissemination of fungi so must be aggressively treat. Infected wounds should be widely excised and most patients treated with fluconazole or amphotericin B.

SOFT-TISSUE INFECTION

Risk factors (other than burns) for soft tissue infection are listed in Table 6.

SPECIAL INFECTIONS

Progressive Bacterial Synergistic Gangrene

Progressive bacterial synergistic gangrene follows abdominal or thoracic wounds with contaminated foreign bodies or sutures. Necrotic ulcers with purple skin and erythema enlarge slowly, but progressively. Wide local excision usually cures the process.

Synergistic Necrotizing Cellulitis

Synergistic necrotizing, cellulitis occurs in diabetics, particularly those with perineal infections. Tenderness and ulceration with vesicles containing "dishwater" pus in a toxic patient with diabetic ketoacidosis is the usual clinical setting. Skin may appear nearly normal and gas in underlying tissues occurs late in the disease. Anaerobic streptococcus and aerobic gram-negative rods are causative. Fluid resuscitation, appropriate broad-spectrum antibiotic coverage, and radical debridement constitute optimal management.

Fournier's Gangrene

Fournier's gangrene is necrotizing fasciitis of the genitalia (Fig. 1). It frequently follows trauma or contaminated operations, initially presenting with decreased sensation, swelling, necrosis,

TABLE 6   Risk Factors for Soft-Tissue Infection

Risk factor	Infection
Diabetes	All
Cancer, congenital agranulocytosis	*Clostridium septicum* gangrene
Omphalitis, urachal cyst, necrotizing enterocolitis, neonatal monitoring devices, varicella, circumcision, anorectal disease	Necrotizing fasciitis Fournier's gangrene
Outdoor puncture wounds	Tetanus
Chronic immunosuppression, i.e., transplant recipient, AIDS	All

and wound drainage. Polymicrobial etiology, particularly streptococci and *Enterobacteriaceae*, is most likely. Dusky discoloration of the skin indicates impending gangrene. Diabetics are more prone to this infection. It may also follow circumcision, insect bites, or burns. Appropriate broad-spectrum antibiotics and radical debridement are necessary.

Clostridial Cellulitis

Clostridial cellulitis presents with pain, swelling, foul-smelling exudate, and subcutaneous emphysema but with little systemic toxicity. Erythema and serosanguinous discharge progress to give bronzed skin with vesicles and crepitation. Underlying fascia and muscle have extensive necrosis. Wide debridement and high-dose penicillin are usually effective.

Clostridial Myonecrosis

Clostridial myonecrosis (gas gangrene) is associated with diabetes, necrotic tissue, and arterial compromise. Infections of extremities have a better prognosis because of the option for amputation. Physical findings include tachycardia, severe local pain (disproportionate to the

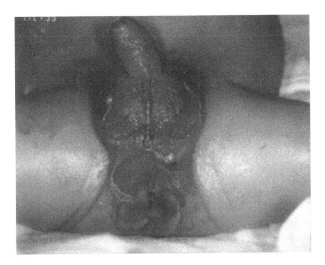

FIGURE 1   Fournier gangrene. Necrotizing fasciitis occurring in the male genital area involving the scrotum and perineum.

appearance of the wound), systemic toxicity, erythema, and discharge. High-dose penicillin is the antibiotic of choice.

Clostridium septicum infection occurs in leukemia, chemotherapy, lymphoma, and congenital agranulocytosis. This organism is more aerotolerant than other clostridial pathogens. Its mode of invasion is translocation across the bowel wall in the absence of neutrophils. Treatment includes bone marrow-stimulating growth factors, aggressive resuscitation, and debridement with high-dose penicillin and clindamycin as the antibiotics of choice.

CARDIAC SURGERY

Patients undergoing open heart surgery, especially with placement of prosthetic heart valves or prosthetic intravascular or intracardiac materials, are at risk for bacterial endocarditis. Endocarditis associated with open heart surgery is most often due to *Staphylococcus aureus*, coagulase-negative staphylococci, or diphtheroids. Streptococci, gram-negative bacteria, and fungi are less common. Vancomycin is most often selected for initial empiric therapy, although the choice of antibiotic should be influenced by each hospital's antibiotic susceptibility data. Prophylaxis should be started immediately before the operative procedure and continued for more than 2 days postoperatively to minimize the emergence of resistant microorganisms. The effects of cardiopulmonary bypass and compromised postoperative renal function on serum antibiotic levels should be considered and doses timed appropriately before and during the procedure.

CHEST INFECTION

Mediastinitis

The limits of the mediastinum are the medial pleura, the sternum, and the vertebral column. Contamination of the mediastinal space occurs by accidental or operative trauma or from spillage from adenopathy (Table 7).

Prompt surgical drainage is necessary to control serious infection and use of continuous antibiotic irrigation can be used to supplement systemic broad-spectrum antibiotics, which provides coverage for gram-positive and gram-negative bacteria. Granulomatous infections including tuberculosis and histoplasmosis can cause superior vena cava syndrome or

TABLE 7   Features and Management of Mediastinitis

Symptoms
Pain
Dyspnea
Tachycardia
High fever
Radiographic signs
Mediastinal and/or subcutaneous emphysema
Mediastinal widening
Mediastinal air/fluid levels
Pericardial effusion on echocardiography
Organisms
Gram-positive cocci
Anaerobes
Treatment
Prompt Drainage
Meropenem plus vancomycin or linezolid

obstruction of the trachea and esophagus secondary to direct compression or fibrosis. The features and management of mediastinitis are summarized in Table 5.

Empyema

The antibiotic era has gradually changed the causal factors, incidence, and seriousness of empyema. Pleural fluid should be aspirated for culture and determination of character. Analysis for pH, white blood cell count, protein level, glucose, lactate dehydrogenase (LDH) and culture should be performed (see Chapter 7, Table 16). Empyema must be regarded as an abscess and treated as such by complete evacuation of purulent material. Following thoracentesis or tube thoracotomy, the patient's clinical condition rather than radiography should guide therapy. The early use of thoracotomy, or preferably thoracoscopy with decortication should be considered if a patient with empyema has persistent difficulty in respiration, multiple loculations with pleural thickening, a febrile course, or persistent leukocytosis despite the use of drainage and antibiotics (see Chapter 8). In addition, empyemas in children with multiple organisms, immunocompromise, an infradiaphragmatic source, or those with empyema secondary to aspiration pneumonia can benefit from decortication if lesser measures are not rapidly effective. Antibiotic therapy for pneumonia-associated empyemas is outlined in Table 8.

Pulmonary Abscess

Pulmonary abscess follows cavitation of suppurative lung infections. Very young, immuno-compromised, or chronically ill children are most frequently affected. Precipitating factors may include aspiration, operation, or coma. Staphylococcus is the most frequently involved organism and α- and β-hemolytic streptococci, *Pseudomonas*, *Escherichia coli*, and *Klebsiella* are also seen. Careful bacteriologic examination for anaerobic organisms may yield *Peptostreptococcus*, *Peptococcus*, *Bacteroides melaninogenicus*, or *Bacteroides fragilis*. The empiric choice of antimicrobial therapy is clindamycin or penicillin G for those with allergy. Antibiotics must be continued for 6 weeks. Bronchoscopic aspiration of contents will allow additional assessment of anatomic pathology, including retained foreign body examination. Lobectomy with thoracostomy drainage may be needed for chronic thick-walled abscesses, which have not responded to 2 weeks of medical management.

ABDOMINAL INFECTION

Peritonitis

Following inflammation or perforation of the gastrointestinal tract, both a chemical and bacterial insult are introduced into the peritoneal cavity. Leukocyte and macrophage congregation into a fibrinopurulent serosal exudate and migration of the omentum usually converts generalized peritonitis into an abscess. Abdominal pain is the response to chemical irritation and cytokine release. This pain, although initially localized, soon spreads throughout

TABLE 8 Antibiotic Therapy for Pneumonia-Associated Empyemas

Organism	Age	Radiologic findings	Treatment
Staphylococcus	<1 year	Patchy bronchopneumonia	Vancomycin, clindamycin, or linezolid
Streptococcus	3–5 years	Diffuse broncho-pneumonia	Penicillin or Ceftriaxone
Unknown	3 months to 3 years	Lobar pneumonia	Ceftriaxone or Cefotaxime plus Clindamycin or Vancomycin

the abdomen. A profound ileus with decreased bowel sounds and vomiting often occur. There is also abdominal guarding and rebound tenderness. The child with peritonitis usually appears toxic and third spacing cause vascular depletion. Fluid repletion and appropriate antibiotics with coverage for *Escherichia coli* and other coliform organisms, enterococcus, and *Bacteroides fragilis* should be provided (see Table 3).

Appendicitis

Appendicitis is the most common surgical problem of the abdomen in children. At least 40% of cases in the pediatric age group have complicated forms of appendicitis. A typical presentation begins with a "seasick" feeling followed by periumbilical pain, and subsequent right lower quadrant pain. Anorexia, nausea, vomiting, and fever may accompany the process. Persistent right lower quadrant tenderness is the most reliable indication of appendicitis. As simple appendicitis is impossible to differentiate from the more complex forms, intravenous fluid repletion and administration of antibiotics (i.e., cefoxitin) should precede operation (Table 9). A single preoperative dose is sufficient for negative exploration or simple acute appendicitis. If perforation has occurred, most authorities would recommend more generalized coverage consistent with gastrointestinal perforation elsewhere in the tract. The length of coverage in these cases is dependent on resolution of fever, leukocytosis, and symptoms.

Stomach and Small Bowel Infection

The stomach and proximal small bowel have low concentrations of organisms and these are generally not pathogenic. However, hypo- or achlorhydria induced by prior operation, H_2 blockers or omeprazole, or intestinal obstruction permits polymicrobial bacterial overgrowth more characteristic of the terminal ileum and colon. Surgical intervention under these circumstances, as well as with associated obesity, malnutrition, high risk of contamination, immunocompromise, or presence of ventricular peritoneal shunt within the abdomen, requires prophylaxis with a first-generation cephalosporin. Cefoxitin, cefotetan, or cefazolin plus metronidazole are the preferred regimens for distal small bowel procedures.

Necrotizing Enterocolitis

Although we are now approaching 30 years of management of necrotizing enterocolitis (NEC), the precise pathophysiology remains debatable. It occurs in 1 in 400 births and 2% of admissions to neonatal intensive care units (typically in stressed, prematurely born babies during the first 2 weeks of life). Initial findings include high gastric residuals, abdominal distention, vomiting, diarrhea, lethargy, apnea, bradycardia, poor perfusion, and blood per rectum. Pneumatosis cystoides intestinalis is the radiographic herald of NEC (Fig. 2). There are multiple associated factors but nearly all neonates are found to have been fed. Many fecal organisms have been recovered but only enterotoxic *Escherichia coli* are associated with clusters. Clostridia-positive neonates have fulminate and highly lethal disease. The child

TABLE 9   Antibiotic Use in Appendicitis

Stage	Antibiotic	Duration

Normal or simple Suppurative	Cefoxitin or cefotetan
	Gentamicin plus clindamycin
	    plus ampicillin
		1 dose preoperatively
		1 dose preoperatively plus
		    2 doses postoperatively

Gangrene, perforation, or abscess	Cefoxitin or cefotetan plus Gentamicin plus Metronidazole	Until afebrile, normalization of leukocytosis, and resolution of symptoms; average 5 days

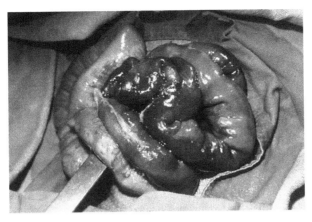

FIGURE 2 Necrotizing enterocolitis involving the distal ileum and ascending colon. There is submucosal hemorrhage, edema, coagulative transmural necrosis, and a large area of necrotic bowel.

culture-negative for *Clostridium* sp. can often be treated with medical therapy alone (nearly 90%). When diagnosis of NEC is entertained, the child is placed non per os (NPO), on gastric suction, and given meropenem, an aminoglycoside, and vancomycin. Stool cultures may help identify abnormal flora. A summary of features of NEC and therapy is given in Table 10.

Elective Colon Surgery

The colon has 10^{11} to 10^{13} bacteria/mm^3 with colonization occurring within hours of birth. A vigorous mechanical preparation with Go-Lytely® (30 mL/kg/hr for 4 hrs) the day before operation can significantly reduce the bacterial count (<10^5/mm^3 ideally). Cefoxitin, cefotetan, or cefazolin plus metronidazole are used for elective prophylaxis. Combination broad-spectrum antibiotics should be used for fecal contamination.

TABLE 10   Features of Necrotizing Enterocolitis and Therapy

Signs
Lethargy
Thermolability
Poor perfusion
Increased gastric aspirate
Radiologic findings
Pneumatosis cystoides intestinalis
Therapy
Fluid and electrolyte repletion
NPO
Gastric decompression
Antibiotics (meropenem, an aminoglycoside and vancomycin); average 10 days
Nutritional support
Operation for pneumoperitoneum, peritonitis, abdominal mass, fixed bowel loop on radiograph, uncorrectable acidosis, or positive findings on paracentesis

Anorectal Infection

The inherent resistance to infection of anorectal tissue means that special bowel preparations are not indicated for perianal operations. However, cefoxitin or cefotetan should be used for prophylactic coverage. Perirectal infections occur with folliculitis in the very young infant and, in the slightly older infant, due to malformation of the anal crypts with resulting persistent "fistula-in-ano." Recurrent perianal abscesses should be treated by fistulectomy or fistulotomy.

Biliary Infection

Biliary Atresia. Biliary atresia is the progressive obliteration of bile ducts in the newborn. Prompt diagnosis of infants presenting with direct hyperbilirubinemia beyond 2 weeks of age permits long-term survival after portoenterostomy. Prophylactic antibiotics for suppressive therapy is continued indefinitely (Table 11). Cholangitis prompted by cholestasis and bacterial contamination from the intestinal conduit presents with fever, leukocytosis, and jaundice. Bile quantity and concentration decreases if the conduit is external. Liver function deteriorates with each attack and cessation of bile flow can occur. Empiric, broad-spectrum, intravenous antibiotic therapy along with tapering dosages of methylprednisolone should be started when symptoms are first recognized. Meropenem or other drugs should be continued for a minimum of 5 days. Steroids act by both increasing bile acid dependent bile flow and anti-inflammatory effect, thus reducing edema at the anastomosis. Failure of response to medical management within several days should prompt consideration for revision of the biliary conduit.

Gallbladder Disease. Gallbladder disease in children consists of hydrops, acalculous cholecystitis, and cholelithiasis of hemolytic or cholesterol origin. Scarlet fever, Kawasaki disease, severe diarrhea, leptospirosis, familial Mediterranean fever, mesenteric adenitis, sepsis, typhoid fever, salmonellosis, a postoperative state, serious trauma, or extensive burns are associated processes causing hydrops of the gallbladder and acalculous cholecystitis. Cholecystectomy or cholecystostomy may be necessary and should be managed prophylactically with cefoxitin.

Hemolytic disorders cause bilirubinate stones and cholecystectomy for symptomatic children requires cefoxitin coverage. Hemoglobin S levels must be below 30% before elective operation in children with sickle cell disease. Nonspecific abdominal pain is the herald for cholesterol cholelithiasis and ultrasonography defines the disease. Cholecystectomy requires cefoxitin prophylaxis.

Hepatic Abscess. Hepatic abscess may be amebic or pyogenic. In the United States, amebic abscess occurs most often in Hispanic males. *Entamoeba histolytica* titers of at least 1:512 are diagnostic. Treatment with metronidazole plus iodoquinol (see Chapter 9) is appropriate. Antibiotics, percutaneous catheter drainage, open drainage, or a combination of these modalities are proper therapies for primary hepatic abscess or superinfection of an amebic

---

TABLE 11   Biliary Atresia Cholangitis

Signs
Fever
Leukocytosis
Decreased bile flow
Increased bilirubin
Suppression
Amoxicillin for first year of life; trimethoprim/
sulfamethoxazole thereafter
Therapy
Meropenem
Steroids

abscess. Antibiotics are used to treat undrainable multiple microabscesses. Cefotaxime, metronidazole, and an extended penicillin (e.g., ticarcillin) is usually adequate therapy.

Trauma

Abdominal Trauma. In cases of intestinal perforation following abdominal trauma, bacterial contamination is present at the time of antibiotic administration. However, lesser therapy is necessary than for patients with longer established peritonitis, as the interval prior to treatment is shorter than for other causes. Antibiotics must be given preoperatively and in proper dosage to cover aerobic cocci, especially enterococcus, anaerobic organisms, and gram-negative rods. Second- or third-generation cephalosporins are effective in preventing intraabdominal abscesses and wound infection following abdominal exploration for penetrating abdominal wounds. Multiple studies show that there is no advantage in giving antibiotics for more than 2 days. Other drug combinations such as ticarcillin/clavulanate, mezlocillin, or ampicillin/sulbactam are also effective.

Splenic Trauma. Splenectomy is associated with overwhelming operative postspenectomy sepsis (OPSS) and is characterized by bacteremia with meningitis or pneumonia. The mortality is nearly 50% even in this day of multiagent antibiotics. The most common pathogen is pneumococcus. There is no increased risk to viral, fungal, or myobacterial infection. The greatest risk for bacterial infection following splenectomy is seen in the following cases: patients under 2 years of age, Wiskott–Aldrich syndrome, thalassemia, and during the first 2 years following splenectomy for trauma. Loss of the spleen causes loss of its dual function as a filter for bacteria and as a locus for antibody production. Nonoperative management, partial splenectomy, or splenorrhaphy can avoid the need for spleen removal in approximately 90% of instances of traumatic rupture of the spleen. Splenic function can then be most conveniently followed by looking for Howell–Jolly bodies, which are present in at least 50% of patients with functional asplenia.

Pneumococcal, *Haemophilus*, and meningococcal vaccination should precede elective splenectomy in children. Currently, recommendations for antibiotic prophylaxis reflect the experience gained in sickle cell disease. Prophylaxis with oral penicillin V is recommended for all asplenic children under 5 years of age (125 mg b.i.d.) and for older children (250 mg b.i.d.). The newer conjugate pneumococcal vaccine is effective in children as young as 2 months of age and is now recommended not only for asplenic patients but routinely in all patients.

Antibiotic prophylaxis is most important in this high-risk group. If a patient presents with a high index of suspicion for overwhelming postsplenectomy sepsis, initial treatment should include antibiotics effective against streptococcus, *Neisseria meningitides*, β-lactamase-producing *H. influenza* type B, and *Staphylococcus*.

POSTOPERATIVE FEVER

Fever is a common complication following operation. Identification of the pyrogenic source (Table 12) begins with physical examination. A preexisting disease process can present in the postoperative period. If the patient has had an inflammatory process preoperatively, bacteremia from manipulation of the infected source can cause a vigorous postoperative fever. Continuation of pre- and intraoperative antibiotics and antipyretics is the appropriate response.

Atelectasis is the usual cause of fever beginning in the 24 hours following operation. Preoperative instruction in the use of incentive spirometry in older children can decrease the incidence. All children should be given analgesics sufficient to relieve postoperative pain. Diminished breath sounds are auscultated. Insufficient therapy may lead to more extensive segmental collapse requiring nasotracheal suction or bronchoscopy for reinflation. Invasive pulmonary infection may occur if this persists.

Pneumonia may also be respiration associated or result from aspiration in those who have altered sensorium while awakening from anesthesia. After the first day, consider other

TABLE 12   Causes of Postoperative Fever

Time of Onset	Etiology
Immediate	Manipulation of infected focus
Day 1	Atelectasis, preexisting illness, streptococcus, *Clostridia*
Day 2–3	Atelectasis, otitis media, phlebitis, urinary tract infection
Day 4	Staphylococcus
Day 5 (or later)	Enteric wound, otitis media, phlebitis, urinary tract infection, abdominal abscess

causes, including otitis media induced from barotitis or irritation from nasogastric tubes, catheter-induced phlebitis, streptococcal wound infection, and catheter or instrument-induced urinary tract infections. Pyuria justifies urine culture, with a positive culture ($>10^5$ bacteria/mL) requiring antibiotic therapy (see Chapter 11).

Intraabdominal infections are difficult to recognize because of the changes produced by the recent abdominal incision. Fever, leukocytosis, ileus, or diarrhea herald purulent collections and ultrasound or computerized tomography can verify clinical suspicion. Occasionally, operative exploration without verification of the locus is necessary for diagnosis. In children, other sources, although unusual, include parotitis, pancreatitis, and cholecystitis.

REFERENCE

1.   Bratzler DW, Houck PM, for the Surgical Infection Prevention Guidelines Writers Workgroup. Clin Infect Dis 2004; 38:1706–1715.

15 | Sexually Transmitted Diseases and Genital Tract Infections

CLINICAL PRESENTATIONS

Sexually transmitted diseases (STDs) can be broadly divided into those characterized by genital ulcers, with or without inguinal adenopathy, infections of epithelial surfaces, and specific well-defined syndromes (Table 1).

ETIOLOGIES

STDs can also be classified by specific pathogens (Table 2), although this is less practical than approaching etiologic diagnosis on the basis of clinical presentations. As an example, urethritis can be caused by bacteria, viruses, or even protozoa. History of previous STD may also alter suspected pathogens. Repeated episodes of pelvic inflammatory disease (PID) are more likely to be produced by coliform bacteria than initial infections. Selection of antimicrobial therapy may therefore vary for reinfection.

DISEASES ASSOCIATED WITH GENITAL ULCERS AND LYMPHADENITIS

Genital ulcers are most commonly associated with herpes simplex, syphilis or, less commonly, chancroid and can be differentiated by the presence or absence of pain. Syphilis is usually painless while herpes and chancroid are painful. Depending on this finding and other features such as adenopathy (syphilis, lymphogranuloma venereum [LGV], and chancroid), evaluation of genital ulcers would include the following: direct immunofluorescence test or dark

TABLE 1 Clinical Presentations of STDs and Genital Tract Infections

Syndrome	Etiologies
Female and male	
Genital ulcers and lymphadenitis	Herpes, syphilis, chancroid, lymphogranuloma venereum
Urethritis	Gonococcus, chlamydia, *Ureaplasma* sp. herpes simplex virus, *Trichomonas* sp.
	Neisseria gonorrhoeae
Arthritis-dermatitis syn.	
Urethritis-arthritis-conjunctivitis syn.	Reiter's syndrome (uncertain etiology), possibly chlamydia
Warts	Human papilloma virus types 6 and 11
Hepatitis	Hepatitis B
AIDS	Human immunodeficiency virus
Female	
Vaginitis	*Trichomonas, Gardnerella vaginalis, Candida* sp.
Cervicitis	Gonococcus, chlamydia, *Mycoplasma hominis*, herpes simplex virus, *Trichomonas* sp.
Pelvic inflammatory disease (PID)	Gonococcus, chlamydia, anaerobic bacteria, *M. hominis*, coliform bacteria
Postabortion, postsalpingitis	Gonococcus, chlamydia, *M. hominis*
Male	
Epididymitis	Gonococcus, chlamydia
Balanitis	*Candida albicans, Trichomonas vaginalis, Gardnerella vaginalis*

TABLE 2   STDs Classified by Pathogen

Disease	Pathogens
Chancroid	*Haemophilus ducreyi*
Genital herpes	Herpes simplex virus type 2 (occasionally type 1)
Genital warts	Human papilloma virus types 6 and 11
Granuloma inguinale	*Calymmatobacterium granulomatis*
Lymphogranuloma venereum (LGV)	*Chlamydia trachomatis* (LGV serovars)
Pelvic inflammatory disease (PID)	Gonococcus, chlamydia, anaerobic bacteria, *Mycoplasma hominis*, coliform bacteria
Pubic lice	*Pthirus pubis*
Syphilis	*Treponema pallidum*
Vaginosis or nonspecific vaginitis	*Gardnerella vaginalis*, *Mobiluncus* sp., anaerobic bacteria
AIDS	HIV-1 and HIV-2 (rare in the United States)

field examination for *Treponema pallidum*; serologic tests for syphilis; culture, Tzanck test or fluorescence stains for herpes simplex virus (HSV); and culture for *Haemophilus ducreyi* (Table 3).

Appearance of skin lesions are often diagnostic. Genital warts (human papilloma virus [HPV]), ecchymoses of the arthritis–dermatitis syndrome (*Neisseria gonorrhoeae*), and the multiple painful ulcers of herpes simplex can be easily recognized.

Herpes Simplex

Primary genital infection is characterized by painful ulcers, which persist for 4 to 15 days until crusting (see Table 4 for treatment of HSV infection). Viral shedding occurs for an average of 12 days. There is then a 90% recurrence rate following HSV type 2 (HSV-2) genital infection, and 60% for HSV-1. The number of reactivation episodes varies considerably, averaging 5 episodes per year for the first 2 years, but decreasing thereafter.

Primary infection is associated with generalized signs and symptoms including fever, malaise, headache, myalgia, and painful inguinal adenopathy. Aseptic meningitis with cerebrospinal fluid (CSF) pleocytosis and positive viral cultures is seen in 1% to 3% of cases but is a benign disease, which should not be confused with herpes encephalitis.

Syphilis

The four presentations of disease commonly occurring in the pediatric population are: congenital syphilis, acquired disease in adolescents, asymptomatic adolescents with positive screening assays, and child sexual abuse. Each requires an understanding and interpretation

TABLE 3   Diagnostic Studies for Genital Ulcers

Treponema pallidum	Specific treponemal serology direct immunofluorescence test or darkfield examination
Herpes simplex virus	Antigen test (fluorescent or Tzanck prep.) or culture
Haemophilus ducreyi	Culture

TABLE 4 Treatment of Genital Herpes Simplex Virus (HSV) Infections

Primary infection
  Acyclovir 80 mg/kg/day p.o. div q 8 hrs (max. 1.2 g/day) for 10 days or until clinical resolution occurs
  Alternatives: Famacyclovir 250 mg p.o. t.i.d. for 7–10 days; valacyclovir 1 g p.o. b.i.d. for 7–10 days;
    acyclovir 5% topical ointment q 3 hrs 6 times per day for 7 days (inferior to oral therapy)
  For HSV meningitis or hospitalized symptomatic patients—acyclovir 15 mg/kg/day i.v. div. q 8 hrs until
    symptoms resolve
Recurrent infection
  Treatment usually unnecessary
  Severe infection—acyclovir 200 mg p.o. 5 times per day for 5 days
  Suppression of HSV reactivation—acyclovir 200 mg p.o. t.i.d. or 400 mg p.o. b.i.d.

of both screening and specific tests for syphilis. Those commonly available are as follows: venereal disease research laboratories (VDRL) test; fluorescent treponernal antibody-absorption test (FTA-ABS); or *T. pallidum* particle agglutination (TP-PA). Screening assays are quite sensitive (95–100%) for secondary syphilis (Fig. 1) but positive in only 70% to 80% of primary, tertiary and latent disease and even lower for incubating and early primary infection (Table 5). Therefore, a history of possible recent exposure warrants retesting up to 90 days after initial negative results. Specific treponemal tests (FTA-ABS or TP-PA) should be routinely ordered for patients in who disease is strongly suspected.

Primary disease may be asymptomatic, particularly in women, since the chancre is usually not readily visible and is painless. Secondary syphilis is characterized by a maculopapular rash, condyloma lata, mucous patches, lymphadenopathy, and fever. Disease tends to be remittent with variable intervals of asymptomatic latent infection. Half of untreated patient's progress to a secondary phase, and half go directly into latency. Treatment depends on the stage of disease at diagnosis (Table 6).

Repeat quantitative nontreponemal tests are indicated until a fourfold decrease in titer is seen (usually measured at 3, 6, and 12 months). Retreatment is recommended if clinical signs persist, a fourfold increase in titer is documented, or the screening syphilis assay does not decrease fourfold by 12 months.

Chancroid

Chancroid is distinguished by a painful genital ulcer accompanied, in about one-half of cases, by painful inguinal lymphadenopathy. Culture for *H. ducreyi* will confirm the etiology.

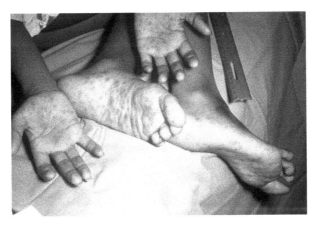

FIGURE 1 (*See color insert.*) Secondary syphilis. Copper-colored papulosquamous rash including the palms and soles in this 9-year-old girl following sexual abuse.

TABLE 5 Percent Sensitivity of Serology Testing for Syphilis

	Test sensitivity (%)			
	Stage of Syphilis			
Assay	Primary	Secondary	Latent	Tertiary
VDRL	72	100	73	77
FTA-ABS	91	100	97	100
TP-PA	60	100	98	100

Chancroid is highly associated with both HIV infection and syphilis, thereby necessitating serologic screens for these conditions.

Following treatment of chancroid (Table 7), symptomatic improvement is expected within 3 days and improvement of lesions and reduction of exudate within 7 days. Adenitis may require needle aspiration.

Lymphogranuloma Venereum

LGV is caused by *Chlamydia trachomatis* (LGV serovars) and should be considered with the clinical presentation of persistent inguinal lymphadenopathy, although it is rare in the United States. Treatment is with doxycycline (100 mg p.o. b.i.d. for 21 days). Alternative regimens are erythromycin (500 mg p.o. q.i.d. for 21 days) or sultisoxazole (500 mg p.o. q.i.d. for 21 days).

DISEASES ASSOCIATED WITH URETHRITIS

Gonococcal Infections

Clinical manifestations can be divided into age-related presentations as summarized in Table 8. *Neisseria gonorrhoeae* are gram-negative diplococci, which cause infections only in humans and are transmitted by intimate sexual contact, parturition, and occasionally in prepubertal children from caregivers, following normal contact.

Treatment decisions are influenced by changing sensitivity patterns of the organism, clinical manifestations, cost of therapy, and presence of other STDs. Uncomplicated gonococcal urethral, endocervical, or rectal infections can be treated with a single-dose regimen in conjunction with therapy for presumed chlamydial disease (Table 9). Ceftriaxone (125 mg) is adequate therapy for incubating syphilis. All patients with gonorrhea should be tested for syphilis (at the time of diagnosis and 1 month later) and, at least, counseled on HIV infection. Persons exposed to active gonorrhea cases within 30 days of diagnosis should be examined, cultured, and routinely treated. Follow-up cultures are not necessary since treatment failures with ceftriaxone/doxycycline are so rare.

TABLE 6 Treatment of Acquired Syphilis in Adolescents and Older Children

Stage	Treatment
Primary, secondary and early latent (<1 year)	Benzathine penicillin G 2.4×10^6 U (50 000 U/kg) i.m., single dose
Late latent syphilis (>1 year), gummas, cardiovascular syphilis (not neurosyphilis); tertiary	Benzathine penicillin G 2.4×10^6 U (50,000 U/kg) i.m. 3 doses, given 1 week apart
Neurosyphilis	Aqueous crystalline penicillin G, $12–24 \times 10^6$ U/day (200,000–300,000 U/kg/day) i.v. div. q 4 hrs for 14 days
Penicillin allergy (nonpregnant)	
Early syphilis	Doxycycline 100 mg p.o. b.i.d. for 14 days
Late syphilis	Doxycycline 100 mg p.o. b.i.d. for 28 days

TABLE 7   Treatment of Chancroid

Ceftriaxone 250 mg i.m. single dose (small children 50 mg/kg)
or
Azithromycin, 20 mg/kg (max. 1 g) p.o. as a single dose
Alternative regimens:
   Ciprofloxacin 500 mg p.o. b.i.d. for 3 days
   Erythromycin base, 500 mg p.o. t.i.d. × 7 days

Nongonococcal Urethritis

Painful urethritis with an exudate containing abundant polymorphonuclear leukocytes but without gram-negative intracellular diplococci, is caused by *C. trachomatis* in approximately 50% of cases and in 10% to 20% by *U. urealyticum, T. vaginalis,* HSV, or other mycoplasmas. Specific etiologies are often difficult to confirm.

Empiric treatment should be offered to adolescents, using azithromycin 1.0 g as a single dose or doxycycline (100 mg p.o. b.i.d.) for 7 days. Children younger than 9 years of age can receive erythromycin (30–50 mg/kg/day p.o. div. q.i.d.) for 14 days. Failures should undergo a second treatment course.

Chlamydia Trachomatis

Most treatment for chlamydia occurs as part of routine therapy in patients with gonorrhea. This recommendation is based on the observation that one-third of patients with gonorrhea are concomitantly infected with *C. trachomatis.*

Diagnosis in infants with conjunctivitis and/or pneumonia also necessitates treatment of the mother and her sexual partner(s). Chlamydia is an STD transmitted to the newborn from

TABLE 8   Clinical Manifestations of Gonococcal Infections

Sexually active adolescents
   Urethritis
   Endocervicitis
   Pelvic inflammatory disease (PID)
   Perihepatitis (Fitz-Hugh and Curtis syndrome)
   Disseminated gonococcal infection (DGI)
      Arthritis-dermatitis syndrome
      Arthritis
      Meningitis
      Endocarditis
      Osteomyelitis
      Pneumonia
      Adult respiratory distress syndrome
Neonates
   Ophthalmia
   Disseminated gonococcal infection (DGI)
   Scalp abscess (from fetal monitoring)
   Vaginitis
Prepubertal children
   Sexual abuse
   Vaginitis
   Pelvic inflammatory disease (PID)
   Perihepatitis (Fitz-Hugh and Curtis syndrome)
   Anorectal infection
   Tonsillopharyngitis

TABLE 9   Treatment of Gonococcal Infections

Uncomplicated genital/anal/oral (adolescent)
  Ceftriaxone 125 mg i.m., single dose
  Alternatives: spectinomycin, 40 mg/kg (max 2 g) IM in a single dose cefixime 400 mg p.o., ciprofloxacin
    500 mg p.o., ofloxacin 400 mg p.o., or levofloxacin 250 mg p.o., all in a single dose
  plus
  Azithromycin 1 g p.o. single dose
  or
  Doxycycline 100 mg p.o. b.i.d. for 7 days or (children <45 kg)
  Erythromycin base or ethylsuccinate, 50 mg/kg/day (max. 2 g/day) p.o. div. q 6 hrs × 14 days
Genital/anal/oral (children)
  Ceftriaxone 25–50 mg/kg/day i.m. or i.v. for 10 days
Neonate
  Ophthalmia: ceftriaxone 25–50 mg/kg i.m. or i.v. (maximum 125 mg) single dose, irrigate eyes with
    saline for 24 hrs
  Mother with gonococcal infection: ceftriaxone 50 mg/kg i.m. or i.v. (maximum 125 mg) single dose
Meningitis
  Ceftriaxone 100 mg/kg/day i.v. div. b.i.d. for 10 days
Endocarditis
  Ceftriaxone 100 mg/kg/day i.v. div. b.i.d. for 28 days

the mother during childbirth, therefore clinical confirmation for infection in the mother already exists. Perinatal infection does not become clinically apparent until 2 to 20 weeks of life, when conjunctivitis and afebrile interstitial pneumonia are the most common manifestations. Failure to thrive is an occasional feature. Colonization rarely occurs after 20 weeks of age, and then only in asymptomatic infants or children.

Sexually active male adolescents present with urethritis or epididymoorchitis while females may develop urethritis, cervicitis, or PID. Both culture and rapid antigen detection assays (ELISA, fluorescence, genetic probe) are available and should be routinely obtained for suspected infection in children and adolescents. Treatment of chlamydia is presented in Table 10.

Ureaplasma Urealyticum

Approximately 25% of nongonococcal, nonchlarnydial urethritis in males is caused by *U. urealyticum*. Disease in women is usually asymptomatic. There is increasing evidence that this organism is associated with spontaneous abortion, sepsis, and bronchopulmonary dysplasia in neonates. This potential pathogen can be cultured in special broth medium containing urea, but since as many as half of sexually active adults are colonized, its presence is difficult to correlate with disease.

Recommended treatment for adolescents and adults is doxycycline (100 mg p.o. b.i.d.) for 7 days. Children younger than 9 years of age, or those allergic to tetracycline, can be treated with erythromycin (30–50 mg/kg/day p.o. div. q.i.d.) for 7 days.

TABLE 10   Treatment of Chlamydia Infections

Age	Site	Therapy
Infants	Conjunctivitis and pneumonia	Azithromycin 20 mg/kg q 24 hrs × 3 or erythromycin 40–50 mg/kg/day p.o. for 14 days
Infants and children	Genital	Azithromycin 20 mg/kg q 24 hrs × 3 or erythromycin 40–50 mg/kg/day p.o. for 14 days
Adolescents and adults	Urethral, endocervical, rectal	Azithromycin 1 g p.o. single dose or doxycycline 100 mg p.o. b. i.d. for 7 days

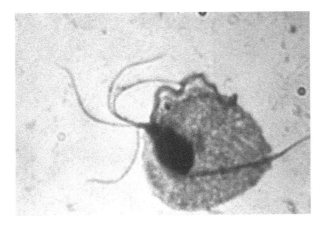

FIGURE 2 Wet mount prep identifying *Trichomonas vaginalis*, a flagellated protozoan whose presence is often asymptomatic in females.

Trichomoniasis

Trichomonas vaginalis is a flagellated protozoan (Fig. 2) often asymptomatic in females. Moderate to heavy colonization produces a yellow-green discharge with a fishy odor associated with pruritic vaginitis, cervicitis, or urethritis. Their presence in postmenarchal girls strongly suggests sexual activity, while in premenarchal children they necessitate careful examination for sexual abuse. Males are more frequently symptomatic, with urethritis or prostatitis. Diagnosis is made by direct microscopic examination (wet preparation) of fresh vaginal discharge; treatment is summarized in Table 11.

DISEASES ASSOCIATED WITH VAGINAL DISCHARGE

Vaginosis

Bacterial vaginosis, also called nonspecific vaginitis, results from the overgrowth of *G. vaginalis* and/or anaerobes such as *Mobiluncus* sp. Diagnosis is suggested by the presence of a homogeneous discharge with a pH > 4.5, positive amine odor test and clue cells. Infection is of greatest concern during pregnancy, since bacterial vaginosis is associated with premature rupture of membranes and premature delivery.

Only symptomatic infection should be treated. The recommended regimen is metronidazole (500 mg p.o. b.i.d.) for 7 days. Alternatives include: metronidazole gel 0.75% intravaginally daily × 5 days; clindamycin cream 2% intravaginally at bedtime × 7 days; clindamycin 300 mg p.o. b.i.d. × 7 days; or clindamycin ovules intravaginally at bedtime

TABLE 11 Treatment of *Trichomonas vaginalis*

Group (plus concurrent treatment of sexual partner)	Treatment
Adolescents	Metronidazole 2 g single dose or tinidazole 2 g single dose
Prepubertal girls	Metronidazole 15 mg/kg (maximum 250 mg) 3 doses q 8 hrs for 7 days
Treatment failures in adolescents	Metronidazole 500 mg b.i.d. for 7 days
Second treatment failures	Metronidazole 2 g/day for 5 days
First trimester of pregnancy	Clotrimazole 100 mg vaginal tablet h.s. for 7 nights
Second and third trimesters of pregnancy	Metronidazole 2 g p.o. single dose, the 7 day regimen or with tinidazole

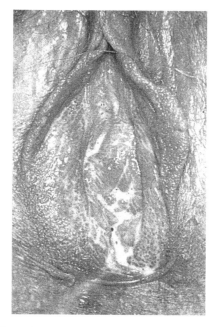

FIGURE 3 (*See color insert.*) Bacterial vaginosis, also called nonspecific vaginitis, results from the overgrowth of *Gardnerella vaginalis* and/or anaerobes such as *Mobiluncus* species. The diagnosis is suggested by the presence of this homogenous discharge with a pH >4.5 and a positive amine odor test.

× 3 days. Because the safety of metronidazole during pregnancy has not been established, pregnant patients should receive clindamycin (300 mg p.o. b.i.d.) for 7 days.

Vulvovaginitis

Prepubertal vaginitis is usually secondary to *C. albicans, T. vaginalis, N. gonorrhoeae*, foreign bodies, or irritation secondary to chemicals or pinworm; it may, however, be the only physical finding in sexual abuse. Gonococcal vaginitis in the prepubertal child is usually mild because it is localized to the superficial mucosa.

Major symptoms in vulvovaginitis include vaginal itching and a minor crusting discharge that discolors the child's underwear. Dysuria and pyuria are common. The character of the vaginal discharge in all patients (Fig. 3), and the speculum examination in postpubertal (especially sexually active) females, are useful in establishing the diagnosis (Table 12). The treatment of vulvovaginitis in pre- and postpubertal females is dependent on the etiologic agent (Table 13).

A thorough speculum examination is important to ascertain whether the discharge emanates from the vagina or the cervical os. The most common etiologies of vaginitis are: *Candida,*

TABLE 12 Clinical Considerations in Vulvovaginitis

Clinical examination	Vaginal discharge
Ectropion	
Oral contraceptives, pregnancy	Clear mucus
Cervicitis (gonococcal infection, *Chlamydia* sp., herpes simplex virus)	Purulent exudate, cervix friable
Vaginitis (*Candida albicans, Trichomonas vaginalis, Gardnerella vaginalis*)	Malodor, yellow to white, frothy discharge; cervicitis may be present

TABLE 13 Etiologic Agents and Treatment in Vulvovaginitis

Candida albicans	Discontinue antibiotics and oral contraceptives, if possible. Topical antifungals: clotrimazole, miconazole, butoconazole, terconazole, or tioconazole intravaginally once daily for 7 days
Trichomonas vaginalis	Metronidazole 10–30 mg/kg/day (maximum 2 g) p.o. single dose, tinidazole 2 g p.o. single dose or metronidazole 250rag p.o. t.i.d. for 10 days
	In pregnancy: topical antifungals as above
	Neonatal trichomoniasis: symptomatic or persistent colonization; metronidazole 10–30 mg/kg/day p.o. for 5–8 days
Nonspecific vaginitis	Metronidazole 10–30 mg/kg/day (maximum 500 mg) p.o. b.i.d. for 7 days
(*Gardnerella vaginalis*)	Alternatives: metronidazole gel 0.75% intravaginally daily × 5 days; clindamycin cream 2% intravaginally at bedtime × 7 days; or clindamycin phosphate cream 2% intravaginally as a single dose
	Sexual partners: controversial; recommend treatment as in the female

Trichomonas spp., and *G. vaginalis*. In *Candida* sp. vaginitis, the following are helpful in diagnosis: itching, dysuria, curds or plaques, 10% KOH (no odor), yeast or pseudomycelia, pH <4.5, and a positive culture for yeast. In vaginitis due to *Trichomonas* sp., the diagnosis is apparent with profuse, yellow-green discharge, 10% KOH (amine odor), motile trichomonads (wet preparation, magnification ×400), and a vaginal pH 5.5 to 6.0. In nonspecific vaginitis due to *G. vaginalis*, the diagnosis is apparent with an adherent homogeneous discharge, also 10% KOH (amine odor), clue cells (Fig. 4), which are vaginal epithelial cells coated with coccobacillary forms of *G. vaginalis*, a pH > 4.5, and a positive culture. In some cases of vaginitis, anaerobes have been isolated but no predominant organism has been demonstrated. For comparison, normal vaginal secretions have no odor with 10% KOH and a pH < 4.5.

Pelvic Inflammatory Disease

The spectrum of acute PID includes endometritis, salpingitis, tubo-ovarian abscess, and pelvic peritonitis. Most infection is caused by *N. gonorrhoeae* and *C. trachomatis* although genital

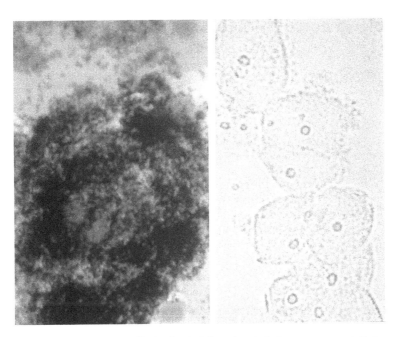

FIGURE 4 Most specific for bacterial vaginosis is the presence of clue cells, which are epithelial cells with clumps of bacteria on their surface.

TABLE 14   Treatment of Acute Pelvic Inflammatory Disease (PID)

Parenteral	
Inpatient	
Regimen A	Cefoxitin 2 g i.v. q.i.d. or cefotetan 2 g i.v. b.i.d. for at least 24 hrs after significant clinical improvement plus doxycycline 100 mg i.v. or p.o. b.i.d. for 14 days or
Regimen B	Clindamycin 900 mg i.v. t.i.d. (40 mg/kg/day) plus gentamicin: loading dose 2 mg/kg i.v., maintenance 1.5 mg/kg i.v. t.i.d.
Outpatient	
Regimen A	Ofloxacin 400 mg p.o. b.i.d. for 14 days or levofloxacin 500 p.o. daily × 14 days plus metronidazole 500 mg p.o. b.i.d × 14 days
Regimen B	Ceftriaxone 250 mg i.m. once or cefoxitin 2 g i.m plus probenecid 1 g p.o. once plus doxycycline 100 mg p.o. b.i.d. for 14 days plus metronidazole 500 mg p.o. b.i.d. × 14 days

colonizing organisms (anaerobes, coliforms, streptococci, and mycoplasmas) are also potential pathogens, particularly for recurrent disease.

Diagnosis can be aided by pelvic ultrasonography or laparoscopy. Clinical findings are lower abdominal pain and tenderness, bilateral adnexal tenderness on motion of the cervix, recent onset vaginal discharge, fever, and abnormal menstrual bleeding. Even a low index of suspicion for infection necessitates early institution of antimicrobial therapy. Specific etiology is usually based on culture and rapid antigen detection assays of exudate from the lower genital tract.

Most adolescents should be hospitalized, not only for inpatient therapy (Table 14) but to assure compliance in follow-up, to offer comprehensive counseling for sexual activity and other potential STDs, and to detect sequelae, which are more severe in this age group. Complications are perihepatitis (Fitz-Hugh and Curtis syndrome), tubo-ovarian abscess, infertility, pelvic adhesions, and ectopic pregnancy. PID is more severe in patients with intrauterine devices in place so these should be removed.

Follow-up of all patients is recommended at 3 to 5 days after beginning therapy and 7 to 10 days after completing antibiotics. Cultures should be obtained 21 to 28 days after completing therapy to document eradication of *C. trachomatis* and *N. gonorrhoeae*. Male sexual partners should be cultured and routinely treated for gonorrhea and chlamydia infection. Both patients and partner(s) should abstain from intercourse until therapy is complete.

MALE STD SYNDROMES

Balanitis

Cellulitis of the glans penis may occur as a consequence of poor hygiene in prepubertal uncircumcised children but is more commonly seen in sexually active males following intercourse with a partner who is colonized with *Candida albicans*, *Trichomonas vaginalis*, or *Gardnerella vaginalis*. Etiology can be determined by direct examination of the first aliquot of a voided urine and, if negative, examination of the female sexual contact. Inflammation may occasionally represent a hypersensitivity reaction from contact with *Candida albicans*; for these patients good hygiene and treatment of the sexual partner are curative. Balanitis may also be related to trauma or postcircumcision wound infections where streptococci and staphylococci are likely pathogens. Treatment of balanitis is summarized in Table 15.

Epididymitis

Epididymitis must be differentiated from testicular torsion, orchitis, or testicular cancer. Acute epididymitis in adolescents often occurs after trauma and/or heavy lifting but is occasionally a primary infection caused by *N. gonorrhoeae* or chlamydia. However, in most cases highly suspected of having infectious etiologies, because of associated scrotal edema and fever, no

TABLE 15 Treatment of Balanitis

Type	Treatment
Candida albicans	Fluconazole 150 mg p.o. single dose; butoconazole or terconazole topical ointment applied q.i.d. for 3–7 days or until resolved; also treat sexual partner
Trichomonas vaginalis	Children—metronidazole 10–30 mg/kg/day p.o. t.i.d. for 7 days or tinidazole 50 mg/kg single dose (max. 2 g)
	Adult—metronidazole 2 g p.o. single dose or 250 mg t.i.d. for 7 days
Gardnerella vaginalis	Children—metronidazole 10–30 mg/kg/day p.o. t.i.d. for 7 days
	Adults—metronidazole 500 g p.o. b.i.d. for 7 days

organism is recovered. There are, therefore, two distinct types of disease; nonspecific bacterial epididymitis and sexually transmitted epididymitis.

In acute epididymitis, ultrasonography shows the swollen epididymis as distinct parallel lines posterolateral to the discrete testicular echo and an enlarged, but separate, epididymal head. In torsion of the testis, the testicular echo is disrupted and the echogenic epididymis is inseparable from the testis. Urine culture may isolate the causative organism if this is an infectious process. Mumps orchitis is suspected by the lack of white blood cells in the urine of these patients, a negative culture, and an elevated serum arnylase.

Scrotal elevation by an athletic supporter or towel across the thighs facilitates drainage and relief of pain. Sexual excitement may exacerbate pain and infection. Antibiotics active against gonococcus, chlamydia, and coliform organisms (ceftriaxone and doxycycline) may be of benefit. Severe pain may be relieved by infiltrating the spermatic cord in the upper scrotum with xylocaine or other anesthetizing agents. Exploration and open biopsy are indicated to distinguish testicular tumors and to avoid spread of malignant cells.

Orchitis

Mumps and group B coxsackieviruses are the most common causes of orchitis in children. These can be differentiated clinically because mumps produces parotitis with elevated serum amylase. One-third to one-fourth of patients with mumps orchitis develops oligo or aspermia in the involved testis. The other testis remains normal and potency is not affected. Treatment is symptomatic with analgesics and elevation of the scrotum.

OTHER SPECIFIC DISEASES

Genital Warts

Exophytic genital and anal warts can be readily diagnosed clinically, only requiring biopsy to exclude dysplasia or carcinoma if lesions are atypical, pigmented, or persistent. Although HPV can cause laryngeal papillomatosis in infants, the method of transmission has not been defined and cesarean section is not recommended to prevent disease in infants born to mothers with active genital warts. Treatment of HPV infection is summarized in Table 16.

HPV Vaccine

A vaccine is now available which prevents genital warts and cervical cancer caused by HPV strain types 6, 11, 16, and 18. It is recommended for routine administration to girls 9 to 26 years of age, and requires 3 doses given at 0, 2, and 6 month intervals. Its greatest benefit is for girls naïve to these strains of HPV so early immunization, i.e., 9 to 11 years of are is highly encouraged.

TABLE 16   Treatment of HPV Infection

```
External anogenital warts
   Patient-applied
      Pidofilox 0.5% solution or gel or
      Imiquimod 5% cream
   Provider-administered
      Cryotherapy with liquid nitrogen or cryoprobe
   Alternatives: podophyllin, podophyllotoxin, trichloracetic acid 80–90%,
      electrodesiccation/electrocautery, interferons, laser therapy
Vaginal warts
   Cryotherapy with liquid nitrogen
   Alternatives: trichloracetic acid (80–90%), podophyllin (10–15%),
      5-fluorouracil cream, laser therapy
Urethral meatus
   Cryotherapy with liquid nitrogen
   Alternatives: podophyllin (10–15%), 5-fluorouracil cream, laser therapy
Anal warts
   Cryotherapy with liquid nitrogen
   Alternatives: trichloracetic acid, (80–90%), surgical removal (cold blade,
      laser therapy)
Oral warts
   Cryotherapy with liquid nitrogen
   Alternatives: electrodesiccation/electrocautery, surgical removal
Laryngeal papillomas
   Laser therapy
   Alternatives: photodynamic therapy, interferons
```

Granuloma Inguinale

Although rare in the United States, granuloma inguinale should be suspected with ulcerated cutaneous lesions, subcutaneous nodules, and granulomas (pseudobuboes) in the genital or anal regions. The demonstration of Donovan bodies on Wright's stain or Giemsa stain of a crush-preparation from a lesion, confirms the diagnosis. Ciprofloxacin is the recommended treatment. Gentamicin should be added if no response is seen in 7 days. Alternatives include doxycycline, trimethoprim/sulfamethoxazole (TMP/SMX), azithromycin and erythromycin. All therapies should be given for 3 weeks, or until lesions have resolved. Response to therapy should occur within 7 days but failures are common.

Pediculosis Pubis

Intense itching in the anogenital region is the most common manifestation of pubic lice but infestation may also involve other hairy areas such as eyelashes, eyebrows, beard, or axillae. A highly suggestive clinical finding is blue-gray macules on the chest, abdomen, or thighs.

Numerous effective treatments are available (Table 17) but permethrin is preferred because it is available over-the-counter, has a high cure rate, and virtually no toxicity. Pediculosis of the eyelashes should be treated by smothering lice and nits with petrolatum ointment 3 to 4 times daily for 10 days.

TABLE 17   Treatment of Pediculosis Pubis

```
Topical malathion 0.5% or topical permethrin 1%
Alternatives
Pyrethrin (A-200, RID, R & C) 10 min shalpoo
Retreatment in 7–10 days
Ivermectin 200 mcg/kg × 3; days 1, 2, and 10
```

TABLE 18   Routine Testing Following Sexual Abuse

	Organism/syndrome	Specimens
All children	*Neisseria gonorrhoeae*	Rectal, throat, urethral, vaginal, and/or endocervical culture(s)
	Chlamydia trachomatis	Throat, rectal, urethral, vulvovaginal culture(s)
	Syphilis	Immunofluorescence examination of chancre (if present), blood for serologic tests
Selected cases	HIV	Serology of perpetrator (if possible), serology of child at time of abuse and 3, 6, and 12 months later
	Hepatitis B	Serology of perpetrator
	Herpes simplex	Culture only if a lesion is present
	Bacterial vaginosis	Wet mount of vaginal discharge
	Human papilloma virus	Biopsy of lesion
	Trichomonas vaginalis	Wet mount of vaginal discharge, culture of discharge

TABLE 19   Empiric Treatment for Sexual Abuse Victim When the Perpetrator Cannot be Examined

Potential disease	Treatment
Gonorrhea and incubating syphilis	Ceftriaxone 125 mg i.m. single dose
Chlamydia	Azithromycin 20 mg/kg (max. 1 g) p.o. as a single dose or erythromycin 40–50 mg/kg/day p.o. for 14 days
Hepatitis B	Hepatitis B immunoglobulin (HBIG) 0.5 mL i.m., hepatitis B vaccine at 0, 1, and 6 months (dose dependent on age and product)
Trichomonas and bacterial vaginosis	Metronidazole 15 mg/kg/day p.o. div. q 8 hrs × 7 days

SEXUAL ABUSE AND RAPE

Suspected sexual abuse requires a forensic as well as medical evaluation that are in some ways different. As an example, rapid diagnostic tests, such as Gram stain, Tzanck test, ELISA, and direct fluorescence techniques, are useful for early medical intervention but cannot be used as legal evidence. Routine tests carried out following suspected sexual abuse are listed in Table 18.

If the perpetrator is unknown or not available for testing, victims of recent abuse should usually be treated for gonorrhea, syphilis, chlamydia, and hepatitis B (Tables 19 and 20).

TABLE 20   Infection and the Likelihood of Sexual Abuse

Disease	Likelihood of sexual abuse
Neisseria gonorrhoeae	Diagnostic
Chlamydia (child older than 2 years)	Diagnostic
Syphilis	Diagnostic
HIV (not perinatal; not transfusion associated)	Diagnostic
Trichomonas vaginalis	Highly suspicious
Genital herpes	Suspicious
Genital warts (after 1 year)	Probable
Vaginosis	Possible
Mycoplasma hominis or *Ureaplasma urealyticum*	Indeterminate

16 | AIDS

The acquired immunodeficiency syndrome was first recognized in children in 1982, one year after the first description in adults. Initially, a large number of pediatric cases were transmitted through blood and blood products but after 1985, when an antibody test for HIV became commercially available, blood bank screening essentially eliminated this as a route of transmission. Almost all infections in children at the present time are the result of maternal disease.

PREVENTION

Without intervention, vertical transmission from HIV-infected mothers to neonates is approximately 25%. With zidovudine treatment of the mother and neonate (Table 1), transmission is reduced to 6% to 8%. This is further decreased to 2% to 3% if the newborn is delivered by Caesarian section. Other antiretroviral agents may be necessary for the treatment of the infected mother to reduce her viral load, better control her infection, and further reduce the likelihood of vertical transmission of HIV to the fetus.

Additional general principles have been developed by the U.S. Public Health service to further define appropriate interventions for pregnant HIV-infected mothers (Table 2), modified according to the gestational age of the fetus, maternal CD4 lymphocyte count, clinical disease stage, and previous antiretroviral therapy.

DIAGNOSIS

Differentiating infected from uninfected infants has been greatly simplified with the development of highly sensitive and specific polymerase chain reaction (PCR) assays. HIV infection can be identified in many infected infants by age 1 month and in virtually all infected infants by age 4 months using viral diagnostic assays (Table 3). A positive virologic test result at birth (i.e., detection of HIV by HIV DNA PCR or culture) indicates probable HIV infection and should be confirmed by a repeat virologic test on a second specimen at 1 to 2 months of age. It is recommended for all infants born to HIV positive mothers to obtain a DNA PCR determination before the infant is 48 hours of age, at 1 to 2 months, and at 4 months. These HIV-exposed infants should be evaluated by or in consultation with a specialist in HIV infection in pediatric patients.

HIV DNA PCR is the preferred virologic method for diagnosing HIV infection during infancy. Of infected children, 38% have positive PCR test results by 48 hours of age. No

TABLE 1   Zidovudine Regimen to Prevent Pediatric AIDS

Routine testing of pregnant women
HIV-infected pregnant women
Zidovudine (AZT) 200 mg p.o. t.i.d. or 300 mg b.i.d. beginning after week 14 of gestation
During labor
Zidovudine 2 mg/kg i.v. over 1 hr, then 1 mg/kg per hour until delivery
Newborn
Zidovudine syrup 2 mg/kg per dose p.o., q.i.d. for 6 weeks

TABLE 2 U.S. Public Health Service Recommendations for Use of Zidovudine to Reduce Perinatal HIV Transmission

Clinical scenario	Recommendations
CD4 ≥200/mm³ 14–34 wks of gestation No maternal clinical indication for zidovudine	Risk vs. benefit discussion Recommend full protocol (Table 1) zidovudine regimen
CD4 ≥200/mm³ >34 wks of gestation No maternal clinical indication for zidovudine No extensive history (>6 mos) of prior zidovudine	Risk vs. benefit discussion Recommend full protocol (Table 1) zidovudine regimen May be less effective because therapy is initiated late

CD4 <200/mm³
 14–34 wks of gestation
 No extensive history (>6 mos) of prior
   zidovudine
	Risk vs. benefit discussion
	Recommend antenatal zidovudine therapy for woman's health
	Recommend intrapartum and neonatal components of
	   zidovudine regimen (Table 1)

Significant prior administration of zidovudine or
   other antiretoviral therapy (>6 mos)
	Risk vs. benefit discussion
	Recommend zidovudine therapy on a case-by-case basis
	Issues to consider
	   Likelihood of resistance to therapy
	   Duration of prior zidovudine therapy
	   Reason alternative therapy was given; if received
	      (intolerance vs. progression of disease despite therapy)

Woman is in labor and has not had antepartum
   zidovudine therapy
	Risk vs. benefit discussion
	Discuss and offer intrapartum and neonatal ZDV if clinical
	   situation permits

Infant is born to a woman who has not received
   intrapartum zidovudine
	Risk vs. benefit discussion
	If ≤24 hrs old and clinical situation permits:
	   Discuss and offer neonatal zidovudine
	   Start zidovudine as soon as possible after birth
	If >24 hrs old: no data support offering zidovudine therapy

substantial change in sensitivity during the first week of life occurs, but sensitivity increases rapidly during the second week, with over 90% of infected children testing PCR-positive by age 14 days. Some experts therefore recommend repeat testing of PCR-negative neonates at two weeks of age.

For infants born to HIV-infected mothers who are not identified until some time after delivery, diagnosis in the infant is usually made by the subsequent clinical course or persistence of antibody beyond 15 months of age. The CDC classification system, outlined in Table 4, was designed both to identify the variable clinical characteristics of AIDS and to categorize patients for future treatment protocols.

HUMAN IMMUNODEFICIENCY VIRUS (HIV) THERAPY

Decisions for HIV-specific antiviral therapy must take into consideration immunologic (Table 5) and clinical (Table 6) parameters as well as quality-of-life issues (1). It should also be remembered that although early intervention is theoretically advantageous, most present medications have significant potential adverse effects and the risk of development of resistance.

Recommendations for antiretroviral therapy (beyond 6 weeks postnasally when used prophylactically) in HIV-infected children have been based on viral load, CD4 lymphocyte count and percentage and clinical conditions. Due to rapidly expanding knowledge concerning the dynamic interaction of the HIV virus with the host's immune system and due to the availability of multiple new antiretroviral drugs, recommendations for

TABLE 3 Laboratory Tests for HIV

Test	Advantages and disadvantages
HIV DNA PCR (polymerase chain reaction)	Preferred diagnostic test for HIV-1 subtype B infection in children younger than 18 mos Rapid, sensitive, and specific by age 2 wks Requires only 1–3 ml of blood False negatives in non-B subtype HIV-1
Viral culture	Highly specific Not routinely available Requires 7–28 days Labor intensive
p24 Antigen assay	Highly specific when positive Lacks sensitivity particularly with high titers of antibody False positives during first month of life

Antibody assays
  ELISA and Western blot
  Latex agglutination
  HIV-IgM, HIV-IgA
Immune function assays
  CD4 quantitation
  CD8 quantitation
  CD4:CD8 ratio
  Mitogen-induced lymphocyte stimulation
  Quantitative immunoglobulins
  Specific antibody responses
	Standard screening assays for older patients; not diagnostic <15 mos of age
	Lacks sensitivity
	Not routinely available
	Surrogate tests (nonspecific)—meet CDC criteria in symptomatic infant for starting antiretroviral therapy

antiretroviral therapy are being revised. Thus, decisions regarding antiretroviral therapy in HIV-infected children should be made in conjunction with a physician with expertise in pediatric HIV infection.

The CD4+ T-lymphocyte count or percentage value is used in conjunction with other measurements to guide antiretroviral treatment decisions and primary prophylaxis of PCP after age 1 year (Table 5). However, measurement of CD4+ cell values can be associated with considerable intrapatient variation. Even mild intercurrent illness or undergoing vaccination can produce a transient decrease in CD4+ cell number and percentage; thus, CD4+ values are best measured when patients are clinically stable. No modification in therapy should be made in response to a change in CD4+ cell values until the change has been substantiated by at least a second determination, with at least one week between measurements.

There are a number of antiretroviral agents approved for use in HIV-infected adults and children in the United States but many of these are not approved at the present time for pediatric patients (Table 8). The agents available fall into three major classes: (1) nucleoside/nucleotide analogue reverse transcriptase inhibitor (NRTI) agents; (2) non-nucleoside analogue reverse transcriptase inhibitor (NNRTI) agents; and (3) protease inhibitor (PI) agents.

INFECTIOUS COMPLICATIONS

Many children initially exhibit HIV-induced changes in immune function by developing unusual infections. Unfortunately, once established, infectious diseases are often difficult to treat because immunosuppression is so severe. Therefore, early recognition and therapy are essential. Some of these opportunistic pathogens are predictable enough to offer prophylaxis.

TABLE 4   Revised HIV Pediatric Classification System: Clinical Categories

---

Category N: Not Symptomatic
Children who have no signs or symptoms considered to be the result of HIV infection or who have only one of the
  conditions listed in Category A

Category A: Mildly Symptomatic
Children with two or more of the conditions listed below but none of the conditions listed in categories B and C
  Lymphadenopathy (≥0.5 cm at more than two sites; bilateral = one site)
  Hepatomegaly
  Splenomegaly
  Dermatitis
  Parotitis
  Recurrent or persistent upper respiratory infection, sinusitis or otitis media

Category B: Moderately Symptomatic
Children who have symptomatic conditions other than those listed for category A or C that are attributed to HIV
  infection. Examples of conditions in clinical category B include but are not limited to:

  Anemia (<8 gm/dL), neutropenia (<1000/mm^3) or thrombocytopenia (<100 000/mm^3) persisting ≥30 days
  Bacterial meningitis, pneumonia, or sepsis (single episode)
  Candidiasis, oropharyngeal (thrush) persisting (>2 mos) in children >6 mos
  Cardiomyopathy
  Cytomegalovirus infection, with onset before 1 mo of age
  Diarrhea, recurrent or chronic
  Hepatitis
  HSV stomatitis, recurrent (more than two episodes within 1 yr)
  HSV bronchitis, pneumonitis, or esophagitis with onset before 1 mo of age
  Herpes zoster (shingles) involving at least two distinct episodes or more than one dermatome
  Leiomyosarcoma
  LIP or pulmonary lymphoid hyperplasia complex
  Nephropathy
  Nocardiosis
  Persistent fever (lasting >1 mo)
  Toxoplasmosis, onset before 1 mo of age
  Varicella, disseminated (complicated chickenpox)

Category C: Severely Symptomatic
  Serious bacterial infections, multiple or recurrent (i.e. any combination of at least two culture-confirmed
    infections within a 2-yr period) of the following types: septicemia, pneumonia, meningitis, bone or joint
    infection, or abscess of an internal organ or body cavity (excluding otitis media, superficial skin or mucosal
    abscesses, and in-dwelling catheter-related infections)
  Candidiasis, esophageal or pulmonary (bronchi, trachea, lungs)
  Coccidioidomycosis, disseminated (at site other than or in addition to lungs or cervical or hilar lymph nodes)
  Cryptococcosis, extrapulmonary
  Cryptosporidiosis or isosporiasis with diarrhea persisting >1 mo
  Cytomegalovirus disease with onset of symptoms at age >1 mo (at a site other than liver, spleen, or lymph
    nodes)
  Encephalopathy (at least one of the following progressive findings present for at least 2 mos in the absence of a
    concurrent illness other than HIV infection that could explain the findings): (1) failure to attain or loss of
    developmental milestones or loss of intellectual ability, verified by standard developmental scale or
    neuropsychological tests; (2) impaired brain growth or acquired microcephaly demonstrated by head
    circumference measurements or brain atrophy demonstrated by CT or MRI (serial imaging is required for
    children <2 yrs of age); (3) acquired symmetric motor deficit manifested by two or more of the following:
    paresis, pathologic reflexes, ataxia, or gait disturbance
  HSV infection causing a mucutaneous ulcer that persists for >1 mo, or bronchitis, pneumonitis, or esophagitis
    for any duration affecting a child >1 mo of age
  Histoplasmosis, disseminated (at a site other than or in addition to lungs or cervical or hilar lymph
    nodes)
  Kaposi's sarcoma
  Lymphoma, primary, in brain

(Continued)

TABLE 4   Revised HIV Pediatric Classification System: Clinical Categories *(Continued)*

Lymphoma, small, noncleaved cell (Burkitt's), or immunoblastic or large cell lymphoma of B-cell or unknown
   immunologic phenotype
Mycobacterium tuberculosis infection, disseminated or extrapulmonary
Mycobacterium, other species or unidentified species infection, disseminated (at a site other than or in addition to
   lungs, skin, or cervical or hilar lymph nodes)
Pneumocystis jiroveci pneumonia
Progressive multifocal leukoencephalopathy
Salmonella (nontyphoidal) septicemia, recurrent
Toxoplasmosis of the brain with onset at after 1 mo of age
Wasting syndrome in the absence of a concurrent illness other than HIV infection that could explain the following
   findings: (1) persistent weight loss >10% of baseline; (2) downward crossing of at least 2 of the following
   percentile lines on the weight-for-age chart (e.g., 95th, 75th, 50th, 25th, and 5th) in a child 1 yr of age or older;
   Or (3) <5th percentile on weight-for-height chart on 2 consecutive measurements, >30 days apart; *plus* (1)
   chronic diarrhea (i.e., at least 2 loose stools per day for >30 days); *or* (2) documented fever (for >30 days,
   intermittent or constant)

Source: Modified from Ref. 2.

Prophylaxis

There are four potential secondary infections in pediatric acquired immunodeficiency syndrome (AIDS) that warrant prophylaxis: bacteremia/sepsis, *Pneumocystis jiroveci* infection, tuberculosis, and *Mycobacterium avium-intracellulare* infection. Table 9 summarizes criteria for these indications and currently recommended treatment.

Intravenous immunoglobulin has been used in infants and children infected with human immunodeficiency virus (HIV), with encouraging reports of its efficacy in preventing bacterial sepsis and decreasing the number of hospitalizations.

Pneumocystis jiroveci pneumonia (PCP), the most common infection in pediatric AIDS and often the first manifestation of disease (Fig. 1), warrants an early primary prevention strategy. Trimethoprim-sulfamethoxazole is currently the drug of choice for prophylaxis, with dapsone or aerosolized pentamidine reserved as alternatives for patients intolerant of TMP/SMX.

Although the incidence of *Mycobacterium tuberculosis* infection in pediatric patients with AIDS is considerably lower than in adults, a prevention strategy should be considered for children living in an environment of high tuberculosis (TB) prevalence. The World Health Organization (WHO) currently recommends that administration of bacilli Calmette-Guerin (BCG) vaccine for HIV-infected patients in high TB prevalence areas. However, disseminated BCG infection has been reported in children with symptomatic HIV infection who have received this vaccine. *Mycobacterium avium-intracellulare* complex (MAC) infection has been recognized with increased frequency and is associated with high morbidity and short survival. Prophylaxis is recommended for adult patients with AIDS, and many experts also recommend treatment for children seen in centers where MAC is commonly encountered. Rifabutin has

TABLE 5   Pediatric HIV Classification System: Immunologic Categories Based on Age-Specific CD4 Lymphocyte Count and Percentage

	Age of child					
	<12 mo		1–5 yr		6–12 yr	
Immune category	Number/μL	%	Number/μL	%	Number/μL	%
Category 1: no suppression	≥1500	≥25	≥1000	≥25	≥500	≥25
Category 2: moderate suppression	750–1499	15–24	500–999	15–24	200–499	15–24
Category 3: severe suppression	<750	<15	<500	<15	<200	<15

Source: Modified from Ref. 3.

TABLE 6   Clinical Classification of HIV Infection for Children Younger Than 13 Years of Age

	No signs or symptoms (N)	Mild signs and symptoms (A)	Moderate signs and symptoms (B)	Severe signs and symptoms (C)
No suppression	N1	A1	B1	C1
Moderate suppression	N2	A2	B2	C2
Severe suppression	N3	A3	B3	C3

been approved for prophylaxis. Additional options currently under investigation include azithromycin, clarithromycin, and biological-response modifiers.

Other clinical syndromes and opportunistic infections in patients with HIV may require suppressive or secondary prevention since recurrence of these diseases is common (Table 11).

Bacteremia and Sepsis

In contrast to adults with AIDS, children are uniquely susceptible to serious bacterial infections early in the course of HIV disease. Pathogens are those that are also the more common etiologies of infection in normal children (Table 11). Infection is common enough that IVIG prophylaxis is recommended as described previously (Table 9).

Empiric therapy for a toxic febrile child can be provided with a broad-spectrum cephalosporin (ceftriaxone, cefotaxime or ceftazidime) as a single agent if there is no central intravenous access line in place. For patients with a central line, it would be prudent to offer additional coverage for *Staphylococci* by adding vancomycin or clindamycin. Antimicrobial therapy can be adjusted as soon as culture results are available. As with any immunocompromised patient, bactericidal antibiotics are preferred to bacteristatic agents, using synergistic combinations when available. Antimicrobial agents should be given in maximum dosages and for maximum durations.

Respiratory Infections

Although pneumonia is the most commonly reported bacterial respiratory tract disease in childhood AIDS, upper respiratory tract infections, particularly otitis media and sinusitis, are far more frequent, and both tend to be recurrent. Oral candidiasis is also quite common, occurring early in the course of HIV disease (Fig. 2). Mucocutaneous herpes simplex can be severe and may produce recurrent or chronic gingivostomatitis. Therefore, intravenous antiviral therapy is sometimes necessary.

Pathogens causing otitis media and sinusitis in childhood AIDS are somewhat different from those causing disease in otherwise normal children in that *Staphylococci* (both *S. aureus* and *S. epidermidis*), enterococcus, and Gram-negative coliform organisms are relatively more common. However, antibiotics routinely recommended for infection in all children are still appropriate for childhood AIDS patients (Tables 12 and 13).

TABLE 7   Clinical Manifestations Warranting HIV Antiviral Therapy

AIDS-definitive infection (see Table 4)
Wasting or failure to thrive (or lower than the 5th percentile)
HIV encephalopathy
AIDS-associated malignancy (see Table 4)
Two episodes of sepsis or meningitis

TABLE 8   Drugs Used in Pediatric HIV Infection

Drug	Dosage
Nucleoside/nucleotide analogue reverse transcriptase inhibitors (NRTI)	
Abacavir (ABC) ZIAGEN®	Not approved <3 mos
Preparations:	>3 mos: 8 mg/kg (max 300 mg) b.i.d.
Oral solution: 20 mg/mL	
Tablets: 300 mg	
Didanosine (ddI) (dideoxyinosine) VIDEX®	Neonatal dose (infants <90 days): 50 mg/m² q 12 hrs
Preparations:	Pediatric usual dose: in combination with other
Pediatric powder for oral solution (when	antiretrovirals, 90 mg/m² q 12 hrs
reconstituted as solution containing	Pediatric dosage range: 90–150 mg/m² q 12 hrs (Note:
antacid, 10 mg/mL)	may need higher dose in patients with CNS disease)
Chewable tablets with buffers, 50, 100,	Adolescent/adult dose:
and 150 mg	>60 kg. 200 mg bid
Buffered powder for oral solution 100, 167,	<60 kg. 125 mg bid
and 250 mg	
Emtricitabine (FTC) EMTRIVA®	Not approved <3 mos
Preparations: capsule 200 mg	>3 mos 6 mg/kg (max. 240 mg) once daily
Oral solution: 10 mg/mL	
Lamivudine (3TC) EPIVIR®	Neonatal dose (infants <30 days): 2 mg/kg bid
Preparations:	Pediatric dose: 4 mg/kg bid
Solution: 10 mg/mL; 5 mg/mL	Adolescent/adult dose:
Tablets: 100, 150, and 300 mg	≥50 kg: 150 mg bid
Tablets: COMBIVIR® (150 mg lamivudine	<50 kg: 2 mg/kg bid
in combination with 300 mg zidovudine)	
Stavudine (d4T) ZERIT®	<14 days: 0.5 mg/kg q 12 hrs
Preparations:	>14 days: 1 mg/kg q 12 hrs (up to body weight of 30 kg)
Solution: 1 mg/mL	Adolescent/adult dose:
Capsules: 15, 20, 30, and 40 mg	≥60 kg, 40 mg bid
	<60 kg, 30 mg bid
Tenofovir (TDF) VIREAD®	Not approved in children <18 yrs
Tablets: 300 mg	Investigational:
	2–8 yrs: 8 mg/kg once daily
	>8 yrs: 210 mg/m² q.d. max 300 mg
Zalcitabine (ddC) HIVID®	Neonatal dose: Not approved
Preparations:	Pediatric usual dose: 0.01 mg/kg q 8 hrs
Syrup, 0.1 mg/mL (investigational; available	Pediatric dosage range: 0.005–0.01 mg/kg q 8 hrs
through compassionate use program)	Adolescent/adult dose: 0.75 mg tid
Tablets, 0.375 mg and 0.75 mg	
Zidovudine (ZDV, AZT) RETROVIR®	Premature neonates (standard neonatal dose may be
Preparations: Syrup, 10 mg/mL	excessive in premature infants)
Capsules: 100 mg	i.v 1.5 mg/kg q 12 hrs from birth to 2 wks of age; then
Tablets: 300 mg	increase to 2 mg/kg q 8 hrs after 2 wks of age
Tablets: COMBIVIR (300 mg zidovudine	Neonatal dose: Oral, 2 mg/kg q 6 hrs
in combination with 150 mg lamivudine)	Intravenous 1.5 mg/kg q 6 hrs
Concentrate for injection, for intravenous	Pediatric usual dose: Oral, 160 mg/m² q 6 hrs
infusion: 10 mg/mL	Intravenous (intermittent infusion), 120 mg/m² q 6 hrs
	Intravenous (continuous infusion), 20 mg/m²/hrs
	Pediatric dosage range: 90 mg/m² to 180 mg/m² q 6–8 hrs
	Adolescent/adult dose: 200 mg tid or 300 mg bid
Non-nucleoside analogue reverse transcriptase inhibitors (NNRTIs)	
Delavirdine (DLV) RESCRIPTOR®	Neonatal dose: Unknown
Preparations:	Pediatric dose: Unknown
Tablets: 100 mg	Adolescent/adult dose: 400 mg tid

(Continued)

TABLE 8   Drugs Used in Pediatric HIV Infection *(Continued)*

Drug	Dosage
Efavirenz (DMP-266, EFV) SUSTIVA® Preparations: Capsules: 50, 100, 200 mg Tablets: 600 mg	10–15 kg: 200 mg 15–20 kg: 250 20–25 kg: 300 25–32.5 kg: 350 32.5–40 kg: 400 >40 kg: 600
Nevirapine (NVP) VIRAMUNE® Preparations: Suspension: 10 mg/mL Tablets: 200 mg, scored	Neonatal dose (through 3 months): 5 mg/kg or 120 mg/m^2 once daily for 14 days, followed by 120 mg/m^2 q 12 hrs for 14 days, followed by 200 mg/m^2 q 12 hrs Pediatric dose: 120 to 200 mg/m^2 12 hrs Initiate therapy with 120 mg/m^2 given once daily for 14 days Increase to full dose administered q 12 hrs if no rash or other untoward effects. Adolescent/adult dose: 200 mg q 12 hrs Initiate therapy at half dose for the first 14 days. Increase to full dose if no rash or other untoward effects
Protease inhibitor (PI) agents Amprenavir (APV) AGENERASE® Preparations: Solution: 15 mg/mL Capsules: 50 mg Indinavir (IDV) CRIXIVAN® Preparations: Capsules: 100, 200, 333, and 400 mg	Solution 4-12 yrs or 13–16 weighing <50 kg 22.5 mg/kg b.i.d. or 17 mg/kg t.i.d. Capsules: 20 mg/kg b.i.d. or 15 mg/kg t.i.d. Neonatal dose: not approved because of side effect of hyperbilirubinemia, should not be given to neonates until additional information available Pediatric dose: under study in clinical trials, 500 mg/m^2 q 8 hrs Adolescent/adult dose: 800 mg q 8 hrs
Nelfinavir (NFV) VIRACEPT® Preparations: Powder for oral suspensions: 50 mg per 1 level scoop (200 mg per 1 level teaspoon) Tablets: 250 and 625 mg Ritonavir (RTV) NORVIR® Preparations: Oral solution: 80 mg/mL Capsules: 100 mg	Neonatal and infants: not approved Age 2–13 years: 45–55 mg/kg b.i.d or 25–35 mg/kg t.i.d. Adolescent/adult dose: 750 mg t.i.d Neonatal dose: under study Pediatric dose: 350–400 mg/m^2 q 12 hrs To minimize nausea/vomiting, initiate therapy at 250 mg/m^2 q 12 hrs and increase stepwise to full dose over 5 days as tolerated. Pediatric dosage range: 350–400 mg/m^2 q 12 hrs Adolescent/adult dose: 600 mg q 12 hrs (single PI therapy) 400 mg q 12 hrs (in combination with SQV) To minimize nausea/vomiting, initiate therapy at 300 mg q 12 hrs and increase stepwise to full dose over 5 days tolerated
Saquinavir (SQV) INVIRASE® (hard gel capsule) FORTOVASE® (soft gel capsule) Preparations: Hard gel capsules: (HGC) 200 mg Soft gel capsules: (SGC), 200 mg	Neonatal dose: Unknown Pediatric dose: SGC: under study: 50 mg/kg t.i.d Adolescent/adult dose: HGC, 600 mg t.i.d SGC, 1200 mg tid (single PI therapy) 400 mg bid (in combination with RTV)
Fusion inhibitors Enfuvirtide FUZEON® Preparation: Injection: 90 mg/mL	Children >6 years 2 mg/kg (max 90 mg) b.i.d

TABLE 9   Routine Prophylaxis for Children Infected with Human Immunodeficiency Virus

Clinical syndrome	Indications	Prophylaxis and dosage
Bacterial sepsis	Hypogammoglobulinemia Abnormal antibody formation Serious bacterial infection or Presumed bacterial pneumonia x 2	IVIG 400 mg/kg/mo

Pneumocystis jiroveci pneumonia	Age (yr) CD4+ cells/mm^3
	<1 <1500 (20% of total lymphocytes)
	1–2 <750 (20%)
	2–6 <500 (20%)
	>6 <200 (20%)
		TMP/SMX
		  150 mg/m^2/day
		TMP p.o. divided bid on 3
		  consecutive days (M, T, W)
		  each week
		or
		Dapsone, 1 mg/kg/day p.o.
		  (max, 100 mg)
		or
		Aerosolized pentamidine

Tuberculosis	At birth (when immune function is near normal)
	  for neonates born to HIV-positive mothers if
	  high risk for TB
		BCG vaccine

MAI/MAC	Same as in PCP	Rifabutin 5 mg/kg/day p.o. (max, 300 mg, once daily)

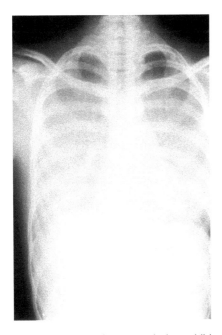

FIGURE 1   *Pneumocystis jiroveci* pneumonia in a child with AIDS. The chest X ray shows diffuse alveolar and interstitial. Patients are often afebrile with tachypnea, peripheral cyanosis, and minimal crackles on lung auscultation.

TABLE 10   Suggested Antimicrobial Therapy for Suppressive or Secondary Prevention of Opportunistic Infections in Patients Infected with Human Immunodeficiency Virus

Clinical syndrome for which initial therapy has been completed	Prophylaxis
Oral and esophageal candidiasis	Clotrimazole, fluconazole, or ketoconazole
Toxoplasma cerebritis	TMP/SMX or pyrimethamoine plus sulfadiazine
Cytomegalovirus	High-dose acyclovir, ganciclovir, or Foscarnet
Herpes simplex	Acyclovir or vidarabine
Cryptococcosis	Fluconazole or ketoconazole

The differential diagnosis of lower respiratory tract disease (Table 13) is unusual, often requiring open lung biopsy for final resolution. One difference as contrasted with adult AIDS is that fungal pneumonias such as histoplasmosis and coccidioidomycosis are extremely rare.

Gastrointestinal Infections

In patients with AIDS, normally nonpathogenic gastrointestinal colonizing parasites may produce prolonged symptomatic disease. For this reason, available treatment should be offered if the clinical course suggests an etiologic relationship (Table 14). Usual stool pathogens such as rotavirus, *Salmonella*, *Shigella*, *Campylobacter*, *Yersinia* spp., and *Giardia lamblia* can be diagnosed and treated in the usual fashion (see Chapter 9).

Additional stool and gastrointestinal studies might include a modified acid-fast or monoclonal antibody stain of stool or duodenal aspirate (*Cryptosporidium* sp. and *Isospora belli*), small bowel biopsy (*Cryptosporidium* and *Microsporidium* spp.), duodenal biopsy (*Isospora belli*, *G. lamblia*, and *Strongyloides stercoralis*), and ELISA of stool for *G. lamblia*.

Tuberculosis

Propensity to mycobacterial disease results both from immunodeficiency and increased exposure to adults with tuberculosis. By definition, all children born to HIV-positive mothers may be at risk because of the high incidence of tuberculosis among their mothers and other family members. Therefore, any child born into this setting would be a candidate for BCG vaccination. Once disease develops, therapy must be continued for a prolonged period of time (Table 15). Atypical mycobacteria are extremely difficult to treat and ideal regimens have really not been determined.

Varicella-Zoster

Primary infection (i.e., chickenpox), can be severe and prolonged in children with AIDS. Therefore, exposure to disease warrants the use of varicella-zoster hyperimmune immuno-globulin (VZIG) within 96 hours of initial contact (see Chapter 3). Once disease has developed, most AIDS patients should be hospitalized and begun on intravenous acyclovir (30 mg/kg/day or 1500 mg/m^2/day div. t.i.d.) for 6 to 14 days, depending on the clinical course. If vesicles continue to erupt but there is no visceral involvement, and cutaneous disease is mild, oral acyclovir (20 mg/kg per dose 5 times per day div. q4h) can be offered. Response to oral therapy is quite variable so duration of treatment should be individualized.

TABLE 11   Bacterial Pathogens Causing Serious Infection in Children with AIDS

Streptococcus pneumoniae	*Pseudomonas* spp.
Haemophilus influenzae	*Klebsiella* sp.
Salmonella spp.	Streptococci, Group A and B
Staphylococcus aureus	Enterococcus
Staphylococcus epidermidis	*Escherichia coli*

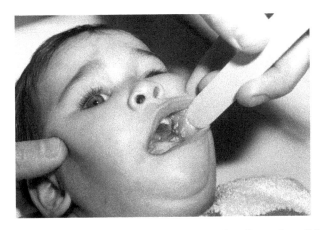

FIGURE 2 Thrush is the common term used to describe oral candidiasis, manifested by the presence of irregular white plaques on the tongue, buccal mucosa, lips, and palate.

Measles

Wild measles is a life-threatening infection in childhood AIDS patients and, unfortunately, there is no antiviral therapy of proven benefit. Early in the course of infection, all cases should be treated with a single oral dose of vitamin A; 200 000 U for children over 1 year and 100 000 U for infants 6 months to 1 year of age. In addition, the antiviral agent, ribavirin, has been shown in vitro to exhibit virucidal activity against measles and, in limited clinical trials, both the aerosolized and intravenous preparations have been used.

Fungal Infections

Systemic mycoses are relatively rare in childhood AIDS but, when present, are managed as for other immunosuppressed pediatric patients (see Chapter 18 and Tables 18 and 19 of Chapter 20).

Oral candidiasis is quite common, often requiring continual suppressive therapy for recurrent or chronic disease. If disease remains uncontrolled with nystatin oral suspension (200 000 U (2 mL) p.o. q.i.d.) for 6 to 12 days, either fluconazole (1–2 mg/kg/day p.o. div. qd) or ketoconazole (3–5 mg/kg/day p.o. div. b.i.d.) may be substituted.

HIV EXPOSURE IN HOSPITAL PERSONNEL

Primary prophylaxis against HIV following exposure to contaminated needles remains controversial. The risk for HIV-1 transmission associated with a single parenteral exposure to

TABLE 12 Treatment of Common Upper Respiratory Infections

Disease	Therapy
Otitis media	Macrolide or cephalosporin
Sinusitis	Macrolide or cephalosporin
Oral candidiasis	Fluconazole, nystatin, clotrimazole, or ketoconazole
Herpes gingivostomatitis	Acyclovir p.o. or i.v.

TABLE 13   Differential Diagnosis and Treatment of Lower Respiratory Tract Infections in Childhood AIDS

Etiology	Treatment
Lymphoid interstitial pneumonitis	Prednisone 2 mg/kg per day p.o. div. qd for 4–12 wks; taper dose to lowest maintenance level
Pneumocystis jiroveci	TMP/SMX 20 mg TMP/100 mg SMX/kg per day p.o. or i.v. div, q6hrs for 21 days plus Prednisone 2 mg/kg per day p.o. div. b.i.d. for 5 days, then 1 mg/kg per day div. qd for 5 days, then 0.5 mg/kg per day div. qd for 11 days Alternative: pentamidine isethionate 4 mg/kg per day i.m. div, qd for 12–14 days
Bacterial: *Streptococcus pneumoniae, Pseudomonas aeruginosa, Staphylococcus aureus, Klebsiella* sp., *Haemophilus influenzae, Enterococcus, Salmonella* sp., *Nocardia* sp., *Listeria* sp., *Pertussis, Legionella* sp., *Moraxella catarrhalis*	See individual pathogen
Tuberculosis and atypical mycobacteria (MAI)	See Tuberculosis section; Chapter 15
Viral: Respiratory syncytial virus (RSV)	Aerosolized ribavirin (20 mg/mL in the reservoir) 18 hrs per day for 5–10 days
Influenza A	Amantadine 5–8 mg/kg per day (max. 200 mg) p.o. div. b.i.d. for 7–14 days Rimantadine 5 mg/kg per day p.o. div. q12–24hrs
Influenza A and B, parainfluenza, measles	Aerosolized ribavirin (as above)
Cytomegalovirus (CMV)	Ganciclovir 7.5 mg/kg per day i.v. div. t.i.d. for 14–21 days then 10 mg/kg per day div. b.i.d. only treat if biopsy is positive for interstitial inflammation with CMV inclusions and no other pathogens

TABLE 14   Treatment of Gastrointestinal Protozoa in Childhood AIDS

Pathogen	Treatment
Balantidium coli	Tetracycline 40 mg/kg/day (max. 2g) div. q.i.d. × 10 days
Blastocystis hominis	Metronidazole 35–50 mg/kg/day p.o. div. T.i.d. × 10 days
Cryptosporidium sp.	Paromomycin 30 mg/kg per day p.o. div. t.i.d. Nitazoxanide 1–3 yr 100 mg b.i.d. × 3 days 4–11 yr 200 mg b.i.d. × 3 days Oral human immune globulin or bovine colostrum Improve antiretroviral therapy to raise CD4 count
Dientamoeba fragilis	Iodoquinol 40 mg/kg/day (max. 2 g) p.o. div. t.i.d. × 20 days
Entamoeba coli	Treatment rarely necessary Metronidazole 35–50 mg/kg per day p.o. div. t.i.d. for 10 days
Isospora belli	TMP/SM× 40 mg TMP/200 mg SM×/kg per day p.o. div. q.i.d. for 10 days (max. 640 mg TMP 3200 mg SM× per day) then 20 mg TMP 100 mg SM×/kg per day (max. 320 TMP 1600 mg SM× per day) for 3 wk
Microsporidiosis.	*E. bieneusi*—Fumagillin 60 mg/d p.o. × 14 days *E. intestinalis*—Albendazole 400 mg b.i.d. × 21 days
Strongyloides stercoralis	Ivermectin 200 mcg/kg/d × 2 days

TABLE 15 Treatment of Tuberculosis and Atypical Mycobacterial Disease

Mycobacterium tuberculosis	Isoniazid, rifampin, and pyrazinamide for 2 months *followed by* Isoniazid and rifampin for 10 months (for dosages see Table 7.14)
Mycobacterium avium—M. intracellulare complex (MAI, MAC)	Clarithromycin 15 mg/kg/day p.o. div. b.i.d. *plus* Rifampin 20 mg/kg/day i.v, or p.o. div. b.i.d. *plus* Amikacin 22.5 mg/kg/day i.v. div. t.i.d. *plus* Ciprofloxacin 30 mg/kg/day i.v. or p.o. div. b.i.d.

a contaminated needle is 0.37%. Zidovudine (AZT) alone or in combination with other antiretroviral agents is currently recommended but efficacy for prophylactic use has not been established.

REFERENCES

1. Working Group on Antiretroviral Therapy and Medical Management of HIV-Infected Children. Guidelines for the Use of Antiretroviral Agents in Pediatric HIV Infection. http://aidsinfo.nih.gov/.
2. Centers for Disease Control and Prevention 1994 Revised classification system for human immunodeficiency virus infection in children less than 13 years of age. MMWR 1994; 43(No. RR-12):1–19.
3. Centers for Disease Control 1994 Revised classification system for human immunodeficiency virus infection in children less than 13 years of age. MMWR 1994; 43(No. RR-12):1–10.

17 | The Immunocompromised Host

NEONATES

The largest group of patients with immunodeficiency are newborn infants who have been shown to exhibit a variety of immune defects that predispose these otherwise healthy neonates to life-threatening illness (Table 1). It is unclear which defects might be relatively more important and which may be related to specific disease processes. The absence of IgM is considered one of the more important deficiencies, and one that at least partially accounts for propensity to gram-negative bacterial meningitis and sepsis (see Chapter 1).

The newborn is particularly vulnerable to treatment modalities that may further depress immune function. Congenital asplenia or splenectomy is associated with a much higher long-term morbidity in the neonate as compared to older children and adults, and steroid therapy, similarly, is fraught with more complications in this age group. The trauma of surgery and thermal burns both suppress immune function in patients of all ages but, in neonates, they may have a more potent influence on immune capabilities with resulting fatal infection.

Most of the basic principles that apply to the management of immunocompromised patients are relevant to neonates. Maximum doses of bactericidal antibiotics should be given with duration of therapy often being longer than for similar disease in infants and children.

IATROGENIC FACTORS

Secondary immunodeficiency is often iatrogenically introduced. Chemotherapeutic regimens for cancer patients, directed at inhibiting tumor replication are, at the same time, toxic to all elements in bone marrow, including immunologically competent white blood cells. In addition, patients with a variety of diseases are kept alive for a longer period of time using extraordinary supportive measures that offer a much greater chance for eventual colonization with multiresistant or unusual microorganisms, and eventual overt infectious disease. The infectious agents which cause such disease are often opportunistic organisms. For each medical intervention in these fragile patients, the physician must calculate risk factors and anticipate complications. Some common complications involve local factors related to diagnostic or therapeutic procedures, and to the placement of indwelling catheters, cannulae,

TABLE 1 Maturational Defects of Immunity in Neonates

Humoral: absent IgM and IgA
Complement levels: 50% adult concentrations
Specific antibody production: poor response to polysaccharide antigens
Cell-mediated immunity: increased CD8 suppressor cells; decreased killer cell function
Skin test responses: decreased reaction to recall antigens
Phagocytosis: particularly with low concentrations of opsonizing antibody
Inflammatory response
Intracellular killing of bacteria
Viral killing by monocytes
Polymorphonuclear leukocyte and monocyte chemotaxis
Random migration of phagocytes
Polymorphonuclear leukocyte deformability
Generation of serum chemotactic factors

TABLE 2   Iatrogenic Predisposition to Infection

Local factors; mucosal and skin lesions
    Drugs (e.g. cyclophosphamide)
    Procedures (i.v. administration, cutdown, bone
        marrow biopsy)
    Surgical wounds
Urinary catheters
Intravascular devices (intravenous, intra-arterial,
    central venous pressure, Swan-Ganz catheters,
    etc.)
Respiratory support (ventilator, intermittent positive
    pressure breathing, etc.)
Transfusion transmitted disease
Splenectomy
Hospital-acquired resistant bacteria (due to
    inadequate handwashing)

TABLE 3   Infections Transmitted by Blood Transfusions

Bacterial
    Bacterial sepsis
    Endotoxemia
    Brucellosis
    Syphilis
    Salmonellosis
Viral
    Cytomegalovirus
    Epstein-Barr virus
    Hepatitis A, B and C viruses (now rare)
    Measles virus
    Rubella virus
    Colorado tick fever virus
    Human immunodeficiency virus (now rare)
Other
    Toxoplasmosis
    Babesiosis
    Malaria
    Leptospirosis
    Filariasis
    Trypanosomiasis
    Chagas' disease
    Creutzfeldt-Jakob variant (not established)

or other foreign bodies. This sets the stage for colonization with opportunistic pathogens, which may then account for significant morbidity and mortality.

Most patients with diseases that result in secondary immunodeficiency receive blood or blood products during the course of their therapy. The transmission of infectious diseases to these patients represents a significant risk, particularly if multiple transfusions are given (Table 3). It should be noted that many of these agents are not routinely screened for in potential blood donors. Hepatitis is the best-understood and most carefully monitored disease, whereas recent literature incriminates cytomegalovirus as an agent that is increasingly likely to cause severe illness. Blood donors are often asymptomatic for infectious agents at the time of phlebotomy. In the compromised host, additional care should be taken in screening donors and in providing follow-up medical examination of donors as a routine aspect of the recipient's care. Additional problems of transfusion therapy are pulmonary edema from volume overload, hemolytic reactions, and other incompletely understood febrile reactions (Tables 2 and 3).

PRIMARY IMMUNODEFICIENCY

It is difficult to determine the incidence of primary immunodeficiency syndromes because many of the more severe forms may result in early infant death before diagnosis is made. In one British study, it was estimated that 1 in 50 child deaths was a result of immune dysfunction. Realistically, the more severe defects are only occasionally encountered by primary care physicians. The more common deficiencies, such as transient hypogamma-globulinemia of infancy and selective IgA deficiency, are familiar to clinicians.

Most primary immunodeficiency syndromes present during infancy or early childhood with the most notable exceptions being common variable hypogammaglobulinemia, cyclic neutrope-nia, and complement deficiencies which may not become clinically apparent until later in life. The deficiencies of the latter components of complement (C5–8) are not seen until adolescence or early adulthood, with the presentation of recurrent meningococcal and gonococcal disease. Immunodeficiency syndromes and their usual age at diagnosis are summarized in Table 4.

TABLE 4 Primary Immunodeficiency Syndromes in Order of Their Frequency

	Usual age at diagnosis	Gender
Transient hypogammaglobulinemia of infancy	6–12 mos	Both
Selective IgA deficiency	4–16 yrs	Both
Common variable hypogammaglobulinemia	All ages	Both
Chronic mucocutaneous candidiasis	1–2 yrs	Both
Cyclic neutropenia	All ages	Both
X-linked hypogammaglobulinemia (Bruton type)	6–12 mos	Male
Ataxia telangiectasia	3–5 yrs	Both
Chronic granulomatous disease	2 yrs	Primarily male
Severe combined immunodeficiency	9 mos	Both
Wiskott-Aldrich syndrome	1–2 yrs	Male
Thymic hypoplasia (DiGeorge syndrome)	3 mos	Both
Complement deficiencies	All ages	Both

The approach to therapy varies according to the specific defects demonstrated (Table 5). The most difficult deficiencies to manage are those with T lymphocyte or combined T and B lymphocyte abnormality where bone marrow transplantation usually represents definitive therapy. Selective B lymphocyte deficiencies with hypogammaglobulinemia are treated with immunoglobulin replacement, and this is best managed by the primary care physician. Intravenous preparations of human serum Ig are readily available for therapy generally given at a dosage of 400 mg/kg monthly. These should be used only for patients with documented hypogammaglobulinemia accompanied by recurrent clinical infection, or with demonstrated inability to produce specific antibody following antigenic challenge (e.g. tetanus). The "physiologic" hypogammaglobulinemia, apparent at 3 to 6 months of age, does not require supplemental Ig and must be distinguished from transient hypogammaglobulinemia of infancy. The latter deficiency represents a delay in normal antibody synthesis after maternal IgG is no longer at protective levels; these infants occasionally require Ig supplementation until approximately 18 months of age.

Defects in neutrophil function are characteristically followed closely with antibiotics especially during acute infectious episodes. Thus, close communication between patient and physician becomes the most important aspect of management.

TABLE 5 Therapeutic Approaches to Immunodeficiency Syndromes

Syndrome	Therapy
T cell deficiency	
DiGeorge syndrome (thymic aplasia)	Bone marrow transplantation
Nezelof syndrome (thymic hypoplasia)	Antimicrobial therapy, bone marrow transplantation
Wiskott-Aldrich syndrome (Fig. 1)	Bone marrow transplantation
Ataxia telangiectasia	Fresh plasma, antibiotics
Chronic mucocutaneous candidiasis (Fig. 2)	Ketoconazole, fluconazole suppressive therapy
B cell deficiency	
Hypogammaglobulinemia	I.v. immunoglobulin replacement
Selective IgA deficiency	Antibiotics
Complement deficiencies	Antibiotics, fresh plasma, meningococcal vaccine
T and B cell deficiency	
Severe combined immunodeficiency	Bone marrow transplantation
Phagocytosis	
Hyper IgE; Job syndrome (Fig. 3)	Antibiotics
Chronic granulomatous disease	Antibiotics, interferon, bone marrow transplantation
Neutropenia	Antibiotics, granulocyte colony stimulating factor; granulocyte transfusions

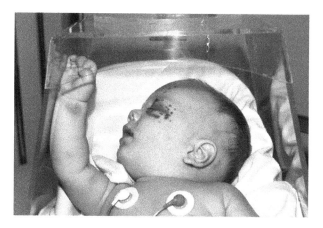

FIGURE 1   This patient with Wiskott-Aldrich syndrome initially presented at 5 months of age with thrombocytopenia and ocular and periorbital herpes simplex infection. By 18 months he had extensive eczema, and at age 3 years, severe chickenpox, which disseminated to the lungs and liver.

SECONDARY IMMUNODEFICIENCY

Suppression of immunologic function with resulting increased susceptibility to infection may occur as a result of a number of primary diseases (Table 6). This circumstance is more common in adults than in children because of the higher incidence of malignancy and greater use of immunosuppressive chemotherapy for a variety of diseases. AIDS is the most common predisposing factor in children and their management is covered in detail in Chapter 16.

Over 2% of all hospitalized children demonstrate secondary immunodeficiency. Recognition and treatment of these host defense abnormalities have therefore become a very

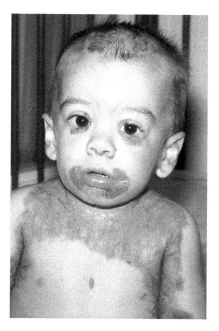

FIGURE 2   (*See color insert.*) Chronic mucocutaneous candidiasis, an inherited defect of T cell and mononuclear phagocyte function, presents with persistent candidal infection of the mouth, scalp, skin, and nails.

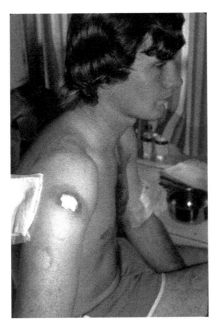

FIGURE 3 Hyperimmunoglobulinemia E, or Job syndrome, is defined by recurrent staphylococcal abscesses involving the skin, lungs, joints, and bones associated with serum IgE levels >1000 IU/ml. Eosinophilia and atypical atopic eczema attributed are often seen. This entity is attributable to an imbalance of TH-1 and TH-2 lymphocytes.

important aspect of hospital practice. Secondary deficiency is actually much more common than primary immunologic disorders, even in infants and children, and is usually managed by primary care physicians with consultative support.

Recognition of associations between specific infectious processes and primary disease offers important guidance to diagnosis and treatment (Table 7). All of these should be well-understood by the physician caring for pediatric patients.

Neutropenia

The congenital neutropenias may present either in childhood or during the adult years and include benign neutropenia with variants thereof, cyclic neutropenia, and what is termed infantile genetic agranulocytosis. These syndromes are secondary to inadequate production of granulocytes and, although a large spectrum of clinical consequences have been described, most patients do not experience a significantly increased propensity to infection. Inadequate production of neutrophil precursors may also be the consequence of nutritional deficiencies, including vitamin B_{12} and folate, or secondary to infectious processes such as typhoid fever, infectious mononucleosis, and viral hepatitis. More common are neutropenic states secondary to cytotoxic drugs used in cancer therapy, autoimmune disease, and excessive destruction of granulocytes (either as inherited disorders, hypersplenism, or as a result of artificial heart valves or hemodialysis).

TABLE 6 The Most Common Causes of Secondary Immunodeficiency in Children

AIDS	Splenectomy
Sickle cell disease	Poor nutrition
Leukemia	Other malignancies
Nephrotic syndrome	Autoimmune disease
Down syndrome	Immunosuppressive chemotherapy

TABLE 7 Unusual Pathogens and Disease Entities Associated with Secondary Immunodeficiency

Leukemia	Disseminated chickenpox
	Pneumocystis carinii pneumonia
	Herpes simplex
	Candida sp. sepsis
	Ecthyma gangrenosum (*Pseudomonas, Aeromonas* spp.)
	Aspergillus sp. pneumonia
Sickle cell disease	Pneumococcal meningitis, bacteremia and pneumonia
	Salmonella sp. osteomyelitis
Nephrotic syndrome	Pneumococcal peritonitis
	Disseminated chickenpox
Down syndrome	Pneumococcal pneumonia
	Hepatitis
Splenectomy	Pneumococcal sepsis
Diabetes	Malignant otitis externa (*Pseudomonas* sp.)
	Phycomycosis (mucormycosis)
	Listeriosis

More recently described, is an autoimmune process where antibodies, directed at neutrophils, produce profound neutropenia. These autoantibodies are often seen in conjunction with autoimmune states such as lupus erythematosus and Felty's syndrome. In such cases, infectious diseases are difficult to manage and account for the observed high mortality. Granulocyte transfusions are of no benefit because antineutrophil antibodies destroy donor cells.

The clinical approach for patients with neutropenia secondary to immunosuppressive chemotherapy is careful monitoring for infectious episodes and early institution of antimicrobial therapy. Once acute infection is documented, these patients must be treated for much longer periods as it is extremely difficult to eradicate bacteria without the help of the host's granulocyte killing capacity.

Normal neutrophil counts are generally in the range of 2 to $5000/mm^3$, with variations accounted for by age, gender, and race. Although neutropenia is defined as an absolute neutrophil count of $<1500/mm^3$, increased infection is not observed until a neutrophil count is below $1000/mm^3$. The absolute neutrophil count is an important objective parameter for making clinical decisions for immunosuppressed patients with fever (Table 8). It has become a fairly standard protocol to offer antibiotics, pending results of culture to febrile patients who have a neutrophil count of $<500/mm^3$.

During periods of anticipated transient neutropenia, such as during induction therapy for cancer, patients may benefit from granulocyte transfusions. This is impractical unless the period of neutropenia is 6 weeks or less but, under these defined conditions, benefits from such transfusions have been demonstrated.

Neutropenia and Fever

The most common clinical circumstance in which the physician must make decisions for the immunocompromised host is fever in the neutropenic patient. In pediatrics this individual is

TABLE 8 Susceptibility Staging for Neutropenia Secondary to Immunosuppressive Chemotherapy

Absolute neutrophil count/mm^3	Predisposition to bacterial infection
>1000	Little
500–1000	Mild
<500	Moderate (50%)
<100	Severe (100%)

most likely a child with leukemia who is neutropenic secondary to chemotherapy administered during treatment of the oncologic process. Such patients are not only neutropenic, but their remaining granulocytes function poorly in mechanisms of phagocytosis and bacterial killing, unlike other neutropenic states (e.g. congenital neutropenia) where remaining neutrophils function normally. This accounts for the increased susceptibility of neutropenic cancer patients over those with neutropenia of other etiologies. More common pathogens causing infection in childhood leukemia are listed in Table 9.

The best indicator of susceptibility to systemic bacterial disease is the absolute neutrophil count. A count of $<500/\text{mm}^3$ in a febrile patient dictates empiric antimicrobial therapy (Table 10). If therapy is not instituted and blood cultures are obtained daily for 5 days, 50% to 80% will eventually demonstrate bacteremia. If antibiotics are not started until a positive culture is obtained, mortality with such delayed therapy is over 80%.

Diagnostic evaluation should include cultures of blood, urine, stool, throat, and any other suspicious focus, with chest X-ray and lumbar puncture if CNS infection cannot be ruled out clinically. Baseline liver enzymes, renal function studies, and serum electrolytes should also be obtained prior to beginning antimicrobial therapy. Selection of antibiotics must obviously provide coverage for the most likely pathogens yet be particularly directed at the most "difficult-to-treat" organisms. In most settings, *Pseudomonas aeruginosa* represents the most resistant potential organism.

There is presently no clinical evidence that one particular combination from the list in Table 11 is more efficacious than another. Monotherapy is preferred unless *Staphylococcus aureus* is a major consideration or absolute neutrophil counts are $<200/\text{mm}^3$.

The final general comment is that the duration of recommended therapy is different from that for routine infections; treatment courses are dependent on the duration of fever and granulocytopenia. If a patient shows return of peripheral neutrophils after three days of therapy, then intravenous antibiotics could be discontinued and the patient changed to oral therapy, particularly if cultures are negative and the patient is afebrile. On the other hand, if fever and granulocytopenia persist, antibiotics are usually continued even after what would normally be considered adequate therapy (Table 12).

Candidemia

Recovery of *Candida* sp. from the blood of immunosuppressed patients has become commonplace, and is usually the result of two predisposing factors: long-term, broad-spectrum antibiotics and the presence of intravascular access lines. In almost all cases, medically placed catheters or other offending "foreign bodies" should be removed to allow eradication of this fungus. Consideration must also be given to limiting the number of broad-

TABLE 9   Documented Etiology of Infection in Childhood Leukemia

Bacteria	(75%)
Staphylococcus epidermidis	50%
Staphylococcus aureus	15%
Escherichia coli	3%
Pseudomonas aeruginosa	2%
Klebsiella/Enterobacter sp.	1%
Others	4%
Viral	(20%)
Varicella-zoster virus	7%
Herpes simplex virus	5%
Cytomegalovirus	5%
Fungal	(5%)
Candida albicans	4%

TABLE 10   Initial Management of the Febrile Neutropenic Patient

Monotherapy (preferred)
 Cefepime
 Ceftazidime
 Meropenem
 Imipenem cilastatin
S. aureus or *S. epidermidis* highly suspected
 Add vancomycin
Gram (−) highly suspected
 Add aminoglycoside
 Other combinations with aminoglycoside
  Ticarillin
  Ticarcillin/clavulanic acid
  Azlocillin
  Mezlocillin
  Piperacillin
Reassess after 3 days (Tables 11 and 12)

TABLE 11 Continued Management of the Neutropenic Patient After 3 Days of I.V. Antibiotics

Afebrile and etiology identified
Adjust to most appropriate management
Afebrile and etiology not identified
Low risk
Oral antibiotics: cefprozil, cefpodoxime, cefixime
ANC >500/mm^3 at day 7: stop
Intermediate risk (ANC <500/mm^3 at day 7)
Clinically well: stop antibiotics when afebrile 5 days
High risk (unstable or ANC <100/mm^3)
Continue same i.v. antibiotic(s)

TABLE 12 Management of Patients with Persistent Fever (5–7 Days)

Reassess
Options for management
Continue initial antibiotics
Stop vancomycin if stable
Change antibiotics for progressive disease
Add i.v. fluconazole or amphotericin B
Duration of therapy
Day 7: afebrile and ANC >500/mm^3
Stop antibiotics
Day 7: afebrile and ANC <500/mm^3
Continue oral or i.v. antibiotics × 14 days; reassess
Day 7: febrile
Continue i.v. antibiotics until afebrile 5 days

spectrum antimicrobial agents used. Table 13 summarizes the management of candidemia. Fluconazole or amphotericin B, in relatively low doses and short duration, is usually effective in the treatment of this infection. In the immunologically normal host with candidemia, removal of the intravascular line is often the only step necessary.

PROPHYLAXIS

Some infections in a well-defined group of immunosuppressed hosts are frequent enough to warrant prophylactic therapy (Table 14).

CUTANEOUS ANERGY

Transient defects in cell-mediated immunity are commonly encountered during the course of acute or chronic illnesses (Table 15). For a variable period of time, patients may fail to demonstrate positive delayed hypersensitivity to intradermal skin testing. This presents an enigma to the clinician using a skin test to diagnose a patient's primary illness. To differentiate global cutaneous anergy, a battery of skin tests might be applied along with the test antigen. A positive skin test to a recall antigen such as tetanus or candida along with a negative skin test to the pathogen in question would reassure the physician that this patient can respond to specific antigens, and then interpret the negative specific skin test as evidence against disease. However, this reactivity is not absolute, particularly when skin testing for tuberculosis, since antigen-specific non-reactivity has been observed.

TABLE 13 Treatment of Candidemia in Neutropenic Patients

Stable patients
Fluconazole 12 mg/kg/day i.v. div b.i.d.
Unstable Patients
Amphotericin B 0.8–1.0 mg/kg/day i.v. div q 24 h
plus
5-fluorocytosine 100 mg/kg/day p.o. div q 6 h
or
Fluconazole 12 mg/kg/day i.v. div b.i.d.
When stable: fluconazole
Empirical therapy (including other fungi)
Fungus unlikely: fluconazole
Fungus likely: amphotericin B

TABLE 14 Prophylaxis for the Immunocompromised Host

Underlying disease	Infectious agent	Prophylactic regimen

Leukemia
Primary immunodeficiency
  SCID
  DiGeorge syndrome
  Nezelof syndrome
	Pneumocystis carinii	Trimethoprim/sulfamethoxazole (TMP/SMX) 5 mg TMP/25 mg SMX/kg per day p.o. div. q 24 h or three times weekly

Asplenia
  Splenectomy
  Sickle cell disease
  Congenital complement deficiencies
    (C2, C3, C3b inhibitor, C5)
	Streptococcus pneumoniae	Conjugate pneumococcal vaccine at age 2, 4, 6 and 12–15 mo; pneumococcal polysaccharide vaccine at 2 years and 5 years later
		PLUS
		Benzathine penicillin G 1.2×10^6 U i.m. q 3 wk (>60 lb); 600 000 U (<60 lb)
		or
		Penicillin V 250 mg p.o. b.i.d. (>60 lb); 125 mg (<60 lb)

Chronic granulomatous disease	*Staphylococcus aureus*	TMP/SMX (for immune augmentation) 4 mg TMP/20 mg SMX/kg per day p.o. div. q 12 h

The phytohemagglutination (PHA) skin test is probably most sensitive for evaluating anergy; therefore a more rapid resolution of the question would be achieved with this mitogen in the initial skin test battery. Placing other skin tests first would create a delay of 2 days while reading these tests before the PHA skin test can be applied as a second step in the diagnostic work-up.

It is always better to have monitored patients with diseases known to be associated with cellular immunodeficiency to alert the physician that a patient is highly predisposed to viral and fungal infectious processes. The degree of cellular immunosuppression can be roughly determined by quantitating T lymphocyte CD4 subpopulations. This testing for clinical management helps direct early and aggressive use of antifungal or antituberculous medication for the severely immunosuppressed individual, often prior to receiving final culture results. Using a staging system (Table 16), patients can be categorized into those who have mild

TABLE 15 Causes of Cutaneous Anergy

Primary immunodeficiency	Infectious
Secondary immunodeficiency	diseases
AIDS	Bacterial
Malignancy	Viral
Immunosuppressive	Fungal
therapy	Rickettsial
Autoimmune disease	Chronic diseases
Surgery (recent)	Sarcoidosis
Trauma	Rheumatoid
Burns	Renal
Poor nutritional status	Alcoholism
Advanced age	Cirrhosis
Acute disease process	Diabetes

TABLE 16 Cellular Immunosuppression and Susceptibility Staging of Patients

Degree of immunosuppression	CD4 cells/mm^3
Severe	
Age (years)	
<1	<700
1–2	<500
2–6	<250
>6	<100
Moderate	
Age (years)	
<1	700–1200
1–2	500–750
2–6	250–500
>6	100–250
Mild	
Age (years)	
<1	1200–1750
1–2	750–1000
2–6	500–750
>6	250–500

suppression of cellular immunity, and those severely immunosuppressed. The latter group of patients are at extremely high risk to infection with opportunistic pathogens, particularly fungi and herpes group viruses.

TRANSPLANT RECIPIENTS

Patients who have recently undergone transplantation, either bone marrow or solid organs, represent a population with moderate to severe immunodeficiency and with a high risk for opportunistic infections. Many are caused by reactivated pathogens present in the host or donor organs at the time of transplant. Etiology varies with timing pre or post transplant and is consistent enough to use this parameter in the initial approach to a differential diagnosis (Fig. 4). Reactivation of herpes group viruses, particularly cytomegalovirus, is so common in these patients that it is critical to obtain serologic data prior to transplant to determine previous infection with these potential pathogens for both recipient and donor. Prophylactic antiviral and antibacterial therapy is often warranted.

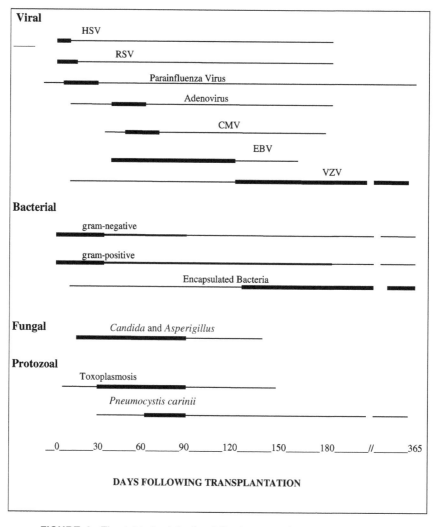

FIGURE 4   Timetable for infection following transplantation.

18 | Systemic Fungal Infections

The incidence of superficial and particularly deep mycotic infections has greatly increased over the last decade primarily attributable to a much larger population of immunosuppressed patients who are frequently on broad spectrum antibiotics and are managed with intravascular catheters and other devices that predispose them to infection.

Invasive fungal infections are now the fifth leading cause of infectious disease deaths in the United States. Most common are infections caused by *Candida* species which is the fourth most frequent pathogen recovered in health care-associated bloodstream infections.

Unfortunately, there are very few pediatric treatment studies with the newer antifungal agents. Most recommendations for treating children are therefore derived from data in adults. In spite of this shortcoming, experience to date has indicated that these antimicrobials are safe and effective in younger patients.

Practice guidelines for the treatment of fungal infections have been published and updated by The Infectious Diseases Society of America and The Mycoses Study Group which is supported by the National Institute of Allergy and Infectious Diseases (1). These references have been used as a primary source for treatment sections in the present chapter.

ASPERGILLOSIS

There are 3 principal manifestations of disease from this organism: (1) invasive aspergillosis involving many organs, particularly the lower respiratory tract; (2) pulmonary aspergilloma; and (3) allergic bronchopulmonary aspergillosis. Aggressive antifungal therapy is essential for invasive disease (Table 1) (2).

Surgical resection is the most frequently recommended therapy for pulmonary aspergillomas but is associated with some morbidity and mortality. Other treatments have included radiation, intracavitary or endobronchial instillation of antifungal agents, inhaled nebulized antifungals, and systemic antifungals.

Corticosteroids represent the primary therapy for allergic bronchopulmonary aspergillosis although well designed clinical trials have not been conducted. Another treatment modality and adjunct with corticosteroids is oral itraconazole. Sixteen weeks of this combination therapy is effective in ameliorating disease, reducing the steroid dose required for maintenance therapy, lowering the serum concentration of IgE, and improving pulmonary function.

TABLE 1   Therapy of Invasive Aspergillosis

Systemic and CNS infections	Voriconazole	IV: 14 mg/kg/day div. q 12 hrs PO: 2–12 yrs: 400 mg/day div. b.i.d. switch when stable Total course minimum 6 wks

	With or without:
	  Caspofungin
	Alternative:
	  Amphotericin B lipid complex
	  or liposomal amphotericin B
		70 mg/m^2 on day 1, then 50 mg/m^2/day q 24 hrs
		5–10 mg/kg IV daily as 3–4 hr infusion
		
		Total course minimum 6 wks

For less severe infections	Itraconazole or Amphotericin B	5–10 mg/kg/day IV or PO div. q 12 hrs 0.25–0.5 mg/kg initially, increase as tolerated to 1.0–1.5 mg/kg/day; infuse as a single dose over 2 hrs

TABLE 2 Therapy for Blastomycosis

Systemic infections	Itraconazole	2.5–5 mg/kg/day IV q 24 hr, or 5–10 mg/kg/day PO q 24 hr
For severe disease	Amphotericin B lipid complex or liposomal amphotericin B	5–10 mg/kg IV daily as 3–4 hr infusion Total course minimum 6 mos
	Alternative: Fluconazole	12 mg/kg/day, single dose
CNS infections	Amphotericin B	0.25–0.5 mg/kg initially, increase as tolerated to 0.5–1.5 mg/kg; infuse as a single dose over 2 hr
For mild to moderate disease	Fluconazole or	3–6 mg/kg/day, single dose
	Itraconazole	5–10 mg/kg/day div. q 12 hr

BLASTOMYCOSIS

Blastomyces dermatitidis is an endemic mycosis in the southeastern and south central states that border the Mississippi and Ohio Rivers, the Midwestern states and Canadian provinces bordering the Great Lakes and portions of New York and Canada adjacent to the St. Lawrence River. Infection results from inhalation of conidia (spores). Some infection is asymptomatic or produces mild self-limited pneumonia but the majority of patients with acute and chronic pulmonary or disseminated disease require antifungal therapy (Table 2) (3). The most frequent presentation is an indolent chronic pneumonia. The skin, bones, and genitourinary system are the most common extrapulmonary sites. Diagnosis requires culture but identification of organisms in clinical specimens is adequate to initiate therapy.

CANDIDIASIS

Candida sp. are by far the most common fungal pathogens. They produce a wide range of infections from thrush and mild diaper rashes to invasive processes involving almost any organ-system. *C. albicans* remains the most common specie causing infection but others have become increasingly frequent requiring that speciation and susceptibilities be obtained on isolates from severe infection. *C. albicans*, *C. tropicalis*, and *C. parapsilosis* are generally susceptible to all classes of antifungals while *C. glabrata* often requires higher dosages of fluconazole or itraconazole, and *C. krusei* is usually resistant to these antifungals as well as flucytosine. *C. lusitaniae* is often resistant to amphotericin B. Initial empiric therapy (Table 3) (4) may require modification based on susceptibility determinations particularly for the latter 3 species.

CHROMOMYCOSIS

Chromomycosis, also referred to as chromoblastomycosis, is caused most frequently by the organism, *Fonsecaea pedrosoi*. Organisms produce unique darkly pigmented flecks within cutaneous lesions. Infection may progress to inflammatory plaques, nodules, and larger masses. Surgical excision is the most effective treatment. If this cannot be accomplished, medical management can be tried (Table 4) but is frequently unsuccessful.

COCCIDIOIDOMYCOSIS

Coccidioidomycosis is endemic in the southwestern U.S. region's San Joaquin Valley. It includes southern Arizona, central California, southern New Mexico, and west Texas. Disease results from the inhalation of arthroconidia (spores) and is usually manifest in the normal host as a self limited localized acute pneumonia. No specific antifungal therapy is necessary unless

TABLE 3   Therapy for Candidiasis

Systemic infections		
Disseminated infection	Amphotericin B	0.5–0.75 mg/kg/day IV q 24 hr
	or	
	Amphotericin B lipid complex	3–5 mg/kg/day IV q 24 hr
	or	
	Fluconazole	6–12 mg/kg IV or PO daily for 2–4 wk
Urinary tract infection	Fluconazole	3–6 mg/kg once daily IV or PO for 7 days
Oropharyngeal, esophageal	Clotrimazole	10 mg troche PO 5 times daily for 7 days
	or	
	Fluconazole	3–6 mg/kg once daily PO for 5 days
	or	
	Itraconazole soln	PO 5 mg/kg/day q 24 hr swished in mouth and swallowed for 5 days
CNS infections	Amphotericin B	0.25–0.5 mg/kg initially, increase as tolerated to 0.5–1.5 mg/kg; infuse as a single dose over 2 hr
	plus	
	Flucytosine	100–150 mg/kg/day PO div. q 6 hr. Maximum 150 mg/kg q24h—adjust for serum levels of 40–60 mcg/mL. Duration: 30 days minimum, guided by enhanced CT or MRI

the pulmonary infection is severe, there is extensive spread of infection, or patients are at high risk for complications because of pregnancy, genetic factors or immunosuppression. Most experts also recommend therapy if the pneumonia becomes chronic. Disseminated disease is most frequently seen in the skin, bones, and central nervous system. Long duration of treatment, weeks to months, is required (Table 5) (5). particularly for immunosuppressed patients, and is best guided by periodic reassessment. Some patients will also benefit from surgical debridement.

CRYPTOCOCCOSIS

Cryptococcus neoformans is ubiquitous, causing a marked increased incidence of disease directly related to the AIDS epidemic and a much larger population of immunosuppressed patients. Pulmonary infection varies from asymptomatic nodular disease that may not require antifungal therapy, to fatal acute respiratory distress syndrome (ARDS) (6). This organism has a particular predilection for causing infection in the CNS (Table 6).

FUSARIUM

Human infections are most frequently caused by 3 species of *Fusarium*: *solani*, *oxysporum* and *moniliforme*.

Keratitis in contact lens wearers is a common manifestation because these organisms readily adhere to plastic type materials. Topical therapy with natamycin or silver sulfadiazine

TABLE 4   Therapy for Chromomycosis

Systemic infections	Itraconazole oral solution	5 mg/kg/day PO q 24 hr for 12 mo
	Alternative:	
	Terbinafine PO	<20 kg: 67.5 mg/day 20–40 kg: 125 mg/day >40 kg: 250 mg/kg/day

TABLE 5   Therapy for Coccidoidomycosis

Systemic infections	Amphotericin B or	1 mg/kg/day IV q 24 hr
	Liposomal amphotericin B or Amphotericin B lipid complex or	5 mg/kg/day IV q 24 hr
	Fluconazole or	6–12 mg/kg IV PO q 24 hr
	Itraconazole soln (osteomyelitis)	5–10 mg/kg/day q 24 hr
CNS infections	Fluconazole	12 mg/kg/day IV div q 24 hr × 30 days

is usually curative but if therapy is delayed, endophthalmitis could occur producing permanent vision loss.

Another common infection caused by *Fusarium* sp. is peritonitis in chronic ambulatory peritoneal dialysis (CAPD) patients. They respond to removal of the catheter alone or catheter removal and a short course of amphotericin B.

The most serious infection with this fungus is disseminated disease in the immunocompromised host, seen most commonly in cancer patients undergoing aggressive chemotherapy or bone marrow transplantation. Neutropenia is the major associated factor. Infection likely begins with inhalation of spores but may follow trauma or contamination of IV catheters.

Fusarium is resistant to older azoles. Amphotericin B has some in-vitro activity and voriconazole appears to be quite promising both in-vitro and in limited clinical experience (Table 7).

HISTOPLASMOSIS

Histoplasma capsulatum is endemic within the Ohio and Mississippi River valleys, producing disease following inhalation exposure. Severity of disease varies dependent on the quantity of organisms inhaled and the immune status of the host. Mild self-limited pulmonary disease, lung calcifications on chest x-rays, and evidence of prior infection in the liver and spleen as an incidental finding during abdominal surgery are common. Most immunocompetent patients

TABLE 6   Therapy for Cryptococcosis

Systemic infections	Fluconazole or	10–12 mg/kg/day IV, PO q 24 hr for 6–12 wk
	Amphotericin B or	1 mg/kg/day q 24 hr
	Liposomal amphotericin B or Amphotericin B lipid complex	3–5 mg/kg/day q 24 hr
CNS infections	Amphotericin B plus	0.5–0.7 mg/kg/day IV div q 24 hr
	Flucytosine	100 mg/kg/day PO div. q 6 hr Duration: 6 wk
	Followed by: Fluconazole	100 mg/kg/day IV/PO div. q 24 hr Duration: 10 wk

TABLE 7 Therapy for Fusarium

Systemic infections	Voriconazole	IV: 6–8 mg/kg q 12 hrs for 1 day then 7 mg/kg q 12 hrs PO: 8 mg/kg q 12 hrs for 1 day, then 7 mg/kg q 12 hrs
	Alternative: Amphotericin B	1–1.5 mg/kg/day

with histoplasmosis recover without specific therapy. Progressive pulmonary infections is likely to occur in patients with underlying pulmonary disease, those who are immunosuppressed or have primary or acquired immunodeficiency (Table 8) (7).

MALASSEZIA

Malassesiafurfur is best known for causing the skin infection, pityriasis versicolor. It is also an occasional pathogen in folliculitis and seborrheic dermatitis, and may cause secondary infection in children with atopic dermatitis. Of particular note is that this organism has caused outbreaks of fungemia in premature neonates and immunocompromised patients who were receiving intravenous intralipids. This is in part a consequence of the lipophilic nature of *Malassezia* (Table 9).

MUCORMYCOSIS

Also called zygomycosis, infection by organisms in the family, *Mucoraceae* (Fig. 1), are rare but can be life threatening and are quite difficult to treat (Table 10). There are 5 clinical forms, in order of frequency: rhinocerebral, pulmonary, gastrointestinal, cutaneous, and disseminated. The unique virulence factor of mucormycosis is vascular invasion which produces thrombosis, infarction, and extensive tissue necrosis. Characteristic predisposing conditions are insulin dependent diabetes mellitus, leukemia, severe malnutrition, and chronic renal failure. Correction of ketoacidosis in diabetic patients is critical for successful management. The presence of black necrotic lesions of the soft palate, hard palate or nasal mucosa in predisposed patients who are febrile and toxic constitute a consistent presentation (Fig. 2).

PARACOCCIDIOIDOMYCOSIS

Formerly called South American blastomycosis because it is only seen in countries of South America, this fungal infection presents as a chronic disease of the lungs, skin, mucous membranes, adrenal glands, and reticuloendothelial system. The etiologic agent,

TABLE 8 Therapy for Histoplasmosis

Systemic infections	Amphotericin B or	1 mg/kg/day q 24 hr
	Liposomal amphotericin B or Amphotericin B lipid complex or	3–5 mg/kg/day q 24 hr
	Fluconazole	5 mg/kg/day PO soln q 24 hr for 6–12 wk
CNS infections	Amphotericin B	0.25–0.5 mg/kg initially, increase as tolerated to 0.5–1.5 mg/kg; infuse as a single dose over 2 hr for 2–3 wk
	Followed by: Fluconazole	12 mg/kg/day PO div. q 24 hr × 6 mo

TABLE 9   Therapy for Malassezia

Systemic infections	Ketoconazole or	400 mg PO qd for 3 days
	Fluconazole	IV 3–6 mg/kg/day single dose
		PO 6 mg/kg once then 3 mg/kg per day

Paracoccidioides brasiliensis, likely causes infection following inhalation; however the natural history has not been well defined. Etiologic diagnosis can be made from histologic examination of tissue with special fungal stains (Grocott silver methenamine) or by culture of biopsy specimens. Measurement of antibodies in serum by many different methodologies is also available. Sulfa drugs are effective for mild disease but combination antifungal therapy is preferred for disseminated cases (Table 11).

PHAEOHYPHOMYCOSIS

This rare infection refers to disease caused by a number of fungi that have in common the production of dark pigment. Severe disease is only seen in immunosuppressed patients. Combined medical and surgical treatment is necessary for most severe infections (Table 12).

PNEUMOCYSTIS JIROVECI

Now classified as a fungus, *P. jiroveci,* causes an afebrile but occasionally febrile pneumonia in children with AIDS or those immunocompromised for other reasons. It has been the most common organism causing serious infection in children with congenital or perinatally acquired HIV infection. More than 85% of otherwise healthy children have antibody to this organism by 20 months of age suggesting that exposure is quite common and that infection is generally asymptomatic unless the child is immunosuppressed.

Disease tends to be subacute in its onset and progression. Patients present with dyspnea, tachypnea and may even be cyanotic. Auscultation of the lungs is often unimpressive. Etiologic diagnosis is made by identifying organisms in bronchoalveolar lavage fluid or lung biopsy.

Treatment (Table 13) is quite effective when offered early in the course of disease and disease is now much less common because of routine prophylactic antibiotics given to all HIV maternally exposed children during early infancy and to those who show evidence of viral infection associated with significant immunosuppression (Chapter 16).

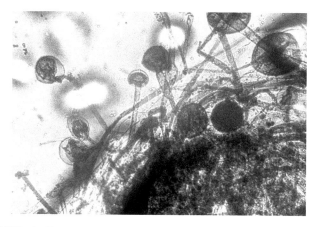

FIGURE 1 Tissue biopsy of the soft palate showing non-septate, irregularly branching hyphal forms of *Rhizopus oryzae.*

TABLE 10   Therapy for Mucormycosis

Systemic infections	Liposomal amphotericin B or Amphotericin B lipid complex	Up to 10 mg/kg/day q 24 hrs for 12 wks or longer
CNS infections	Surgical debridement Amphotericin B	Amphotericin B 1.5 g/kg/day IV div q 24 hrs until completing a total dose of 50 mg/kg
	Topical Amphotericin B Hyperbaric oxygen	

PSEUDALLESCHERIA BOYDII

This ubiquitous fungus causes mycetomas, trauma-related osteomyelitis, and near-drowning pneumonia in immunocompetent persons. *P. boydii* is the most common organism causing pulmonary infection in patients following prolonged submerging in contaminated water. Infections with this organism are increasingly recognized in immunocompromised hosts and include endocarditis, endophthalmitis, pulmonary abscesses, and CNS and disseminated disease. *P. boydii* is sensitive to imidazoles (Table 14) but generally resistant to amphotericin B.

SPOROTRICHOSIS

Sporothrix schenckii generally produces localized infection of the skin and skin structure tissues that is responsive to oral antifungal agents. Intraconazole, the preferred therapy must be given for 3 to 6 months for cutaneous or lymphocutaneous disease and at least 12 months for osteoarticular involvement. Lung infection responds poorly to antifungal agents. Severe infection should be treated with IV amphotericin B while mild to moderate infection can be treated orally with itraconazole (Table 15) (8).

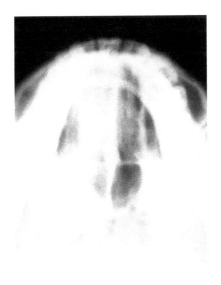

FIGURE 2   Maxillary sinusitis with bone destruction and extension into the central nervous system in an insulin-dependent diabetic, characteristic of mucormycosis.

TABLE 11   Therapy for Paracoccidioidomycosis

Systemic infections	Amphotericin B	0.25–0.5 mg/kg initially, increase as tolerated to 0.5–1.5 mg/kg; infuse as a single dose over 2 hrs for 2–3 wks
	plus	5 mg/kg/day PO q 24 hrs
	Itraconazole	Minimum treatment 6 mos
	or	
	Ketoconazole	PO 5 mg/kg/day, q 24 hrs
	or	
	Bactrim	TMP 8–10 mg/kg daily for minimum 3 yrs

TABLE 12   Therapy for Phaeohyphomycosis

Systemic infections	Surgery	
	plus	
	Amphotericin B	1.5 mg/kg/day; duration determined by clinical course

TABLE 13   Therapy for *Pneumocystis jiroveci*

Systemic infections	Bactrim	TMP: 15–20 mg/kg/day
		SMX: 75–100 mg/kg/day PO or IV in 3 doses for 14 days
	Alternative:	
	Pentamidine	3–4 mg/kg IV daily for 14 days
	or	1–3 mos: 30 mg/kg/day
	Atovaquone	4–24 mos: 45 mg/kg/day
		>24 mos: 30 mg/day

TABLE 14   Therapy for *Pseudallescheria boydii*

Systemic infections	Voriconazole	14 mg/kg/day IV div. q 12 hrs
	or	
	Itraconazole	IV or PO 5–10 mg/kg/day div. q 12 hrs
CNS infections	Voriconazole	6–8 mg/kg IV q 12 hrs on day one, then 7 mg/kg IV q 12 hr

TABLE 15   Therapy for Sporotrichosis

Systemic infections		
Mild to moderate	Itraconazole	5 mg/kg/day PO soln q 24 hrs for 3–6 mos
Severe	Amphotericin B	0.25–0.5 mg/kg initially, increase as tolerated to 1.0–1.5 mg/kg/day; infuse as a single dose over 2 hrs

REFERENCES

1. Sobel JD, Mycoses Study Group. Practice guidelines for the treatment of fungal infections. Clin Infect Dis 2000; 30:652–718.
2. Stevens DA, Kan VL, Judson MA, et al. Practice guidelines for diseases caused by *Aspergillus*. Clin Infect Dis 2000; 30:696–709.
3. Chapman SW, Bradsher RW, Campbell GD, et al. Practice guidelines for the management of patients with blastomycosis. Clin Infect Dis 2000; 30:679–83.
4. Rex JH, Walsh TJ, Sobel JD, et al. Practice guidelines for the treatment of candidiasis. Clin Infect Dis 2000; 30:662–78.
5. Galgiani JN, Ampel NM, Catanzaro A, et al. Practice guidelines for the treatment of coccidioidomycosis. Clin Infect Dis 2000; 30:658–61.
6. Saag MS, Graybill RJ, Larsen RA, et al. Practice guidelines for the management of cryptococcal disease. Clin Infect Dis 2000; 30:710–8.
7. Wheat J, Sarosi G, McKinsey D, et al. Practice guidelines for the management of patients with histoplasmosis. Clin Infect Dis 2000; 30:688–95.
8. Kauffman CA, Hajjeh R, Chapman SW. Practice guidelines for the management of patients with sporotrichosis. Clin Infect Dis 2000; 30:684–7.

19 | Infection Control

INFECTIONS IN PEDIATRIC HOSPITAL PERSONNEL

The hospital provides an environment that contains unique, antibiotic resistant micro-organisms and susceptible, immunosuppressed individuals. In such a setting, hospital personnel are exposed to multiple agents and many patients, and may serve as vectors for disease transmission. The infections for which pediatric hospital personnel are at particular risk are given in Table 1.

MECHANISMS OF DISEASE TRANSMISSION

Hospital infections are transmitted by airborne dissemination, exposure to a contaminated common vehicle, and person-to-person contact. Because the pediatric patient is usually an ineffective aerosolizer, hands of hospital personnel become the primary vehicle for carrying microorganisms from one patient to another.

CONTROL MEASURES

Prevention of infection acquired during hospitalization is a goal of all physicians. A firm understanding of the mechanisms of disease transmission is foremost in infection control (Table 2).

ISOLATION POLICIES

Isolation policies must be modified to meet the needs of individual hospitals. For the purposes of this book, representative diseases, as outlined in the Centers for Disease Control manual *Guidelines for Prevention and Control of Nosocomial Infections*, have been selected to illustrate disease-specific isolation techniques.

All infection control groups now recommend standard—blood and body fluid—precautions (Table 3) since medical history and examination cannot identify all patients

TABLE 1   Infections for Which Pediatric Personnel Are at Special Risk

Bacteria	Viruses	Parasites
Meningococcus	Cytomegalovirus	Pediculosis
Pertussis	Enteroviruses (e.g. hand-foot-mouth disease)	Scabies
Staphylococcus (methicillin-resistant MRSA)	Hepatitis A, B and C	Tinea capitis and corporis
Tuberculosis	HIV	
	Influenza A and B	
	Parvovirus B19	
	Rotavirus	
	Rubella	
	Varicella-zoster	

TABLE 2   Control Measures to Prevent Hospital-Acquired Infection

Hand hygiene
Recognition of infectious processes
Appropriate treatment of infection
Proper handling of patient and body secretions
Isolation

TABLE 3   Standard Infection Control Precautions

Hand hygiene: after touching blood, body fluids, secretions, excretions, and contaminated items. Hands should be washed immediately after removing gloves, between patient contacts, and when otherwise indicated to avoid transfer of microorganisms to other patients or environments

Gloves: worn when touching blood, body fluids, secretions, excretions, and items contaminated with these fluids. Clean gloves should be used before touching mucous membranes and non-intact skin. Gloves should be promptly removed after use, before touching noncontaminated items and environmental surfaces, and before going to another patient

Masks, eye protection, and face shields: should be worn to protect mucous membranes of the eyes, nose, and mouth during procedures and patient care activities to generate splashes or sprays of blood, body fluids, secretions, or excretions

Nonsterile gowns: will protect skin and prevent the soiling of clothing during procedures and patient care activities likely to generate splashes or sprays of blood, body fluids, secretions, or excretions. Soiled gowns should be promptly removed.

Patient care equipment: that has been used should be handled in a manner that prevents skin and mucous membrane exposures and contamination of clothing.

Linen: soiled with blood and body fluids, secretions, and excretions should be handled, transported, and processed in a manner that prevents skin and mucous membrane exposure and contamination of clothing

Blood-borne pathogen exposure: should be avoided by taking all precautions to prevent injuries when using, cleaning, and disposing of needles, scalpels, and other sharp instruments and devices

Mouthpieces, resuscitation bags, and other ventilation devices: should be readily available in all patient care areas and used instead of mouth-to-mouth resuscitation

TABLE 4   Infection Control Categories for Hospitalized Children

Category of precautions	Hand washing before and after contact	Negative pressure room	Private room	Masks	Gowns	Gloves
Standard	Yes	No	No	During procedures	During procedures	When touching blood and body fluids
Airborne	Yes	Yes	Yes	At all times	No	No
Droplet	Yes	No	Yes	If within 3 feet of patient	No	No
Contact	Yes	No	Yes	No	At all times	At all times

TABLE 5 Disease-Specific Isolation Precautions

Agent	Category	Duration of precautions
Adenovirus	Both droplet and contact	Duration of illness
Abscess, etiology unknown		
(Major draining)	Contact	Duration of illness
Comments: Major—no dressing or dressing does not adequately contain the pus		
(Minor or limited draining)	Contact	Duration of illness
Comments: Minor or limited—dressing covers and adequately contains pus, or infected area is small (e.g., stitch abscess).		
Bronchiolitis, usual etiology respiratory syncytial virus	Contact	Duration of illness
Comments: Various etiologic agents (e.g., respiratory syncytial virus, parainfluenza viruses, adenoviruses, influenza viruses) have been associated with this syndrome.		
Bronchitis, infective etiology unknown		
Infants and young children	Contact	Duration of illness
Other	Standard	Duration of illness
Chickenpox (varicella)	Both airborne and contact	Minimum 5 days after onset of rash in the normal host; in immunocompromised patients, as long as the rash is vesicular
Comments: Persons who are not susceptible need not wear a mask. Susceptible persons should, if possible, stay out of room. Special ventilation for the room, if available, may be advantageous, especially for outbreak control. Neonates of mothers with active varicella should be placed in isolation precautions at birth. Exposed susceptible patients should be placed in isolation precautions beginning 10 days after exposure and continuing until 21 days after last exposure. (See *CDC Guideline for Infection Control in Hospital Personnel* for recommendations for exposed susceptible personnel.)		
Common cold		
Infants and young children	Contact	Duration of illness
Comments: Although rhinoviruses are most frequently associated with the common cold, which is mild in adults, severe infections may occur in infants and young children. Other etiologic agents (e.g. respiratory syncytial viruses) may also cause this syndrome.		
Croup	Contact	Duration of illness
Comments: Viral agents (e.g. parainfluenza A virus) have been associated with this syndrome.		
Cytomegalovirus	Standard	Hospital stay
Comments: Pregnant personnel may need special counseling. (See *CDC Guideline for Infection Control in Hospital Personnel.*)		
Diphtheria	Droplet	Until 2 cultures are negative
Enterovirus	Contact	Duration of hospitalization
Epiglottitis	Droplet	24 hrs after start of effective therapy
Gastroenteritis		
Campylobacter sp.; *Clostridium difficile*; *Escherichia coli* (enteropathogenic, enterotoxic, or enteroinvasive); *Giardia lamblia*; *Salmonella* sp; *Vibrio parahaemolyticus*; viral; *Yersinia enterocolitica*; unknown etiology	Contact for diapered or incontinent children	Duration of illness
Rotavirus	Contact	Duration of illness
Shigella sp.	Contact in diapered or incontinent children	Duration of illness
Haemophilus influenzae	Droplet	24 hrs after start of effective therapy

(Continued)

TABLE 5   Disease-Specific Isolation Precautions *(Continued)*

Agent	Category	Duration of precautions
Hepatitis A	Contact for diapered or incontinent children	Duration of illness
Herpes simplex	Contact for primary neonatal disease	Duration of illness
Influenza	Droplet	Duration of illness
Lice	Contact	24 hrs after effective therapy
Measles	Airborne	Duration of illness
Meningitis		
Aseptic nonbacterial or viral meningitis (also see specific etiologies)	Contact	Duration of hospitalization

Comments: Enteroviruses are the most common cause of aseptic meningitis.

Agent	Category	Duration of precautions
Bacterial, gram-negative enteric in neonates	Standard	Duration of hospitalization

Comments: During a nursery outbreak, cohort ill and colonized infants, and use gowns if soiling likely and gloves when touching feces.

Agent	Category	Duration of precautions
Haemophilus influenzae	Droplet	24 hrs after start of effective therapy
Meningococcus	Droplet	24 hrs after start of effective therapy
Meningococcemia	Droplet	24 hrs after start of effective therapy

Comments: See Chapter 5 for recommendation for prophylaxis after exposure.

Agent	Category	Duration of precautions
Metapneumovirus	Contact	Single room or cohort with MPV-infected patients
Mumps	Droplet	9 days after onset of disease
Mycoplasma pneumoniae	Droplet	Duration of illness
Parainfluenza	Contact	Duration of illness
Parvovirus B 19	Droplet	7 days after onset of disease
Pertussis	Droplet	5 days after start of effective therapy
Respiratory syncytial virus	Contact	Duration of illness
Rubella	Droplet	7 days after onset of rash
Scabies	Contact	24 hrs after effective therapy
Staphylococcal disease	Contact	Duration of illness
Streptococcal disease	Contact	24 hrs after start of effective therapy
Tuberculosis, only pulmonary with cavitation	Airborne	Individually based
Zoster (in immunocompromised host)	Both airborne and contact	Duration of illness

Comments: See Chapter 5 for recommendations for prophylaxis after exposure.

infected with HIV. These precautions are especially relevant to blood and blood-containing fluids.

General isolation categories are summarized in Table 4 and disease-specific recommendations are listed in Table 5. Many hospitals use color-coded cards that list requirements for each category and post these on doors of patient rooms. Standard precaution cards are unnecessary since they apply to all patients.

20 | Antimicrobial Therapy

EMPIRIC THERAPY

Initial selection of antimicrobial agents is usually made before definitive cultures and sensitivities are available. The physician must, therefore, first have an understanding of the pathogens that commonly cause the specific infectious process under consideration. Other chapters in this book discuss in greater detail anticipated etiologic agents. This understanding must then be translated into initial empiric therapy (Tables 1 and 2). With the increasing number of new pharmaceutical products entering the market; there are now many alternatives for this selection.

It is, of course, essential to first obtain all necessary Gram stain and culture specimens before beginning treatment. In many cases, Gram stains of body fluids (buffy coat, joint aspiration, cerebrospinal fluid (CSF), urine, pleural effusion, etc.) will guide selection of antimicrobial agents (Table 3).

ADVERSE EVENTS

An appreciation of untoward side-effects is as important as a knowledge of the therapeutic potential of antibiotics. Many antibiotics are of equal efficacy. Therefore, selection is often determined on the basis of relative toxicity (Tables 3 and 4). Third-generation cephalosporins (ceftriaxone, cefotaxime, etc.) are desirable because they circumvent the potential toxicity of aminoglycosides when treating gram-negative coliform infection. Similarly, oxacillin is preferred over nafcillin, because phlebitis is relatively less common. Oxacillin should be used in neonates because nafcillin serum and tissue levels are erratic in this age group. Tetracyclines should be avoided in children less than 8 years of age, as this drug can be deposited in teeth and bones.

There is a narrow margin between therapeutic and toxic levels of chloramphenicol and aminoglycosides. Therefore, monitoring of peak and trough levels is essential for individual dosage adjustment. For most other antibiotics, toxic levels far exceed usual therapeutic ranges.

HOST FACTORS RELATED TO ANTIBIOTIC SELECTION

The Compromised Host

Selection of antibiotics for the compromised host, particularly the granulocytopenic patient, requires three major alterations in prescribing practices. Firstly, two agents rather than one

---

TABLE 1 Initial Empiric Therapy for Serious Neonatal Infections (Birth to Two Months)

Disease	Antibiotics
Sepsis or meningitis (Chapter 1)	Ampicillin plus gentamicin, cefotaxime, or ceftriaxone
Necrotizing enterocolitis (Chapter 14)	Clindamycin or metronidazole plus ampicillin plus cefotaxime, ceftriaxone, gentamicin, or amikacin
Osteomyelitis (Chapter 10)	Clindamycin or vancomycin
Peritonitis (Chapter 14)	Ampicillin, plus clindamycin, plus cefotaxime, ceftriaxone, or gentamicin
Pneumonia	Vancomycin or clindamycin plus cefotaxime, ceftriaxone, or gentamicin
Septic arthritis (Chapter 10)	Clindamycin or vancomycin plus ceftriaxone
Urinary tract infections (Chapter 11)	Ceftriaxone, cefotaxime, or gentamicin

TABLE 2   Initial Empiric Therapy for Infants and Children (>2 Months)

Disease	Antibiotics
Sepsis or meningitis (Chapter 2)	Ceftriaxone or cefotaxime plus vancomycin (add clindamycin if Group A streptococcus is considered)
Cellulitis (Chapter 3)	
Facial, orbital, preseptal	Ceftriaxone or cefotaxime
Facial (following trauma)	Clindamycin or vancomycin
Trunk or extremities	Ceftriaxone or cefotaxime
Osteomyelitis (Chapter 10)	Nafcillin or oxacillin
Foot (following trauma)	Ticarcillin plus gentamicin plus clindamycin or vancomycin
Otitis media (Chapter 3)	Cephalosporin or macrolide
Pneumonia (Chapter 8)	
<5 years	Ceftriaxone
>5 years	Macrolide
Severe or with empyema	Vancomycin plus ceftriaxone, cefotaxime, or cefuroxime
Septic arthritis (Chapter 10)	Clindamycin or vancomycin
Shunt infections (ventriculoperitoneal) (Chapter 13)	Vancomycin plus ceftriaxone or cefotaxime
Sinusitis (Chapter 8)	Cephalosporin or macrolide
Urinary tract infections (Chapter 12)	
Cystitis	Amoxicillin, TMP/SMX,[a] sulfisoxazole, or cephalosporins
Pyelonephritis	Third-generation. Cephalosporin or gentamicin; add ampicillin for adolescents

[a] TMP/SMX, trimethoprim/sulfamethoxazole.

should be given and these should be chosen for their potential synergism against the presumed or identified pathogen (Table 5). Secondly, maximum dosages and duration of therapy should be employed. Finally, where alternatives are available, bactericidal rather than bacteriostatic agents should be given (Table 6). This is necessary because bacteriostatic agents primarily inhibit bacterial growth while relying on host factors for complete killing of the organisms. Following therapy with these agents in the compromised host, relapse is frequent. Bactericidal agents are much more effective in totally eliminating pathogens in the absence of adequate mechanisms of host defense.

Renal Failure

In patients with abnormal renal function, dosages of many antibiotics must be altered relative to the degree of renal impairment. In some circumstances an antibiotic can be chosen that is excreted by extrarenal mechanisms—avoiding potential increased toxicity (Table 7).

However, most antibiotics require some adjustment calculated on the basis of creatinine clearance (Table 8A) and its percentage of normal (Table 8B); if such a selection is made, it becomes more important to monitor drug serum levels when this can be done.

TABLE 3   Relative Frequency of Allergic Reactions to Commonly Used Antibiotics

Highest frequency	Tetracyclines
	Sulfonamides
	Penicillins
	Cephalosporins
	Aminoglycosides
	Quinolones
	Chloramphenicol
Lowest frequency	Oxazolidinones (linezolid)
	Erythromycin

TABLE 4   Important Adverse Reactions Associated with Antibiotics

Antibiotic	Reaction
All antibiotics	Gastrointestinal symptoms most common
	Overgrowth of resistant bacteria and fungi (*Candida albicans*)
	Hypersensitivity skin rashes
	Serum sickness
	Anaphylaxis
	Bone marrow toxicity
	Nephrotoxicity
	Pseudomembranous colitis
	Drug fever
Aminoglycosides	Nephrotoxicity (reversible)
	Ototoxicity (permanent)
Cephalosporins	Nephrotoxicity
	Direct Coomb's reaction (probably of no clinical significance)
Cefaclor	Phlebitis and phlebothrombosis
	Serum sickness-like reaction
Cefamandole	Antabuse (disulfiram) effect
Chloramphenicol	Aplastic anemia
	Circulatory collapse (gray syndrome)
	Hypoplastic bone marrow
Erythromycin	Nausea
	Abdominal pain
	Cholestatic hepatitis
Linezolid	Phlebitis
	Thrombocytopenia, anemia and neutropenia
Penicillins	
Ampicillin	Diarrhea
Ticarcillin, piperacillin	Platelet dysfunction
Quinolones	Unlikely to produce changes in developing cartilage in children (only seen in animals)
Rifampin	Gastrointestinal distress
	Thrombocytopenia
Sulfonamides	Stevens-Johnson syndrome
Tetracycline	Decreased bone growth and staining of teeth in children under 8 years of age, but only if multiple courses given
	Photosensitivity
	Abdominal pain
	Diarrhea
	Pseudotumor cerebri
	Angioedema
	Brown tongue
	Glossitis
	Anal pruritis
Minocycline	Fanconi's syndrome
	Vestibular toxicity
	Hypersensitivity skin rashes
Trimethoprim/sulfamethoxazole	Stevens-Johnson syndrome

After estimating creatinine clearance for patients with renal impairment and determining the percent of CrCl compared to normal values as given in Table 8B, adjustments in antibiotic dosing can be determined using Table 9.

There are two basic approaches to dosage modification: (i) increasing the dosing interval or (ii) decreasing the individual dosage. For severe infections, particularly with bacteremia, many experts recommend the latter approach, which best assures longer intervals with high serum levels of antibiotic. This approach, however, is more likely to result in higher trough levels, which may increase the risk of nephrotoxicity for aminoglycosides. For most other

TABLE 5   Antibiotic Synergism for the Immunocompromised Patient

Pathogens	Synergistic Combinations		
Pseudomonas aeruginosa	Aminoglycoside	plus	a broad-spectrum penicillin, a broad-spectrum cephalosporin, or a carbapenem
Staphylococcus aureus	Gentamicin	plus	nafcillin/oxacillin/vancomycin
Enterococci	Gentamicin	plus	ampicillin, penicillin, or vancomycin
Klebsiella pneumoniae	Aminoglycoside	plus	cephalosporin
Coliforms (*Escherichia coli, Enterobacter proteus*, and *Providencia*)	Gentamicin	plus	ampicillin, broad-spectrum penicillins, or cephalosporins
Mycobacterium tuberculosis	Isoniazid	plus	rifampin

TABLE 6   In Vitro Classification of Antibiotics

Bactericidal
  Aminoglycosides
  Carbapenems (imipenem, meropenem)
  Cephalosporins
  Monobactams (aztreonam)
  Penicillins
  Quinolones
  Vancomycin
Bacteriostatic
  Chloramphenicol
  Clindamycin
  Erythromycin
  Tetracyclines
Both Oxazolidinones (linezolid)

TABLE 7   Antimicrobial Agents Not Requiring Dosage or Dosing Interval Adjustments for Renal Impairment

Antibacterials

Azithromycin	Moxifloxacin
Ceftriaxone	Nafcillin
Clindamycin	Oxacillin
Doxycycline	Pyrimethamine
Linezolid	Rifabutin
Minocycline	Rifaximin

Antifungals

Caspofungin p.o. voriconazole
  (not i.v.)
Itraconazole

infections, it is more prudent to increase the dosing interval and obtain peak and trough levels to further guide therapy.

Hepatic Failure

For patients with severe hepatic disease, antibiotics that are metabolized by the liver, or excreted through the biliary tract, should be avoided (Table 10). Adequate guidelines for dosage modification are simply not available. The only approach, which might assure safe administration, is frequent measurement of serum drug levels.

Penicillin Allergy and Desensitization

In patients with documented allergic reactions to penicillins, one of these classes of antibiotics may still have to be given for certain life-threatening infections. The most common clinical circumstance is streptococcal or staphylococcal endocarditis. For most other severe infections (meningitis, pneumonia, etc.) cephalosporins represent adequate alternatives.

Penicillin allergy skin testing may first be undertaken to confirm hypersensitivity in a patient with a questionable history. Such testing is time consuming and, with currently available reagents, yields a 5% false-negative and 80% false-positive reaction rate. Limitations of this testing are primarily attributable to the absence of a reliable minor determinant mixture (MDM). Major determinant, benzylpenicilloyl/polylysine (PPL), can be obtained through commercial sources (Pre-pen; Kremers-Urban, Milwaukee, Wisconsin, U.S.). Some studies

TABLE 8A   Estimated Creatinine Clearance (CrCl) for Renal Impairment

CrCl calculation (mL/min/1.73 m^2): Crcl = $k \times L$/Pcr, where k, proportionally constant; L, height (cm); Pcr, plasma creatinine (mg/dL)	
k-values	
LBW during first year of life	0.33
Term AGA during first year of life	0.45
Children and adolescent girls	0.55
Adolescent boys	0.70

have used a fresh solution of crystalline penicillin G as the source of MDM. If the antibiotic to be given is a derivative of penicillin, skin testing should include this derivative in addition to testing with PPL and penicillin G. With each product, scratch testing should be followed by intradermal injection (0.01–0.02 mL). For scratch testing, a drop of the test solution is placed on the forearm and a 3 to 5 mm scratch made at this site with a 20-gauge needle. For penicillin G or penicillin derivative testing, serial scratch tests followed by serial intradermal injections with solutions of 0.25, 2.5, and 25 mg/mL are recommended. Each test should be observed for 15 min before proceeding to the next. A positive reaction is a wheal greater than 5 mm. Normal saline and histamine (1 mg/mL) should be included as negative and positive controls.

When a penicillin must be given to an allergic patient, desensitization, beginning with oral administration, should be accomplished—this can be done with penicillin G or any derivative (Table 11). Desensitization should be undertaken in the hospital where careful monitoring and treatment for allergic reactions are available.

DOSAGES OF ANTIBIOTICS

Neonates

There are actually very few antibiotics commonly used for the treatment of neonatal infection. Pharmacokinetics, however, change rapidly during the first weeks of life and differ between prematurely born and full term neonates. Dosages and intervals of administration (Tables 12 and 13) must therefore be adjusted frequently during the course of treatment, and this requirement represents the most unique feature of therapy in the neonatal patient. Selection of

TABLE 8B   Normal Glomerular Filtration Rate (GFR) by Age

Age	GFR—mean (mL/min/1.73 m^2)
Neonates <34 weeks gestational age	
2–8 days	11
4–28 days	20
30–90 days	50
Neonates >34 weeks gestational age	
2–8 days	39
4–28 days	47
30–90 days	58
1–6 months	77
6–12 months	103
12–19 months	127
2–12 years	127

TABLE 9   Dosages of Antimicrobial Agents for Patients with Renal Impairment

Antibiotic	Adjustment for CrCl mL/min (% of normal)		
	50–90%	10–50%	10%
Aminoglycosides (except streptomycin)	75% (q 12 h)[a]	50% q 12 h	20% q 24 h
Streptomycin	50% q 24 h	50% q 48 h	50% q 72 h
Carbapenems			
Imipenem	75% q 8 h	50% q 8 h	25% q 12 h
Meropenem	100% q 8 h	75% q 12 h	25% q 24 h
Cephalosporins	100%	100%	100%
Cefazolin	q 8 h	q 12 h	q 24 h
Cefepime	q 12 h	q 16 h	q 24 h
Cefotaxime	q 8 h	q 12 h	q 24 h
Cefoxitin	q 8 h	q 12 h	q 24 h
Ceftazidime	q 12 h	q 24 h	q 48 h
Ceftriaxone	–	No adjustment	–
Cefuroxime	q 8 h	q 12 h	q 24 h
Fluconazole	100% q 24 h	100% q 24 h	100% q 48 h
Macrolides			
Azithromycin	–	No adjustment	–
Clarithromycin	100% q 12 h	75% q 12 h	50% q 12 h
Erythromycin	100% q 6 h	100% q 6 h	75% q 6 h
Metronidazole	100% q 6 h	100% q 6 h	50% q 6 h
Monobactams			
Aztreonam	100% q 8 h	50% q 8 h	25% q 8 h
Penicillins			
Amoxicillin	100% q 8 h	100% q 8 h	100% q 24 h
Ampicillin	100% q 6 h	100% q 6 h	100% q 12 h
Mezlocillin	100% q 6 h	100% q 6 h	100% q 8 h
Penicillin G	100% q 6 h	75% q 6 h	50% q 6 h
Piperacillin	100% q 6 h	100% q 6 h	100% q 8 h
Ticarcillin	50% q 6 h	50% q 8 h	50% q 12 h
Ticarcillin/clavulanate	100% q 6 h	75% q 6 h	75% q 12h
Tetracycline	100% q 8 h	100% q 12 h	100% q 24 h
TMP/SMX[b]	100% q 12 h	100% q 18 h	100% q 24 h
Vancomycin	50% q 12 h	25% q 24 h	25% q 48 h

[a] % of dosage for children with normal renal function (with dosing interval).
[b] TMP/SMX, trimethoprim/sulfamethoxazole.

an aminoglycoside in a particular institution is more predicated on resistance patterns of coliforms for that institution than on pharmacokinetic differences. It is always necessary to monitor peak and trough levels of aminoglycosides, so laboratory capabilities may influence choices among these agents.

Infants and Children

After 28 days of age, pharmacokinetic patterns are quite constant although different from adult patterns, which have a relatively smaller volume of distribution. This simply means that relatively higher amounts of antibiotics must be given to children to achieve the same serum concentrations. Dosages can be calculated according to weight for most children (Table 14), exceptions being those with excessive obesity or malnutrition (cystic fibrosis and cancer patients). In these cases, dosages should be calculated by body surface area (see Table 17). For children over 12 years of age or weighing more than 40 kg, maximum dosage limitations should be reviewed (see Table 16).

Monitoring of drug levels for aminoglycosides, vancomycin, and chloramphenicol should be undertaken for patients who will be on these antimicrobial agents for more than 48 h

TABLE 10 Antibiotics Requiring Dosage Adjustment in Patients with Hepatic Disease

Cefoperazone
Chloramphenicol
Clindamycin
Isoniazid
Macrolides
Nitrofurantoin
Rifampin
Tetracyclines

(after initial culture information is available). Other antibiotic concentrations may be indirectly measured by performing serum bactericidal assays with the recovered pathogen. These assays should be considered for any patient with serious infection who demonstrates a poor clinical response to apparently appropriate therapy.

For the three most common minor infections requiring antibiotic therapy, otitis media, streptococcal pharyngitis, and skin infections, a maximum dosage of 1 g of a penicillin, cephalosporin, or erythromycin is recommended. In the case of ampicillin, this maximum dosage is reached as early as 1 year of age or in children weighing 10 kg.

Dosage calculations need not be exact but should be calculated so that a convenient individual dose is prescribed (½ teaspoon, 1 teaspoon, etc.). Whenever possible q.d. or b.i.d. rather than t.i.d. or q.i.d. dosing intervals should be used as these are more realistic for patients' and parents' nighttime compliance. Oral antibiotic dosages for infants and children are given in Table 15.

Maximum (Adult) Dosages

For many antibiotics, maximum dosage limitations (Table 16) are reached by approximately 12 years of age (40–50 kg). In these older children, the volume of distribution is decreased, thereby increasing the possibility of overdosing with accompanying toxicity if calculations are made by body weight as with younger patients. Maximum dosages of oral antibiotics are reached even earlier in life, and amounts of antibiotic in tablets and capsules (commonly 250 and 500 mg) reflect this limitation.

(Text continues on page 269)

TABLE 11 Penicillin Desensitization

Time	Dose (mg)	Units	Route
0	0.05	100	p.o.
15 min	0.10	200	p.o.
30 min	0.25	400	p.o.
45 min	0.5	800	p.o.
1 h	1	1,600	p.o.
1 h 15 min	2	3,200	p.o.
1 h 30 min	4	6,400	p.o.
1 h 45 min	8	12,500	p.o.
2 h	15	25,000	p.o.
2 h 15 min	30	50,000	p.o.
2 h 30 min	60	100,000	p.o.
2 h 45 min	125	200,000	p.o.
3 h	250	400,000	p.o.
3 h 15 min	125	200,000	s.c.
3 h 30 min	250	400,000	s.c.
3 h 45 min	500	800,000	s.c.
4 h	625	1,000,000	i.m.
4 h 15 min	Begin full dose i.v.		

TABLE 12   Daily Dosages of Intravenous Antibiotics for Neonates with Serious Infections

Antibiotic	Gestational Age (weeks)	Dose (mg/kg/dose)	Interval (h) (Postnatal Age)
Acyclovir	>34	20	8
	<34	20	12
Amikacin	≤29	18	48 (0–7 days)
		15	36 (8–28 days
		15	24 (>29 days
	30 to 34	18	36 (0–7 days)
		15	24 (>8 days)
	≥35	15	24
	0–4 weeks	7.5	18–24
Amphotericin B	All	0.5–1	24
Amphotericin B liposome	All	5–7	24
Ampicillin	≤29	25 to 50	12 (0–28 days)
			12 (0–14 days)
	30 to 36		8 (>14 days)
			8 (>7 days)
	37 to 44		12 (0–7 days)
			8 (>7 days)
	>45	6	
		100 (meningitis)	
		(severe Group B strep)	
		(sepsis)	
Aztreonam	≤29	30	12 (0–28 days)
			8 (>28 days)
	30 to 36		12 (0–14 days)
			8 (>14 days)
	37 to 44		12 (0–7 days)
			8 (>7 days)
	≥45		6
Cefazolin	<29	25	12 (0–28 days)
			8 (>28 days)
	30 to 36		12 (0–14 days)
			8 (>14 days)
	37 to 44		12 (0–7 days)
			8 (>7 days)
	>45		6
Cefotaxime	≤29	50	12 (0–28 days)
			8 (>28 days)
	30 to 36		12 (0–14 days)
			8 (>14 days)
	37 to 44		12 (0–7 days)
			8 (>7 days)
	≥45		6
Ceftazidime	≤29	30	12 (0–28 days)
			8 (>28 days)
	30 to 36		12 (0–14 days)
			8 (>14 days)
	37 to 44		12 (0–7 days)
			8 (>7 days)
	≥45		8
Ceftriaxone	All	100 (loading)	
		80	24
Chloramphenicol	All	20 (loading)	
	<37	2.5 (<1 mo.)	6
		5.0 (>1 mo.)	

(Continued)

TABLE 12 Daily Dosages of Intravenous Antibiotics for Neonates with Serious Infections (*Continued*)

Antibiotic	Gestational Age (weeks)	Dose (mg/kg/dose)	Interval (h) (Postnatal Age)
	>37	5.0 (<7 days) 12.5 (>7 days)	6
Clindamycin	<29	5–7.5	12 (0–28 days) 8 (>28 days)
	30 to 36		12 (0–14 days) 8 (>14 days)
	37 to 44		8 (0–7 days) 6 (>7 days)
	>45		6
Erythromycin	All	5–10	6
Fluconazole	All	12 (loading)	
	≤29	6	72 (0–14 days) 48 (>14 days)
	30 to 36		48 (0–14 days) 24 (>14 days)
	37 to 44		48 (0–7 days) 24 (>7 days)
	≥45		24
Gentamicin	≤29	5 4 4	48 (0–7 days) 36 (8–28 days) 24 (>29 days)
	30 to 34	4.5 4	36 (0–7 days) 24 (≥8 days)
	≥35	4	24
Imipenem/cilastatin	All	20–25	12
Linezolid	All	10 10	8 12 (<7 days)
Meropenem	All	20 (sepsis) 40 (meningitis) 40 (*Pseudomonas* sp.)	12 8 8
Methicillin	≤29	25–50	12 (0–28 days) 8 (>28 days)
	30 to 36		12 (0–14 days) 8 (>14 days)
	37 to 44		12 (0–7 days) 8 (>7 days)
	≥45		6
Metronidazole	All	15 (loading)	
	≤29	7.5 (maintenance)	48 (0–28 days) 24 (>28 days)
	30 to 36		24 (0–14 days) 12 (>14 days)
	37 to 44		24 (0–7 days) 12 (>7 days)
	≥45		12 (>0–7 days)
Mezlocillin	≤29	50 to 100	12 (0–28 days) 8 (>28 days)
	30 to 36		12 (0–14 days) 8 (>14 days)
	37 to 44		12 (0–7 days) 8 (>7 days)
	≥45		6
Nafcillin	All	50 (meningitis)	
	≤29	25 to 50	12 (0–28 days) 8 (>28 days)

(*Continued*)

TABLE 12   Daily Dosages of Intravenous Antibiotics for Neonates with Serious Infections (*Continued*)

Antibiotic	Gestational Age (weeks)	Dose (mg/kg/dose)	Interval (h) (Postnatal Age)
	30 to 36		12 (0–14 days) 8 (>14 days)
	37 to 44		12 (0–7 days) 8 (>7 days)
	≥45		6
Oxacillin	All	50 (meningitis)	
	≤29	25 to 50	12 (0–28 days) 8 (>28 days)
	30 to 36		12 (0–14 days) 8 (>14 days)
	37 to 44		12 (0–7 days) 8 (>7 days)
	≥45		6
Penicillin G	All	75–100,000 IU/dose (meningitis) 25–50,000 IU/dose (bacteremia) 200–450,000 IU/day (Group B strep)	
	≤29		12 (0–28 days) 8 (>28 days)
	30 to 36		12 (0–14 days) 8 (>14 days)
	37 to 44		12 (0–7 days) 8 (>7 days)
	≥45		6
Piperacillin	≤29	50 to 100	12 (0–28 days) 8 (>28 days)
	30 to 36		12 (0–14 days) 8 (>14 days)
	37 to 44		12 (0–7 days) 8 (>7 days)
	≥45		6
Rifampin	All	5–10	12
Tobramycin	≤29	5 4 4	48 (0–7 days) 36 (8–28 days) 24 (≥29 days)
	30 to 34	4.5 4	36 (0–7 days) 12 (>14 days)
	≥35		24
Vancomycin		15 (meningitis) 10 (bacteremia)	
	≤29		18 (0–14 days) 12 (>14 days
	30 to 36		12 (0–14 days) 8 (>14 days)
	37 to 44		12 (0–7 days) 8 (> 7 days)
	≥45		6
Zidovudine	All	1.5	
	<29		12 (0–28 days) 8 (>28 days)
	30–34		12 (0–14 days) 8 (>14 days)
	>35		6

TABLE 13   Dosages of Oral Antibiotics for Neonates

Antibiotic (Trade name)	Daily dosage
Amoxicillin (numerous trade names)	20–30 mg/kg div. q 12 h
Ampicillin (numerous trade names)	50–100 mg/kg div. q 8 h
Cefaclor (Ceclor®)	40 mg/kg div. q 8 h
Cephalexin (Keflex®)	50 mg/kg div. q 6 h
Clindamycin (Cleocin®)	10–30 mg/kg div. q 8 h
Cloxacillin (Tegopen®)	50–100 mg/kg div. q 6 h
Dicloxacillin (Dycill®, Dynapen®, Pathocil®)	>2.5 kg; 50–100 mg/kg div. q 6 h
	<2.5 kg; 50 mg/kg div. q 8 h
Erythromycin (numerous trade names)	12.5 mg/kg div. q 6 h
Flucytosine (Ancobon®)	12.5–37.5 mg/kg div. q 6 h
Metronidazole (numerous trade names)	Loading dose 15 mg/kg
	Maintenance dose: 7.5 mg/kg q 24 h
Nystatin (Mycostatin®)	100,000 U div. q 6 h
	Premature 200,000 U div. q 6 h
Penicillin V (numerous trade names)	25–50 mg/kg div. q 8 h
Rifampin (Rifadin®, Rimactane®)	10–20 mg/kg div. q 24 h
Zidovudine (Retrovir®)	2 mg/kg/dose
	Premature infants <14 days 4 mg/kg div. q 12 h
	Premature infants >14 days 8 mg/kg div. q 6 h

TABLE 14   Intravenous and Intramuscular Antibiotic Dosages for Serious Infections in Infants and Children

Antibiotic (Trade name)	Daily dosage
Aminoglycosides	
Amikacin (Amikin®)	22 mg/kg div. q 8 h
Gentamicin (numerous trade names)	7.5 mg/kg div. q 8 h
Kanamycin (Kantrex®, Klebcil®)	22.5 mg/kg q 8 h
Netilmicin (Netromycin®)	7.5 mg/kg div. q 8 h
Streptomycin	20–30 mg/kg div. q 12 h
Tobramycin	3–7.5 mg/kg div. q 8 h
Aztreonarn (Azactam®)	90–120 mg/kg div. q 6 h
Cephalosporins	
Cefamandole (Mandol®)	150 mg/kg div. q 6 h
Cefazolin (Ancef®, Kefzol®)	100 mg/kg div. q 8 h
Cefepime (Maxipime®)	>2 months: 150 mg/kg div q 8 h
Cefoperazone (Cefobid®)	>12 years; 150 mg/kg div. q 8 h
Cefotaxime (Claforan®)	150–200 mg/kg div. q 6 h (300 mg/kg for CNS infection)
Cefoxitin (Mefoxin®)	80–160 mg/kg div. q 6 h
Ceftazidime (Fortax®, Tazicef®, Tazidime®)	125–150 mg/kg div. q 8 h; 300 mg/kg for CNS infection and serious *Pseudomonas* disease
Ceftizoxime (Cefizox®)	>6 months; 150–200 mg/kg div. q 6 h
Ceftriaxone (Rocephin®)	50 mg/kg div. q 24 h (80–100 mg/kg for CNS)
Cefuroxime (Zinacef®)	100–150 mg/kg div. q 8 h
Cephalothin (Keflin®)	100 mg/kg div. q 6 h
Cephradine (Anspor®, Velosef®)	100 mg/kg div. q 6 h
Ciprofloxacin (Cipro®)	18–30 mg/kg div. q 12 h
Clindamycin (Cleocin®)	25–40 mg/kg div. q 6 h
Erythromycin (numerous trade names)	15–50 mg/kg div. q 6 h
Fluconazole (Diflucan®)	12 mg/kg div q 12 h
Imipenem/Cilastatin (Primaxin®)	>4 weeks: 100 mg/kg div. q 6 h
Meropenem (Merem®)	60 mg/kg div 8 h (120 mg/kg for CNS)
Metronidazole (Flagyl®)	30 mg/kg div. q 6 h

(Continued)

TABLE 14 Intravenous and Intramuscular Antibiotic Dosages for Serious Infections in Infants and Children (*Continued*)

Antibiotic (Trade name)	Daily dosage
Penicillins	
Ampicillin (numerous trade names)	200 mg/kg div. q 6 h (400 mg/kg for CNS)
Mezlocillin (Mezlin®)	200 mg/kg div. q 6 h
Nafcillin (Nafcil®, Unipen®)	100–150 mg/kg div. q 6 h
Oxacillin (Bactocill®, Prostaphlin®)	150–200 mg/kg div. q 6 h
Penicillin G	400,000 U/kg div. q 6 h for CNS (250,000 units/kg q4 h)
Penicillin G benzathine i.m.	25,000–50,000 U/kg single dose i.m.
Penicillin G procaine i.m.	25,000–50,000 U/kg div. q 12 h i.m.
Piperacillin (Pipracil®)	200–300 mg/kg div. q 6 h
Ticarcillin (Ticar®)	200–300 mg/kg div. q 6 h
Ticarcillin/clavulanate (Timentin®)	200–300 mg/kg div. q 6 h
Rifampin (Rifadin®, Rimactane®)	10–20 mg/kg div. q 12 h
Streptomycin i.m.	20–30 mg/kg div. q 12 h i.m.
Tetracyclines	
Doxycycline (numerous trade names)	2–4 mg/kg div. q 24 h
Minocycline (Minocin®)	4 mg/kg div. q 12 h
TMP/SMX[a] (Bactrim®, Septra®)	20 mg TMP/100 mg SMX/kg div. q 6 h
Vancomycin (Vancocin®)	40 mg/kg div. q 6 h

[a] TMP/SMX, trimethoprim/sulfamethoxazole.

TABLE 15 Dosages of Oral Antibiotics for Infants and Children

Antibiotic (Trade name)	Daily dosage
Azithromycin (Zithromax®)	>6months: 10 mg/kg loading dose then 5 mg/kg/d × 4 days; strep throat 12 mg/kg for 5 days
Cephalosporins	
Cefaclor (Ceclor®)	20–40 mg/kg div. q 8 h
Cefadroxil (Duricef®, Ultracef®)	30 mg/kg div. q 12 h
Cefdinir (Omnicef®)	14 mg/kg div. q 24 h
Cefixime (Suprax®)	8 mg/kg single daily dose
Cefpodoxime (Vantin®)	10 mg/kg div. q 12 h
Cefprozil (Cefzil®)	30 mg/kg div. q 12 h
Ceftibuten (Cedax®)	9 mg/kg single daily dose
Cefuroxime (Ceftin®)	20–30 mg/kg div. q 12 h
Cephalexin (Keflex®)	25–50 mg/kg div. q 6 h
Cephradine (Velosef®)	25–50 mg/kg div. q 6 h
Ciprofloxacin (Cipro®)	20–30 mg/kg div. q 12 h
Clarithromycin (Biaxin®)	15 mg/kg div. q 12 h
Clindamycin (Cleocin®)	10–20 mg/kg div. q 6 h
Dapsone	1 mg/kg single daily dose
Erythromycin (numerous trade names)	30–50 mg/kg div. q 6 h
Linezolid (Zyvox®)	20 mg/kg div. q 12 h
Isoniazid (INH®, Nydrazid®)	10–20 mg/kg div. q 12–24h
Loracarbef(Lorabid®)	15–30 mg/kg div. q 12 h
Methenamine mandelate (Mandelamine®, Thiacide®, Uroquid®)	50–75 mg/kg div. q 8 h
Metronidazole (Flagyl®, Metric®, Protostat®)	15–35 mg/kg div. q 8 h

(Continued)

TABLE 15   Dosages of Oral Antibiotics for Infants and Children (*Continued*)

Antibiotic (Trade name)	Daily dosage
Nalidixic acid (NegGram®)	>3 months: 55 mg/kg div. q 6 h
Neomycin (Mycifradin®, Neobiotic®)	100 mg/kg div. q 6 h
Nitrofurantoin (Furadantin®, Macrodantin®)	5–7 mg/kg div. q 6 h
	1–2 mg/kg div. q 24 h (for urinary tract suppressive therapy)
Penicillins	
Penicillin V (numerous trade names)	25–50 mg/kg div. q 8 h
Amoxicillin (numerous trade names)	25–50 mg/kg div. q 8 h
Amoxicillin/clavulanate (Augmentin®)	20–40 mg/kg div. q 8 h
Ampicillin (numerous trade names)	50–100 mg/kg div. q 6 h
Bacampicillin	25–50 mg/kg div. q 12 h
Carbenicillin (Geocillin®)	30–50 mg/kg div. q 6 h
Cloxacillin (Tegopen®)	50–100 mg/kg div. q 6 h
Cyclacillin (Cyclapen-W®)	50–100 mg/kg div. q 8 h
Dicloxacillin (Dycill®, Dynapen®, Pathocil®)	25–50 mg/kg div. q 6 h
Hetacillin (Versapen®)	50–100 mg/kg div. q 6 h
Nafcillin (Nafcil®, Unipen®)	50–100 mg/kg div. q 6 h
Oxacillin (Bactocil®, Prostaphlin®)	50–100 mg/kg div. q 6 h
Pyrazinamide®	20–40 mg/kg div. q 24 h
Rifampin (Rifadin®, Rimactane®)	20 mg/kg div. q 12 h
Sulfonamides	
Sulfadiazine	100–150 mg/kg div. q 6 h
Sulfamethoxazole (Gantanol®)	50 mg/kg div. q 12 h
Sulfisoxazole (Gantrisin®, SK-Soxazole®)	120–150 mg/kg div. q 6 h
Tetracyclines	
Tetracycline (numerous trade names)	25–50 mg/kg div. q 6 h
Demeclocycline (Declomycin®)	8–12 mg/kg div. q 12 h
Doxycycline (Vibramycin®)	2–4 mg/kg div. q 12 h
Methacycline (Rondomycin®)	10 mg/kg div. q 6 h
Minocycline (Minocin®)	Initial: 4 mg/kg followed by 2 mg/kg div. q 12 h
Oxytetracycline (Terramycin®)	25 mg/kg div. q 6 h
TMP/SMX[a], (Bactrim®, Septra®, Cotrim®, Sulfatrim®)	8–12 mg TMP/40–60 mg SMX/kg div. q 12 h
	4 mg TMP/25 mg SMX/kg div. q 12 h for *Pneumocystis* prophylaxis
Vancomycin[b] (Vancocin®)	50 mg/kg div. q 6 h

[a] TMP/SMX, Trimethoprim/sulfamethoxazole.
[b] Vancomycin is not absorbed.

Body Surface Area

Patients who are excessively obese or malnourished will be overdosed or underdosed, respectively, if antibiotic dosages are calculated by body weight. For these patients, body surface area may be determined using scales or by equation (Fig. 1). Table 17 lists antibiotic dosages calculated for body surface area.

ANTIBIOTICS FOR SPECIFIC PATHOGENS

For many patients, a clinical syndrome is apparent at presentation. Pending results of cultures and their antibiotic sensitivities, therapy should be instituted based on reported susceptibility or efficacy data. Table 18 summarizes recommended initial antimicrobial therapy. Antibiotic therapy should be reevaluated once culture information is available.

TABLE 16 Maximum (Adult) Dosages of Parenteral Antibiotics

Antibiotic	Maximum daily dosage
Aminoglycosides	
Amikacin	1.5 g
Gentamicin	300 mg
Kanamycin	1–1.5 g
Netilmicin	300 mg
Streptomycin	1.5 g
Tobramycin	300 mg
Aztreonam	8 g
Cephalosporins	
Cefamandole	6 g
Cefepime	4 g
Cefazolin	6 g
Cefonicid	2 g
Ceforanide	2 g
Cefotaxime	10 g
Cefoxitin	12 g
Ceftazidime	6 g
Ceftizoxime	6 g
Ceftriaxone	4 g
Cefuroxime	6 g
Cephalothin	12 g
Meropenem	6 g
Chloramphenicol	4 g
Clindamycin	3.6 g
Erythromycin	4 g
Metronidazole	2 g
Penicillins	
Penicillin G	24×10^6 U
Penicillin G benzathine	2.4×10^6 U
Penicillin G procaine	4.8×10^6 U/ 24 h
Ampicillin	12 g
Azlocillin	24 g
Mezlocillin	24 g
Nafcillin	12 g
Oxacillin	12 g
Piperacillin	18 g
Ticarcillin	24 g
Spectinomycin	4 g
Tetracycline	2 g
Vancomycin	4 g

TABLE 17 Dosages of Antibiotics by Body Surface Area

Antibiotic	Daily dosage/m^2
Aminoglycosides	
Amikacin	600 mg div. q 8 h
Gentamicin	180 mg div. q 8 h
Kanamycin	600 mg div. q 8 h
Netilmicin	180 mg div. q 8 h
Tobramycin	180 mg div. q 8 h
Aztreonam	3.2 g div. q 6 h
Cephalosporins	
Cefamandole	4.2 g div. q 8 h
Cefazolin	2.4 g div. q 8 h
Cefonicid	1.1 g div. q 12 h
Ceforanide	1.1 g div. q 12 h
Cefotaxime	4.2 g div. q 8 h
Ceftazidime	4.2 g div. q 8 h
Ceftizoxime	4.2 g div. q 8 h
Ceftriaxone	2.8 g div. q 24 h
Cefuroxime	2.4 g div. q 8 h
Cephalothin	5.6 g div. q 6 h
Chloramphenicol	2.8 div. q 6 h (CNS)
	1.8 div. q 6 h
Imipenem	2.2 g div. q 6 h
Metronidazole	840 mg div. q 8 h
Penicillins	
Penicillin G	10.5×10^6 U div. q 6 h (CNS)
	2.7×10^6 U div. q 6 h
Ampicillin	5.6 g div. q 6 h
Azlocillin	10 g div. q 6 h
Methicillin	5.6 div. q 6 h
Mezlocillin	10 g div. q 6 h
Nafcillin	4.2 div. q 6 h
Oxacillin	5.6 div. q 6 h
Piperacillin	10 g div. q 6 h
Ticarcillin	10 g div. q 6 h
TMP/SMX[a]	300 mg TMP/1.5 g SMX div. q 8 h
Vancomycin	1.7 g div. q 6 h (CNS)
Zidovudine	640 mg div. q 6 h

[a] TMP/SMX, Trimethoprim/sulfamethoxazole.

ANTIVIRAL AGENTS

Antiviral therapy of proven efficacy is currently available for the treatment of the following viruses: cytomegalovirus, hepatitis B, hepatitis C, herpes simplex types 1 and 2, HIV, influenza A, respiratory syncytial virus (RSV), and varicella-zoster. For herpes-group virus infections, therapy is initiated only for certain well-defined infections. Many other antiviral agents are currently under investigation. Table 19 offers a summary of therapy for viral infections.

ANTIFUNGAL AGENTS

Systemic fungal infections are being seen with increased frequency as a result of longer survival for patients with severe disease and compromised immune function. Broad-spectrum

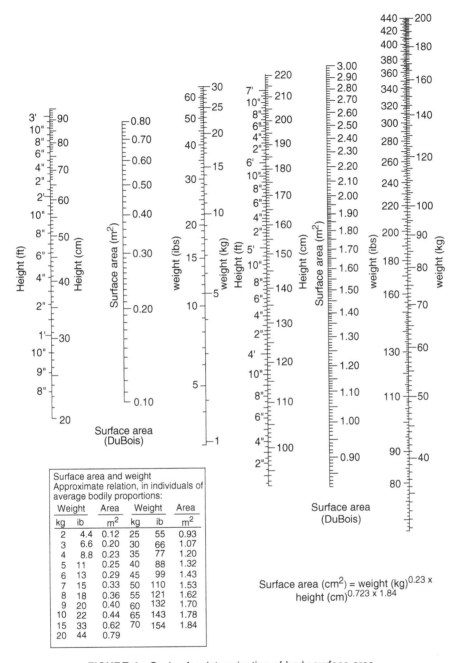

FIGURE 1 Scales for determination of body surface area.

antibiotics and indwelling foreign bodies (central i.v. lines, urinary catheters, and arterial monitoring devices) are the most significant predisposing factors, particularly for infection with *Candida albicans*. Therefore, strong consideration must be given to discontinuing these antibiotics and removing any indwelling source of fungal colonization.

Amphotericin B was previously the most commonly recommended agent for invasive *Candida albicans* infection but because of its toxicity has been largely replaced by fluconazole (see Chapter 18, Table 13).

TABLE 18   Therapy for Defined Clinical Syndromes or Specific Microorganisms

Infection	Drug of choice	Alternatives
Acinetobacter baumanii	Meropenem	Ciprofloxacin, amikacin
Actinobacillus	Ampicillin + gentamicin	Doxycycline
Actinomycosis	Penicillin G	Tetracycline, clindamycin
Adenitis (Chapter 3)	Clindamycin;TMP/SMX Linezolid	Cephalexin
Aeromonas spp	Ceftriaxone	TMP/SMX
Anthrax	Ciprofloxacin	Doxycycline
Arcanobacterium hemolyticum	Erythromycin	Doxycycline
Bacillary angiomatosis	Azithromycin	TMP/SMX
Bacillus spp	Vancomycin	Clindamycin
Bacteroides spp.	Metronidazole	Clindamycin
Bartonellosis	Penicillin	Doxycycline
Borrelia spp.	Ceftriaxone	Doxycycline
Botulism (Chapter 2)	Penicillin	Tetracycline
Brucellosis	Gentamicin *plus* doxycycline	TMP/SMX, rifampin
Burkholderia cepacia	Meropenem	Cefazidime
Burkholderia pseudomallei	Meropenem	Doxycycline
Campylobacter enteritis (Chapter 9)	Erythromycin	Tetracycline
Capnocytophaga canimorsus	Penicillin	Ceftriaxone
Cat-scratch disease	Azithromycin	Gentamicin, TMP/SMX, Rifampin
Chancroid (Chapter 15)	Ceftriaxone	Azithromycin
Chlamydia trachomatis (Chapter 8)	Azithromycin	Doxycycline
Chlamydophila pneumoniae	Azithromycin	Tetracycline
Cholera	Doxycycline	TMP/SMX
Chromobacterium	TMP/SMX + ciprofloxacin	Chloramphenicol
Chryseobacterium	Vancomycin + rifampin	Ciprofloxacin
Citrobacter spp.	Meropenem	Cefepime
Clostridium difficile	Metronidazole	Vancomycin
Diphtheria (Chapter 2)	Penicillin and antitoxin	Erythromycin
Ehrlichiosis	Doxycycline	Chloramphenicol
Eikenella corrodens	Ampicillin	Ceftriaxone
Endocarditis (Chapter 2)	Vancomycin plus gentamicin	
Enterobacter spp.	Cefepime	Meropenem
Enterococcus spp.	Ampicillin + gentamicin	Vancomycin + gentamicin
Erysipelas (Chapter 3)	Penicillin	A macrolide
Erysipeloid	Ampicillin	Ceftriaxone
Erythrasma	Topical clindamycin	Erythromycin
Fusobacterium spp.	Metronidazole	Clindamycin
Gardnerella vaginalis	Metronidazole	Clindamycin
Gas gangrene	Penicillin	Clindamycin
Glanders	Gentamicin plus tetracycline	Chloramphenicol
Gonorrhea (Chapter 15)	Ceftriaxone	Cefixime, ofloxacin, ciprofloxacin, tetracycline, spectinomycin, cefoxitin, or cefotaxime
Granuloma inguinale (Chapter 15)	TMP/SMX	Doxycycline
Haemoplilus aphrophilus	Ceftriaxone	Ampicillin + gentamicin
Helicobacter pylori	Amoxicillin + clarithromycin + omeprazole	Amoxicillin + metronidazole + Pepto-Bismol
Impetigo (Chapter 12)	Cephalexin	Mupirocin (topical)

(Continued)

TABLE 18 Therapy for Defined Clinical Syndromes or Specific Microorganisms (*Continued*)

Infection	Drug of choice	Alternatives
Kingella kingae	Ampicillin	Ceftriaxone
Legionnaires'disease (Chapter 8)	Azithromycin and rifampin	Doxycycline
Leprosy	Clofazimine plus dapsone plus rifampin	Clarithromycin, sparfloxacin; minocycline
Leuconostoc	Ampicillin	Clindamycin
Leptospirosis	Penicillin	Doxycycline
Listeriosis	Ampicillin plus gentamicin	TMP/SMX; vancomycin
Ludwig's angina (Chapter 12)	Ceftazidime plus clindamycin	
Lyme disease (early) (severe)	Doxycycline Ceftriaxone	Amoxicillin
Melioidosis	Meropenem	Ceftazidime
Meningococcemia (Chapter 2)	Ceftriaxone	Penicillin
Morganella morganii	Cefepime	Meropenem
Mycobacterium (atypical)		
avium complex	Clarithromycin + amikacin	Clofazimine
fortuitum/chelonae	Amikacin + cefoxitin	Azithromycin
marinum/balnei	minocycline	Clarithromycin
Mycoplasma pneumoniae	Azithromycin or clarithromycin	Doxycycline
Necrotizing fasciitis	Clindamycin *plus* penicillin or ceftriaxone	
Nocardiosis	Sulfisoxazole or TMP/SMX plus amikacin (for first 7 days)	Meropenem
Oerskovia spp.	Vancomycin	
Otitis externa (Chapter 3)	Antibiotic-steroid eardrops	
Otitis media (Chapter 3)	Cephalosporin, azithromycin or amoxicillin	
Parotitis, suppurative	Clindamycin or vancomycin plus gentamicin	
Pasteurella multocida	Penicillin	Doxycyline
Peptostreptococcus	Penicillin	Clindamycin
Pertussis (Chapter 8)	Azithromycin	TMP/SMX
Plague (Chapter 8)	Gentamicin plus doxycycline	Ciprofloxacin
Plesiomonas shigelloides	TMP/SMX	Ciprofloxacin
Pneumocystis jiroveci (Chapters 16 & 18)	TMP/SMX	Pentamidine
Prevotella melaninogenicus	Metronidazole	Clindamycin
Proprionibacterium acnes	Penicillin	Clindamycin
Pseudomembranous colitis (Chapter 9)	Metronidazole p.o.	Vancomycin p.o.
Psittacosis	Azithromycin	Doxycycline
Q fever	Doxycycline	Ciprofloxacin
Rat-bite fever	Penicillin	Doxycycline
Relapsing fever	Penicillin	Doxycycline
Rhodococcus equi	Meropenem + vancomycin	Amikacin
Rickettsial	Doxycycline	Chloramphenicol
Salmonellosis (Chapter 9)	Ceftriaxone	TMP/SMX; ampicillin (if susceptible)
Scarlet fever	Penicillin	Erythromycin
Shigellosis (Chapter 9)	TMP/SMX	Ceftriaxone, ciprofloxacin
Sinusitis (Chapter 8)	A cephalosporin or azithromycin	Amoxicillin/clavulanate
Staphylococcal scalded skin syndrome	Clindamycin	Vancomycin
Stenotrophomonas maltophilia	TMP/SMX	Ceftazidime

(Continued)

TABLE 18   Therapy for Defined Clinical Syndromes or Specific Microorganisms (*Continued*)

Infection	Drug of choice	Alternatives
Syphilis (Chapter 15)	Penicillin	Tetracycline, ceftriaxone
Tetanus (Chapter 2)	Metronidazole	Penicillin
Toxoplasmosis (Chapter 1)	Pyrimethamine plus sulfadiazine	Spiramycin
Traveler's diarrhea (Chapter 5)	Azithromycin	Ciprofloxacin
Tuberculosis (Chapter 2)	Isoniazid plus rifampin plus pyrizinamide plus streptomycin or ethambutol (older child)	
Tularemia	Gentamicin	Doxycycline
Typhoid fever	Ceftriaxone	Ciprofloxacin
Typhus	Doxycycline	Chloramphenicol
Ureaplasma urealyticum	Azithromycin	doxycycline
Vaginosis (bacterial)	Metronidazole	Clindamycin
Vibrio vulnificus	Doxycycline + ceftazidime	Ciprofloxacin + cefotaxime
Vincent's angina	Penicillin	Erythromycin
Yersiniosis	TMP/SMX	Ciprofloxacin

TABLE 19   Therapy for Viral Infections

Viral Infection	Drug of choice	Dosage
Cytomegalovirus		
Pneumonia	Ganciclovir plus IVIG	2.5 mg/kg q 8 h i.v. × 20 days 500 mg/kg q.o.d. × 10 doses then ganciclovir 5 mg/kg/day 3–5 × /week for 20 doses plus IVIG 500 mg/kg 2×/week × 8 doses
Retinitis	Ganciclovir or foscarnet	5 mg/kg i.v. b.i.d. for 14–21 days 60 mg/kg i.v. q 8 h for 14–21 days
Hepatitis B virus		
Chronic hepatitis	Interferon α-2b	5×10^6 U/day s.c. for 4 months
Hepatitis C virus		
Chronic hepatitis	Interferon α-2b *plus* ribavirin	3×10^6 U s.c. or i.m. 3 times per week for 24 weeks
Herpes simplex virus		
Bell's palsy	Acyclovir *plus* prednisone	20 mg/kg p.o. q.i.d. × 10 days; 0.5–1 mg/kg/day div. q 12 h × 10 days
Conjunctivitis	Trifluridine	1 drop of 1% solution topically q 2 h, up to 9 times per day
Encephalitis	Acyclovir	30 mg/kg/day i.v. div. q 8 h i.v. q 8 h for 14–21 days
Genital herpes (see Chapter 16)	Acyclovir	
Mucocutaneous disease in immunocompromised host	Acyclovir	5 mg/kg i.v. q 8 h or 400 mg p.o. 5 times per day for 7–14 days
Neonatal	Acyclovir	30 mg/kg/day i.v. div. q 8 h for 14–21 days
Acyclovir-resistant	Foscarnet	40 mg/kg i.v. q 8 h
HIV	(See Chapter 17)	
Influenza A virus	Rimantadine Amantadine	5 mg/kg/day p.o. div. q 12–24 h (maximum 200 mg/day) 5–8 mg/kg/day p.o. div. q 12 h (maximum 200 mg/day)
Respiratory syncytial virus	Ribavirin	Aerosol treatment 12–18 h/day for 3–7 days (20 mg/mL in the reservoir)
Rotavirus—gastrointeritis in immunocompromised host	Immunoglobulin p.o.	

TABLE 19   Therapy for Viral Infections (*Continued*)

Viral Infection	Drug of choice	Dosage
Varicella-zoster virus		
Chickenpox	Acyclovir	20 mg/kg p.o. q.i.d. for 5 days (800 mg maximum)
Varicella zoster	Acyclovir	
Varicella or zoster in immunocompromised host	Acyclovir	1500 mg/m^2/day i.v. div. q 8 h until improved then p.o. as above
Acyclovir-resistant	Foscarnet	40 mg/kg i.v. q 8 h

TABLE 20   Therapy for Systemic Fungal Infections

Infection	Drug of choice

Aspergillosis	Amphotericin B 30 days
	Alternative: itraconazole
	For patients with decreased renal function:
	    Amphotericin B lipid complex (Abelcet, ABLC)
	    Liposomal amphotericin B (AmBisome)
	    Amphotericin B cholesteryl complex (Amphotec)
	    Amphotericin B colloidal dispersion (ABCD)

Blastomycosis	Moderate infection: itraconazole p.o. × 3–6 mo Severe infection amphotericin B i.v. × 2 weeks followed by itraconazole p.o. × 6–12 mo
Candidiasis Oropharyngeal	Fluconazole x 5–14 days or nystatin × 14 days or coltrimazole troche × 7–14 days
Systemic	Fluconazole p.o. or i.v. × 14–28 days or amphotericin B i.v. × 14 days
Chromomycosis	Itraconazole × 18 mo.
Coccidioidomycosis	Fluconazole × 12–18 mo Alternative: itraconazole × 12–18 mo
Cryptococcosis Nonmeningeal	Amphotericin B until response then fluconazole p.o. × 8 weeks or fluconazole × 8 weeks
Meningitis	Amphotericin B plus flucytosine × 6 weeks
Chronic suppression	Fluconazole Alternative; amphotericin B
Histoplasmosis	Itraconazole
Pulmonary or non CNS	Amphotericin B
CNS involvement	Alternative: itraconazole
Chronic suppression	Itraconazole
Mucormycosis	Amphotericin B No dependable alternative
Paracoccidioidomycosis	Itraconazole × 6 months Alternative: Ketoconazole 6–18 mo
Pseudallescheriasis	Surgery plus itraconazole
Sporotrichosis	Itraconazole

Therapy for fungal infections is summarized in Tables 20 and 21. Renal function must be carefully monitored and, whenever possible, both dosage and duration of therapy should be minimized.

ANTIPARASITIC AGENTS

Parasitic infections are much less commonly encountered in medical practice today as contrasted with just one generation ago. This change is attributed primarily to improved urban

(Text continues on page 281)

TABLE 21 Antifungal Therapy

Agent (Trade name)	Dosage
Amphotericin B (Fungizone®)	1 mg test dose, followed after 4 h by 0.25 mg/kg i.v. Increase dosage each day by 0.25 mg/kg to a maximum of 1 mg/kg/day given as a single daily infusion. For most systemic infections, a total dose of 30 mg/kg is required. When combined with flucytosine, the daily dose is 0.3 mg/kg
Amphotericin B lipid complex (Abelcet®, ABLC®)	5.0 mg/kg/day
Amphotericin B—liposomal (AmBisome®)	3–5 mg/kg/day
Amphotericin B—colloidal dispersion (ABCD®)	2–6 mg/kg/day
Amphotericin B—cholesteryl (Amphotec®)	3–4 mg/kg/day
Clotrimazole	10 mg troche p.o. 5 times per day for 7 days
Fluconazole	i.v.: 12 mg/kg/day div. q 12 h p.o.:3–6 mg/kg single daily dose
Flucytosine (Ancobon®)	150 mg/kg/day p.o. div. q 6 h
Griseofulvin (numerous trade names)	25 mg/kg/day p.o. div. q 24 h
Itraconazole	2–5 mg/kg/day p.o. div. b.i.d.
Ketoconazole (Nizoral®)	5–10 mg/kg/day p.o. div. q 24 h
Nystatin (Mycostatin®, Nilstat®)	200,000 U (2 mL) p.o. q.i.d. for 6–12 days

TABLE 22 Therapy for Common Parasitic Infections

Infection	Drug	Dosage
Amebiasis (*Entamoeba histolytica*) (see Chapter 10)		
Amebic meningoencephalitis		
Naegleria fowleri	Amphotericin B	1 mg/kg/day i.v. plus intraventricular for 30 days
Acanthamoeba	Unknown	
Ancylostoma duodenale	(See hookworm)	
Angiostrongyliasis		
Angiostrongylus cantonensis	Mebendazole	100 mg b.i.d. for 5 days
Angiostrongylus costaricensis	Thiabendazole	75 mg/kg/day in 3 doses for 3 days (maximum 3 g/day)
Anisakiasis (*Anisakis*)	Surgical or endoscopic removal	
Ascariasis (*Ascaris lumbricoides*)	Albendazole or mebendazole	400 mg 1 dose; 100 mg b.i.d. for 3 days
	Pyrantel pamoate	11 mg/kg single dose (maximum 1 g)
Babesiosis (*Babesia microti*)	Clindamycin	20–40 mg/kg/day in 3 doses for 7 days
	Quinine	plus 25 mg/kg/day in 3 doses for 7 day
Balantidiasis (*Balantidium coli*)	Tetracycline	40 mg/kg/day in 4 doses for 10 days (maximum 2 g/day)
	Alternative: metronidazole	35–50 mg/kg/day in 3 doses for 5 days
Baylisascariasis (*Baylisascaris procyonis*)	Diethylcarbamazine or levamisole or fenbendazole	
Blastocystis hominis infection	Metronidazole	35–50 mg/kg/day in 3 doses for 10 days
Capillariasis (*Capillaria philippinensis*)	Mebendazole	200 mg b.i.d. for 20 days
	Alternative: albendazole	200 mg b.i.d. for 10 days
Chagas' disease	(See trypanosomiasis)	
Clonorchis sinensis	(See fluke infection)	

(Continued)

TABLE 22   Therapy for Common Parasitic Infections (*Continued*)

Infection	Drug	Dosage
Cryptosporidiosis (*Cryptosporidium parvum*)	Paromomycin and/or azithromycin	500–750 mg t.i.d.; 600 mg/day
Cutaneous larva migrans (creeping eruption)	Thiabendazole or ivermectin	Topically and/or 50 mg/kg/day in 2 doses (maximum 3 g/day) for 2–5 days; 150 μg/kg p.o. × one dose
Cyclospora cayetanensis	TMP/SMX	1 double strength tab b.i.d. × 7 days
Cysticercosis	(See tapeworm infection)	
Dientamoeba fragilis infection	Iodoquinol or paromomycin or tetracycline	40 mg/kg/day in 3 doses for 20 days; 25–30 mg/kg/day in 3 doses for 7 day; 40 mg/kg/day in 4 doses for 10 days (maximum 2 g/day)
Diphyllobothrium latum	(See tapeworm infection)	50–75 mg/kg/day in 2 doses for 3 days
Dracunculus medinensis (guineaworm) infection	Surgical removal Alternative: thiabendazole	
Echinococcus	(See tapeworm infection)	
Entamoeba histolytica	(See Chapter 10)	
Enterobius vermicularis (pinworm infection)	Albendazole or mebendazole or pyrantel pamoate	400 mg p.o. × 1; repeat in 2 weeks; single dose of 100 mg; repeat after 2 weeks; 11 mg/kg single dose (maximum 1 g); repeat after 2 weeks
Fasciola hepatica	(See fluke infection)	
Filariasis		
Wuchereria bancrofti, Brugia malayi		
	Ivermectin plus albendazole Alternative: Diethylcarbamazine	100–440 μg/kg × 1 dose; 400 mg × 1 dose Day 1: 1 mg/kg oral, after meal Day 2: 1 mg/kg t.i.d. Day 3: 1–2 mg/kg t.i.d. Day 4–21: 6 mg/kg per day in 3 doses
Loa loa	Diethylcarbamazine	Day 1: 1 mg/kg oral, after meal Day 2: 1 mg/kg t.i.d. Day 3: 1–2 mg/kg t.i.d. Days 4–21: 9 mg/kg/day in 3 doses
Mansonella ozzardi	Ivermectin	25–200 μg/kg × 1 dose
Mansonella perstans	Mebendazole	100 mg b.i.d. for 30 days
Tropical pulmonary eosinophilia (TPE)	Diethylcarbamazine	6 mg/kg/day in 3 doses for 21 days
Onchocerca volvulus	Ivermectin	150 μg/kg single oral dose, repeated every 6–12 months
Flukes hermaphroditic infection		
Clonorchis sinensis (Chinese liver fluke)	Praziquantel	25 mg/kg × 3 doses
Fasciola hepatica (sheep liver fluke)	Bithionol	30–50 mg/kg on alternate days for 10–15 doses
Fasciolopsis buski (intestinal fluke)	Praziquantel or niclosamide	75 mg/kg per day in 3 doses for 1 day; 11–34 kg: 2 tablets (1 g); >34 kg: 3 tablets (1.5 g)
Heterophyes heterophyes (intestinal fluke)	Praziquantel	75 mg/kg/day in 3 doses for 1 day
Metagonimus yokogawai (intestinal fluke)	Praziquantel	75 mg/kg/day in 3 doses for 1 day
Nanophyetus salmincola	Praziquantel	60 mg/kg/day in 3 doses for 1 day
Opisthorchis viverrini (liverfluke)	Praziquantel	75 mg/kg/day in 3 doses for 1 day
Paragonimus westermani (lungfluke)	Praziquantel	75 mg/kg/day in 3 doses for 2 days

(*Continued*)

TABLE 22 Therapy for Common Parasitic Infections (*Continued*)

Infection	Drug	Dosage
Giardiasis (see Chapter 10)		
Gnathostomiasis (*Gnathostoma spinigerum*)	Surgical removal plus Albendazole	400 mg p.o. daily or b.i.d. × 21 days
Hookworm infection (*Ancylostoma duodenale, Necator americanus*)	Albendazole or mebendazole or pyrantel pamoate	400 mg single dose; 100 mg b.i.d. × 3 days; 11 mg/kg (max. 1 g) for 3 days
Hydatid cyst (see tapeworm infection)		
Hymenolepis nana (see tapeworm infection)		
Isosporiasis (*Isospora belli*)	Trimethoprim/ sulfamethoxazole (TMP/SMX)	40 mg TMP/200 mg SMX/kg/day q.i.d. for 10 days then 20 mg TMP/100 mg SMX/kg/day b.i.d. for 3 weeks
Leishmaniasis (*L. mexicana, L. tropica, L. major,* or *L. braziliensis, L. donovani–Kala-azar*)	Stibogluconate sodium or meglumine antimoniate or amphotericin B	20 mg Sb/kg/day i.v. i.m. for 20–28 days; 20 mg Sb/kg/day for 20–28 days; 0.25–1 mg/kg by slow infusion daily, or every 2 days, for up to 8 weeks
Lice infestation (*Pediculus humanus, P. capitis, Phthirus pubis*)	1% Permethrin or 0.5% Malathion Pyrethrins with piperonyl butoxide Lindane Ivermectin (see filariasis)	Topically Topically Topically 200 µg/kg single dose p.o.
Loa loa [*]		
Malaria, Treatment of (*Plasmodium falciparum, P. ovale, P. vivax,* and *P. malariae*)		
All Plasmodium except chloroquine-resistant *P. falciparum*		
Oral	Chloroquine phosphate	10 mg base/kg (maximum 600 mg base), then 5 mg base/kg at 24 and 48 h
Parenteral	Quinidinegluconate or quinidine dihydrochloride	10 mg/kg loading dose (maximum 600 mg) in normal saline slowly over 1 h followed by continuous infusion of 0.02 mg/kg/min for 3 days maximum; 20 mg salt/kg loading dose in 10 mL/kg 5% dextrose over 4 h followed by 10 mg salt/kg over 2–4 h q 8 h (maximum 1800 mg/day) until oral therapy can be started
Chloroquine-resistant *P. falciparum*		
Oral	Quinine sulfate *plus*	25 mg/kg per day in 3 doses for 3 days (7 days with doxycycline)
	Pyrimethamine–sulfadoxine (single dose given on last day of quinine) or, plus	<1 year: 1/4 tablet; 1–3 years: 1/2 tablet; 4–8 years: 1 tablet 9–14 years: 2 tablets
	Doxycycline or, plus	100 mg b.i.d. for 7 days
	Clindamycin Alternatives:	20–40 mg/kg/day in 3 doses for 3 days
	Mefloquine Halofantrine	(<45 kg) 25 mg/kg single dose (<40 kg) 8 mg/kg q 6 h for 3 doses
Parenteral	Quinidine gluconate or Quinine dihydrochloride	Same as for nonresistant stains Same as for nonresistant stains

[*]CDC malaria information: prophylaxis (888)-232-3228; treatment (770)-488-7788   (*Continued*)

TABLE 22 Therapy for Common Parasitic Infections (*Continued*)

Infection	Drug	Dosage
Prevention of relapses (*P. vivax* and *P. ovale* only)	Primaquine	0.3 mg base/kg/day for 14 days
Malaria, Prevention in		
Chloroquine-sensitive areas	Chloroquine phosphate	5 mg/kg base (8.3 mg/kg salt) once per week, up to adult dose of 300 mg base
Chloroquine-resistant areas	Mefloquine	15–19 kg: 1/4 tablet; 20–30 kg: 1/2 tablet; 31–45 kg: 3/4 tablet; >45 kg: 1 tablet (250 mg) oral once per week
	or doxycycline	>8 years of age: 2 mg/kg/day orally, up to 100 mg/day
	or chloroquine phosphate	as above
	plus Pyrimethamine-sulfadoxine (for presumptive-treatment)	<1 year: 1/4 tablet; 1–3 years: 1/2 tablet; 4–8 years: 1 tablet; 9–14 years: 2 tablets for self-treatment of febrile illness
	or, plus Proguanil (in Africa south of the Sahara)	<2 years: 50 mg daily; 2–6 years: 100 mg daily; 7–10 years: 150 mg daily; >10 years: 200 mg daily and for 4 weeks after exposure
Moniliformis moniliformis infection	Pyrantel pamoate	11 mg/kg single dose, repeat twice, 2 weeks apart
Roundworm	(See ascariasis)	
Scabies (*Sarcoptes scabiei*)	5% Permethrin	Topically, repeat in 1 week
	Alternatives: lindane	Topically
	10% Crotamiton	Topically
Schistosomiasis (bilharziasis)		
Schistosoma haemotobium	Praziquantel	40 mg/kg/day in 2 doses for 1 day
S. japonicum	Praziquantel	60 mg/kg/day in doses for 1 day
S. mansoni	Praziquantel	40 mg/kg/day in 3 doses for 1 day
	Alternative: oxamniquine	20 mg/kg/day in 2 doses for 1 day
S. mekongi	Praziquantel	60 mg/kg/day in 3 doses for 1 day
Strongyloidiasis (*Strongyloides stercoralis*)	Ivermectin	200 µg/kg/day for 2 days
	or	
	Albendazole	400 mg daily for 7 days
	Alternative: thiabenazole	50 mg/kg/day in 2 doses (maximum 3 g/day) for 2 days
Tapeworm infection—adult (intestinal stage)		
Diphyllobothrium latum (fish), *Taenia saginata* (beef), *Taenia solium* (pork), *Dipylidium caninum* (dog)	Praziquantel or niclosamide	10 mg/kg single dose; 11–34 kg: single dose of 2 tablets (1 g); >34 kg: single dose of 3 tablets (1.5 g)
Hymenolepis nana (dwarf tapeworm)	Praziquantel	25 mg/kg single dose
	Alternative: niclosamide	11–34 kg: single dose of 2 tablets (1 g) for 1 day, then 1 tablet (0.5 g)/day for 6 days; >34 kg: single dose of 3 tablets (1.5 g) for 1 day, then 2 tablets (1 g)/day for 6 days
Tapeworm infection, larval (tissue stage)		
Echinococcus granulosus (hydatid cyst)	Albendazole	15 mg/kg/day for 28 days, repeated as necessary
Echinococcus multilocularis	Treatment of choice: Surgical excision	

(*Continued*)

TABLE 22 Therapy for Common Parasitic Infections (*Continued*)

Infection	Drug	Dosage
Cysticerus cellulosae (cysticercosis)	Albendazole	15 mg/kg per day in 3 doses for 8 days, repeated as necessary
	or praziquantel Alternative: surgery	50 mg/kg/day in 3 doses for 15 days
Toxocariasis (see visceral larva migrans)		
Toxoplasmosis (*Toxoplasma gondii*)	Pyrimethamine	2 mg/kg/day for 3 days, then 1 mg/kg/day (maximum 25 mg/day) for 4 weeks
	plus Sulfadiazine plus prednisone	100–200 mg/kg/day for 3–4 weeks; 1 mg/kg/day
	Alternative: spiramycin	50–100 mg/kg/day for 3–4 weeks
Trichinosis (*Trichinelia spiralis*)	Albendazole plus steroids for severe symptoms Alternative: Mebendazole	400 mg × 14 days 200–400 mg t.i.d. for 3 days, then 400–500 mg t.i.d. for 10 days
Trichomoniasis (*Trichomonas vaginalis*)	Metronidazole	1 dose: 40 mg/kg (max 2 g) p.o.; or 15 mg/kg/day orally (maximum 1g/day) div. b.i.d. for 7 days
Trichostrongylosis	Mebenadazole or albendazole	100 mg b.i.d. for 3 days; 400 mg single dose
	or pyrantel pamoate	11 mg/kg single dose (maximum 1 g)
Trichuriasis (*Trichuris trichiura*, or whipworm)	Albendazole or mebendazole	400 mg single dose 100 mg b.i.d. for 3 days
Trypanosomiasis (*Trypanosoma cruzi*, South American trypanosomiasis, Chagas' disease)	Nifurtimox	1–10 years: 15–20 mg/kg/day in 4 doses for 90 days; 11–16 years: 12.5–15 mg/kg/day in 4 doses for 90 days
	Alternative: benznidazole	5–7 mg/kg/day for 30–120 days
T. brucei gambiense, *T. b. rhodesiene* (African trypanosomiasis, sleeping sickness)	Suramin or Pentamidine isethionate	20 mg/kg on days 1, 3, 7, 14, and 21 4 mg/kg/day i.m. for 10 days
Late disease with CNS involvement	Melarsoprol or Elfornithine	18–25 mg/kg total over 1 month; initial dose of 0.36 mg/kg i.v., increasing gradually to maximum 3.6 mg/kg at intervals of 1–5 days for total of 9–10 doses
	Alternatives: tryparsamide	1 injection of 30 mg/kg (maximum 2 g) i.v. q 5 d to total of 12 injections; may be repeated after 1 month
	plus Suramin	1 injection of 10 mg/kg i.v. every 5 days to total of 12 injections; may be repeated after 1 month
Visceral larva migrans (Toxocariasis)	Diethylcarbamazine	6 mg/kg/day in 3 doses for 7–10 days
	Alternatives: Albendazole or mebendazole	400 mg po b.i.d. × 5 days 100–200 mg b.i.d. for 5 days
Whipworm	(See trichuriasis)	
Wuchereria bancrofti	(See filariasis)	

sanitation. Moreover, few cities have retained soil conditions necessary for maintenance of the life cycle of most parasites. Pinworm remains the most common parasitic infestation in the United States and therapy is indicated only when symptoms are of clinical significance or the worm burden is excessive since recurrence is almost universal. Giardiasis is being seen with greater frequency as a result of increased use of daycare centers, where disease is readily transmitted. Therapy for parasitic infections is contained in Table 22.

For unusual parasitic infections, telephone consultation should be obtained from the Centers for Disease Control, Atlanta, Georgia, where many of the preferred therapeutic agents are available. The telephone number is +1-770-488-7760.

Index

[Antimicrobial therapy]
maximum (adult) dosages of parenteral antibiotics, 270
penicillin allergy and desensitization, 260–261
renal failure, 258–260
for specific pathogens, 269–270
for systemic fungal diseases, 275
for viral infections, 274–275
compromised host, 257–258
in vitro classification of antibiotics, 260
Antiparasitic agents, 275–281
Antipyretic therapy, 57
Antitoxin, 31, 43
Antiviral agents, 270
Appendicitis, 200
antibiotic use in, 200
Arcanobacterium hemolyticum, 57, 110
Arnold-Chiari malformation, 185
Ascariasis, 66
Aspergillosis, 196, 243–244
invasive aspergillosis
therapy of, 243
Aspirate of cellulites, 89
Aspiration of middle ear fluid, 94
Aspiration pneumonia, 123
organisms causing, 123
Aspirin, 57
Azithromycin, 122, 272–274

Bacille Calmette-Guerin (BCG) Vaccine, 85, 223
BACTEC 460 system, 101
Bacteremia, 15–18, 52–53, 224
associated with intravascular catheters, etiology, 16
fever and occult bacteremia, 54–55
in infants, 53
intravascular catheter-related bacteremia, 16–18
occult bacteremia, 15–16
Bacterial infections, 1–4
etiology, 2
Group B streptococcal disease, prevention, 2–3
infections associated with fetal scalp electrodes, 2
neonatal infection, 3
neonatal sepsis, 1. *See also separate entry*
perinatal risk factors for infection, 2
Bacterial tracheitis, 114–115
epidemiology and presenting symptoms, 115
etiology, 115
Bacteroides fragilis, 191, 199
Bacteroides melaninogenicus, 199
Balanitis, 214
treatment of, 215
Candida albicans, 215
Gardnerella vaginalis, 215
Trichomonas vaginalis, 215
Benzathine penicillin G, 38
Benznidazole, 280
Biliary atresia, 202
Biliary infection, 202–203
biliary atresia, 202
gallbladder disease, 202
hepatic abscess, 202
Bites
animal and human bites, 51–52. *See also separate entry*
Black-dot ringworm, 56
Bladder tap, 89
Blastomyces dermatitidis, 244
Blastomycosis, therapy for, 244
Blepharitis, 173

Blood culture technique, 89–90, 101–102
quantitative blood cultures, procedure for, 90
Blood transfusions, infections transmitted by, 234
Blueberry muffin rash, 4–5
Bone and joint infections, 147–158
discitis, 151–152
hematogenous osteomyelitis, 147–150.
See also separate entry
lyme disease, 157. *See also separate entry*
non hematogenous osteomyelitis, 150.
See also separate entry pelvic
osteomyelitis, 150–151
septic arthritis, 153–155. *See also separate entry*
vertebral osteomyelitis, 151
Bordetella pertussis, 114
Botulism, 18
infant botulism
clinical diagnosis of, 18
differential diagnosis, 18
laboratory diagnosis, 18
prevention, 19
treatment, 18
Brain abscess, 179–181
antibiotics dosage, 183
bacterial organisms causing, 182
echoencephalography, 180–181
electroencephalography, 180–181
management of, 182
predisposing factors for, 180
signs and symptoms of, 181
Bronchiolitis, 115–116
afebrile pneumonia of infancy, 116
Bronchitis, 115
Burns, 195–196

Caesarian delivery, 10
Campylobacter infection, 127–129
clinical characteristics, 128
extraintestinal manifestations of, 128
gastrointestinal manifestations of, 128
symptoms, 128
treatment of, 129
Candida species, 12–13, 155–156, 169, 196,
213, 243
Candidemia, 239–240
Candidiasis, 53–56, 244
treatment, 245
Candiduria, 169
Cardiac infections, 18–20
endocarditis, 19–20. *See also separate entry*
myocarditis, 20
pericarditis, 20
Cardiac surgery, 198
Cat scratch disease, 51
Cean intermittent catheterization, 168
Cefazolin, 23
Cefepime, 27, 272–273
Ceftazidime, 273
Ceftriaxone sodium, 21, 26, 34
Ceftriaxone, 22, 34, 272–274
Cellulitis, 53
clinical features, 54
ascending lymphangitis, 54
erysipelas, 54
infant cellulites, 54
neonatal cellulites, 54
predisposing trauma, 54

About the Author

RUSSELL W. STEELE is Division Head, Pediatric Infectious Diseases, Ochsner Children's Health Center, and Clinical Professor of Pediatrics, Tulane University School of Medicine, New Orleans. He is an editor of journals *Clinical Pediatrics* and *Infections Season Medicine*, and is a past member of the editorial board of the *Red Book*. He has authored over 300 journal publications. Dr. Steele received the M.D. degree from Tulane University School of Medicine, New Orleans, and completed fellowships in infectious disease and immunology at the National Institutes of Health.

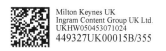